The Myth of the Chemical Cure

The Myth of the Chemical Cure

A Critique of Psychiatric Drug Treatment

Joanna Moncrieff

*Senior Lecturer, Department of Mental Health Sciences,
University College London*

and

*Honorary Consultant Psychiatrist,
North East London Mental Health Trust*

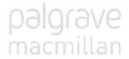

First published 2008 by
PALGRAVE MACMILLAN
Houndmills, Basingstoke, Hampshire RG21 6XS and
175 Fifth Avenue, New York, N.Y. 10010
Companies and representatives throughout the world

PALGRAVE MACMILLAN is the global academic imprint of the Palgrave Macmillan division of St. Martin's Press, LLC and of Palgrave Macmillan Ltd. Macmillan® is a registered trademark in the United States, United Kingdom and other countries. Palgrave is a registered trademark in the European Union and other countries.

ISBN-13: 978–0–230–57431–1   hardback
ISBN-10: 0–230–57431–9   hardback

This book is printed on paper suitable for recycling and made from fully managed and sustained forest sources. Logging, pulping and manufacturing processes are expected to conform to the environmental regulations of the country of origin.

A catalogue record for this book is available from the British Library.

A catalog record for this book is available from the Library of Congress.

2007051221

10   9   8
17   16   15   14   13   12   11   10   09

Printed and bound in Great Britain by
CPI Antony Rowe, Chippenham and Eastbourne

To Martin and Ann Moncrieff for being wonderful parents

Contents

Illustrations, Figures and Tables

Illustrations

Figures

Tables

Acknowledgements

Many people have helped me over the years with the formation of the ideas presented in this book. In particular I would like to mention David Cohen, David Healy and Peter Breggin. I am also grateful to the many service users and carers, mental health professionals, academics and junior and senior psychiatrists who have debated with me at meetings over the years. I would like to thank my head of department Paul Bebbington for allowing me the time and space to develop my ideas and write this book. I would like to thank the Wellcome Trust for funding my historical research; my supervisor for this work, Virginia Berridge; and all members of the Centre for History and Public Health at the London School of Hygiene and Tropical Medicine for making me so welcome. I am very grateful to Duncan Double for reading the whole manuscript, and to Paul Higgs and Martin Moncrieff for reading parts of it. I would like to thank all members of the Critical Psychiatry Network and especially Phil Thomas for his comments at various stages of this project. I could not have done the research for this book without the help of the fantastic librarians at the Aubrey Keep Library, Maureen Rouse and Christine Stephens and I am very grateful to them both. I am also indebted to Michelle Blythe for her efficient administrative support and encouragement. I must also mention Vera Sharav, who has kept me and others up to date with developments concerning research and the pharmaceutical industry. I would like to thank my colleagues Dinesh Kumar and Andreas Fonseca for covering me while I was on research leave. I would like to mention Robin Murray, Colin Drummond, Simon Wessely, Graham Scambler, Peter Tyrer and Bob Clarke, who have all encouraged me in my career and my thinking in different ways. My family including my Mum and Dad, sisters and brother, my partner and children have all been helpful and understanding. Finally, I would like to commend all the staff of Woodside Villa for their patience and hard work.

Abbreviations

CATIE	Clinical antipsychotic trial of intervention effectiveness
D_1, D_2	Dopamine 1 and 2 receptors
ECT	Electroconvulsive therapy
MAOI	Monoamine oxidase inhibitor
NICE	National Institute of Clinical Excellence
NIMH	National Institute of Mental Health
PET	Positron emission tomography
RCT	Randomised controlled trial
SSRI	Selective serotonin reuptake inhibitor

Note on Nomenclature

I have had to use several terms in this book that I am not comfortable with, but they are in common use and better ones do not exist or are not widely understood. I have not always put them in parentheses because if I did, there would be so many inverted commas that the text would be difficult to read. Thus I refer sometimes to 'mental illness', although I do not consider that psychiatric conditions are usefully or validly regarded as illnesses. I have tried to avoid this term where possible with terms such as psychiatric condition, disorder, disturbance or problem, but none of these terms adequately covers the range of problems that psychiatry deals with. I have frequently used the term 'patient' to describe people who have psychiatric problems because it seems less clumsy than the term 'psychiatric service user' and terms such as 'consumer' have their own particular implications, but this does not mean that I accept all its connotations. I have also referred to psychiatric interventions as 'treatments', which has medical implications that I think would be better avoided, but there is no readily understandable alternative. Although I have used alternatives where possible, I have had to refer to some drugs by names that imply disease specificity, which the whole book is disputing. Thus I have used the term 'antidepressant', for example, because there is no other common designation for these drugs.

1
The Disease-Centred Model of Drug Action in Psychiatry*

Conceptions and misconceptions about psychiatric drugs

Since the 1960s we have lived in an age characterised by the idea that drugs can cure the problems that are now referred to as 'mental illness', but have previously been known as insanity, madness, lunacy and neurosis, among other terms. By 'cure' I mean the idea that drugs can improve symptoms by helping to rectify the underlying pathological mechanism that is presumed to give rise to the symptoms in the first place. Increasingly this way of thinking has spread outside psychiatry and drugs have also come to be seen as having a curative role in all sorts of situations in which people feel they are not performing or functioning as well as they should. Such situations are 'diagnosed' as depression, dysthymia, anxiety, social phobia, substance misuse, compulsive shopping, menstrual dysphoric disorder, etc. and drugs are prescribed for their treatment. The story by which drugs first came to be seen in this way, as specific treatments for specific mental disorders or collections of symptoms, and whether or not this way of thinking about drugs and their actions is justified are the subjects of this book.

I shall argue that there is no real demarcation between previous eras' psychiatric treatments and the theories that justified them and our own; that the need to believe in a cure for psychiatric conditions that drove and sustained people's faith in insulin coma therapy, ECT, radical surgery, sex hormone therapy and many other bizarre interventions is the strongest impetus behind the use of modern-day psychiatric drugs. I shall suggest that the belief that modern drug treatments represent

* Parts of this chapter and the next one are based on two papers I wrote with David Cohen: Moncrieff & Cohen (2005, 2006).

specific cures for specific illnesses is just as mistaken as the belief that insulin coma treatment was an effective and specific treatment for schizophrenia. That is not to say that psychiatric drugs are not sometimes useful and I shall try and outline a way of thinking about them that helps to determine when they might be useful and when they might not be. But viewing the history of modern psychiatric drugs as a continuation of previous psychiatric practice should sound a cautionary note. We have only to look to the relatively recent past to see the proclivity of psychiatrists to subject their patients to invasive, degrading, harmful and not unusually fatal procedures in the name of therapy and to blind themselves to the real nature of their activities (Braslow 1997).

Over the following pages I hope to convince readers that the modern understanding of what drugs do in psychiatry, the basis of psychopharmacology, is fatally flawed; that most knowledge about psychiatric drugs is, at best, only a partial account. This is because it is based on a misconception about the nature of drug action, one that has been inspired and promoted by professional, commercial and political interests. This misconception has led to the misdirection of research, the misinterpretation of available evidence and the obstruction of a fuller and more accurate understanding of what psychiatric drugs do.

The place of drug treatment in psychiatry

It is difficult to overstate the central role that drug treatment plays in modern-day psychiatry. Psychiatric hospitals and community mental health team activities revolve around the various rituals of drug treatment. A United Kingdom survey of psychiatric hospitals found that 98–100% of inpatients were prescribed drugs and that most take several different ones at the same time (Healthcare Commission 2007). Drugs have become the focus of hospital life in a way that ECT and other physical procedures were in the 1940s and 1950s (Braslow 1997). The hospital day is punctuated by the regular 'drug rounds', where patients obediently cue up at a drug trolley to be handed their pills. Then there are the dramatic emergency situations where disturbed people are held down and forcibly injected with drugs. Much discussion and energy among staff is devoted to whether patients are on the right sorts of drugs and to whether or not they are actually taking them. When doctors do hospital 'ward rounds', drug regimens are tweaked, doses increased and new drugs added. Less often some drugs are reduced or discontinued, but drugs are rarely stopped without starting another one. Outside hospitals over 90% of patients in contact with psychiatric services are prescribed medication (Healthcare Commission 2007). Again, issues about medication are a central feature of meetings between staff and patients. Administering 'depots' (long-acting psychiatric drugs given by intramuscular injection) is one of the main tasks of community psychiatric nurses, and there is much concern among all staff about whether patients are being 'compliant' with their prescribed medication. When patients develop problems of almost any sort, it is invariably suggested that patients have been non-compliant, whether or not there is any evidence of this.

Since the early 1990s, psychiatric drugs have become much more widely prescribed and increasingly familiar to the general public. Drugs such as Prozac and Ritalin have become household names, and books about them have become best-sellers. This is part of a more general increase in consumption of all types of medicines, indicated by the fact that prescriptions issued increased by 56% between 1988 and 2001 in the United Kingdom. However increases in the use of psychotropic drugs have contributed disproportionately to this increase, with prescriptions of antidepressants rising by 243% in the ten years up to 2002 (National Institute for Clinical Excellence 2004). The rise in cost has been even more marked since the majority of the increases in prescribing have been for expensive new classes of psychiatric drugs. Thus costs of antidepressants in the United Kingdom rose by 700% between 1991 and 2002. In the United States, expenditure on psychotherapeutic drugs rose by 2.5 times between 1997 and 2004. The number of purchases rose by 72% and the number of people making a purchase by 55% (Stagnitti 2007). In 2001 antidepressants were the top-selling class of prescription drugs and continue to rank highly along with antipsychotics, anti-anxiety agents and stimulants (National Institute for Health Care Management 2002). Patterns of drug use have also changed. Use of benzodiazepines, such as Valium and Librium, once the best-selling class of psychotropic drugs, has declined relative to other drugs, and the use of antidepressants, antipsychotics and stimulants has risen (Pincus et al. 1998). However the most recent survey of drug use in the United States showed increased use of sedatives, anxiolytics and hypnotics as well as other sorts of drugs (Stagnitti 2007). The most dramatic increases have occurred among young people and children (Cohen et al. 2001).

This increase in use of prescribed drugs has been achieved firstly by extending the boundaries of well-established conditions such as depression and psychosis. Secondly, lesser-known diagnoses such as panic disorder and social phobia have been promoted, and thirdly, drug treatment has started to colonise areas where it was previously thought to be unhelpful, such as substance misuse and personality disorder. There is also a strong emphasis on the long-term nature of the need for drug treatment in severe mental disorders. For the major psychiatric disorders, such as schizophrenia and manic depression, it is generally suggested that drug treatment is required for life. Even for other less-serious conditions, such as depression treated in General Practice, it is recommended that drug treatment is taken for at least six months after resolution of symptoms (Royal College of Psychiatrists 2007).

Almost all drugs in current use have been introduced into psychiatry since the 1950s. Although drug treatment was common before that time, with extensive use of barbiturates and other sedatives and some use of stimulants, it was rarely given much attention. This was because drugs were generally regarded as having only crude effects, usually acting as chemical forms of restraint (Braslow 1997). However from the 1950s, psychiatric drugs started to arouse considerable interest. Drug treatment changed from something that was given little attention to an exciting activity that was seen as making psychiatry truly scientific (Moncrieff 1999). Part of this transformation consisted of a metamorphosis of the theories about what drugs actually do. Instead of being seen as substances that induced effects that were crude but useful, they came to be seen as specific treatments for specific illnesses. They became 'cures'.

The disease-centred model of drug action

Despite the ubiquity and importance of drugs in psychiatry, very little attention has been paid to the theoretical assumptions that underpin conventional views about what they do and how they work. A certain way of understanding drug action has come to be accepted without any consideration that there might be alternative explanations. Why this should be so is one of the major concerns of this book. But first let us unpick what this mode of understanding consists of.

I have called the current standard view of psychotropic drug action the 'disease-centred model' and its characteristics are outlined in Table 1.1 (Moncrieff & Cohen 2005). This view refers to the idea that drugs are thought to act on the underlying physical disease process. Drugs help to reverse this abnormal process, thus moving the body towards a more normal biological state. As two leading American psychiatrists put it in a rare contemporary discussion of the mechanisms of drug action, 'pharmacotherapeutic agents produce their clinically beneficial effects in an abnormal nervous system' and these effects

Table 1.1   Alternative models of drug action

Disease-centred model	Drug-centred model
Drugs help correct an abnormal brain state	Drugs create an abnormal brain state
Therapeutic effects of drugs derive from their effects on presumed disease pathology	Therapeutic effects derive from the impact of the drug-induced state on behavioural and emotional problems
Drug effects may differ between patients and volunteers	Effects do not differ
Outcomes of drug research consist of effects of drugs on measures of the 'disease' and its manifestations or symptoms	Outcomes are the global state produced by drug ingestion and how this interacts with behaviours and experiences
Paradigm: insulin for diabetes	Paradigm: alcohol for social phobia/social anxiety

'counter or compensate for the abnormal pathophysiology' (Hyman & Nestler 1996, 1997) (quotation 1997, p. 440).

The disease-centred model exists in two related forms. One suggests that drugs act on the underlying causes of a disease or condition, such as schizophrenia. The other suggests that drugs act on the pathology responsible for producing certain sets of psychiatric symptoms. Early versions of this model, for example, suggested that neuroleptic drugs were 'anti-schizophrenic in the broad sense' (The National Institute of Mental Health Psychopharmacology Service Center Collaborative Study Group 1964). More recent commentators have suggested that these drugs target the specific basis of psychotic symptoms, but not necessarily the ultimate cause of the condition. For example, antipsychotics are suggested to redress a hypothesised dopamine imbalance responsible for symptoms of acute psychosis without necessarily affecting the underlying cause of this imbalance (Kapur 2003).

Because the disease model is rarely articulated, its existence has to be largely inferred from the way that psychiatric drugs are described and investigated. For example, the way psychiatric drugs are currently named and classified according to the disease they are thought to act upon reflects the disease-centred model of drug action. Thus there are 'antipsychotics' thought to act specifically on the pathology underlying psychosis, 'antidepressants' thought to act on the pathology of depression, 'anxiolytics' thought to act on the pathological basis of anxiety, antimanic drugs thought to act on the pathology of mania, lithium and other 'mood stabilisers' thought to act on the pathological basis of abnormal mood, and 'hypnotics', whose name suggests they are deemed to work on the mechanisms of abnormal sleep. There is even a drug, clozapine, for the specific condition or situation of 'treatment-resistant schizophrenia'. Coverage of drugs in textbooks of psychiatry and psychopharmacology reflects this system of nomenclature, being organised according to the diseases drugs are meant to treat, not according to the chemical nature or physiological actions of different drugs. In reality, standard drug classification is a little more complex. There are some examples of drugs that are named according to their profile of physiological effects, such as stimulants, although they are now generally discussed under the heading of 'treatments for attention deficit disorder'. Drugs for insomnia are referred to as 'hypnotics', but most of these drugs are benzodiazepines, which are also classified as 'anxiolytics', and it is doubtful that anyone really thinks that they act by reversing the physical disturbance leading to insomnia. Nevertheless, the basic rules consist of classification of drugs by the disease or symptomatology they are thought to treat.

The disease-centred model can also be inferred by the absence of descriptions of characteristic drug-induced effects. In other words, the lack of a drug-centred model or explanation of drug action, described further in Chapter 2, implies a disease-centred understanding of how drugs work. For example, because there is no attempt to describe what sorts of effects are produced by different sorts of antidepressants, there is no acknowledgement that these effects exist and no consideration of how they might impact on someone experiencing emotional distress. Therefore, the 'improvement' or 'response' that antidepressants are thought to produce is suggested by implication to be due to an action on a presumed disease process. Similarly, without an account of the drug-induced state produced by taking the second-generation neuroleptic drugs, there is no rationale for their use apart from the idea that they counteract a disease process.

The disease-centred model also forms the basis on which research on drug efficacy is conducted. In randomised controlled trials (RCT), effects of psychiatric drugs are inferred from patients' scores on symptom measurement scales, which are presumed to measure the manifestations of the underlying disease state. All other effects that drugs produce are designated as 'side effects' and disregarded, unless they are so unpleasant or dangerous that this is impossible. Similarly animal research is conducted by constructing animal 'models' of psychiatric disorders and measuring drug effects on animal behaviours that are thought to be analogous to psychiatric symptoms in humans. Although there are many other questions about the validity of psychiatric research, the point

I want to stress here is that research on psychiatric drugs is predicated on the idea that psychiatric drugs exercise their effects on the manifestations of an abnormal biological state.

The disease-centred model has been imported from general medicine, where, in contrast to what I will suggest about psychiatric drugs, most drug action can be appropriately understood in this way. The purest version of the disease-centred theory of drug action is the idea of the 'magic bullet', a phrase coined by the scientist Paul Ehrlich at the end of the 19th century. Ehrlich first worked on developing antitoxins against infectious diseases such as tetanus and diphtheria, and later developed an arsenic-type drug treatment for syphilis. He used the term 'magic bullet' to describe a drug that acted only against the organism that caused the disease and had no effects on the human body itself. In this ideal sense, even anti-infectious agents are not truly magic bullets. There are no medical drugs whose effects are restricted entirely to correcting the disease process. However the concept illustrates the fact that modern drugs are disease-centred treatments in the sense that they are aimed at the specific pathology of individual diseases. They impact on the body in other ways, but their interaction with a particular disease process is what determines their therapeutic efficacy.

A paradigm case, often referred to by orthodox psychiatrists, is that of insulin treatment for diabetes. Insulin clearly helps to correct the abnormal functioning of glucose regulation that has been identified to be the core of the condition of diabetes. It does not target the ultimate biological cause of diabetes, the failure of the pancreatic glands, but it acts to reverse the consequences of this pathology, the lack of insulin, that produces the symptoms of diabetes. If the disease is understood as a process leading from the original pathology to the symptoms, insulin can be seen as acting directly on a part of this process, albeit not at its original point. The action of many other drugs can be understood in a similar way. Anti-angina drugs act on the pathophysiological pathways that produce angina, bronchodilators act on the physiological basis of reversible airways obstruction. Non-steroidal anti-inflammatory drugs and steroids suppress different parts of the inflammatory process, thus helping to return the body to normal functioning when this process is overreacting. The action of painkilling drugs can also be understood from their action at different points of the processes involved in generating pain. Opiates inhibit nociceptive (pain) stimuli along the fibres that take messages back to the brain, and non-steroidal anti-inflammatory drugs such as aspirin inhibit the production of prostaglandins involved in producing pain and the inflammatory reaction. Thus all these drugs act on biological processes that are considered to be pathological by virtue of causing symptoms of pain, discomfort, dysfunction and death. Some drugs, such as antihypertensives, act on mechanisms that control blood pressure, which reduces the risk of developing other diseases such as heart disease and strokes. None of these drugs acts on the ultimate underlying cause of the disease process. In this sense they might not be technically be classified as 'cures'. However I am using the term cure in the sense of drugs that have a disease-centred action. In this sense these drugs are all cures, albeit for symptoms rather than diseases. Some medical drugs do act directly on the causative agent of disease. Antibiotics and antivirals target the bacteria or viruses responsible for specific diseases and in this sense they come closer to the notion of a 'magic bullet'. Chemotherapy drugs used in cancer target rapidly proliferating cells, which is what distinguishes cancer cells. Again in the sense that chemotherapy often fails to eliminate the cancer completely, it may not always be considered a 'cure'. However regardless of its ability to remove the pathology completely, it qualifies as a 'cure' in the sense of being a disease-centred treatment that acts on the biological basis of the disease.

The disease-centred model implies that the basic action of a drug can usefully be divided into therapeutic effects and side effects. The therapeutic effects are the drugs' effects on the pathological process and the side effects are manifestations of the same effects on other parts of the body. For example, chemotherapy drugs attack proliferating cancer cells but also attack other cells, especially other rapidly proliferating cells such as in the bone marrow and reproductive system, with harmful consequences. Aspirin and other non-steroidal anti-inflammatory drugs inhibit the synthesis of chemicals called prostaglandins. This process is responsible for their analgesic effect and also, through reducing platelet aggregation, it is probably responsible for aspirin's efficacy in preventing recurrence of heart attacks and ischaemic stroke. However since prostaglandins are involved in protecting the stomach lining, this process can also lead to the well-recognised side effects of increased gastric irritation and bleeding.

The fact that most drugs used in general medicine act in a disease-centred way should come as no surprise since they are usually developed using knowledge about the pathophysiology of particular diseases. Even drugs whose actions were discovered serendipitously can be analysed and understood according to their action on a pathological process. What constitutes pathology or disease in general medicine and where the division between pathology and normality lies are, of course, not always clear-cut. But for the purposes of this argument what is important is that the action of a drug is understood with reference to the biological process that is involved in generating the state that needs to be rectified and, as such, is considered to be a disease. This is not to suggest that actions of all drugs thought to act in a specific way are completely understood, but enough drugs have been shown empirically to act in a disease-specific way that the disease-centred model can be considered to be a valid guide to drug action in most cases.

Some effects of some medical drugs can be understood as resulting from non-specific effects (that is, effects that are not directed against the disease pathology), consistent with the drug-centred model of drug action outlined in the next chapter. For example, antihistamines may reduce itching in the inflammatory condition of eczema by causing sedation as well as through their specific anti-inflammatory effect. Alcohol may reduce pain primarily because of its sedative and euphoriant effects, although it may also have some direct action on pain pathways. However more powerful specific drugs have largely replaced the use of non-specific agents in physical medicine.

'Chemical imbalances' and psychiatric drug action

The disease-centred model of drug action begs the question of what is the abnormal biological state that drugs correct. The predominant psychiatric theory about this is colloquially referred to as the 'chemical imbalance' theory of psychiatric disorder. This theory suggests that psychiatric disorders or their symptoms are caused by abnormalities in the chemicals in the brain that are involved in transmission of nerve signals, known as neurotransmitters. Examples of neurotransmitters are dopamine, serotonin, adrenalin and noradrenalin (the catecholamines), acetylcholine and many others such as gamma-aminobutyric acid (GABA), glutamate, glycine, opioid peptides and substance P. The list is being added to all the time as scientists reveal the complexity of the process of neurotransmission. The theory goes that abnormalities of different neurotransmitters cause different psychiatric disorders. Dopamine has long been held to be implicated in schizophrenia. In the different versions of this theory that have been propounded over the years, overactivity of the dopamine system has been proposed to cause schizophrenia itself (Meltzer & Stahl 1976; Rossum 1966), positive symptoms of schizophrenia (Davis et al. 1991) or acute psychosis (Kapur 2003). The monoamine theory of depression suggests that depression is caused by a deficiency of the monoamine neurotransmitters, namely serotonin and noradrenalin (Schildkraut 1965). As I shall discuss in more detail later, these theories are intimately related to the presumption that psychiatric drugs exert their clinical effects according to a disease-based model of drug action. Although biochemical theories are less well established in other disorders, the dopamine theory of schizophrenia and the monoamine hypothesis of depression have a diffuse influence by providing a template for the idea that disorders have a specific biochemical correlate and origin. Discussions about drug treatment for other disorders usually proceed on the assumption that a biochemical basis exists, without feeling the need to state what this is in explicit terms.

Occasionally there are attempts to produce more sophisticated versions of this basic theory. In a rare discussion of mechanisms of drug action in psychiatry, Hyman and Nestler (1996) suggested that therapeutic effects of psychiatric drugs result from brain adaptations to their effects, which 'likely produce therapeutic responses by altering the functional activity of critical neural circuits in the brain'. They do not reject the idea that psychiatric drugs work on specific neurotransmitters, but suggest that this is not simply through effects on neurotransmitter receptors, but through effects on synaptic transmission and complex interacting neural circuits. They still also presuppose that there are underlying abnormalities involving neurotransmitter systems (Hyman & Nestler 1997).

Despite being so rarely acknowledged, the disease-centred model of drug action and its counterpart, the chemical imbalance model of psychiatric disorder, are deeply ingrained in psychiatric culture. I have heard many psychiatrists explain to patients that their symptoms are due to a chemical imbalance, that taking psychiatric medication is like taking insulin for diabetes, that the drugs will help rectify this chemical imbalance and that without the drugs the condition will rapidly recur. The comparison with physical conditions such as diabetes emphasises the presumed physical basis of the problem. It is also employed to reassure depressed patients who are reluctant to take medication for fear of its addictive nature and to frighten patients after psychotic breakdowns into believing that they must take drugs long term.

Official information produced by the psychiatric profession demonstrates the same themes. The British Royal College of Psychiatrists' public information sheet on 'Depression' suggests that 'two ... neurotransmitters (serotonin and noradrenalin) are particularly affected' in depression and claims that 'antidepressants increase the concentrations of these two chemicals at nerve endings, and so seem to boost the function of those parts of the brain that use serotonin and noradrenalin' (Royal College of Psychiatrists 2006). The American Psychiatric Association (APA) says that 'antidepressants may be prescribed to correct imbalances in the levels of chemicals in the brain' (American Psychiatric Association 2005). On psychosis or schizophrenia the Royal College of Psychiatrists (RCP) claims that there are 'abnormalities in the biochemistry of the brain' and 'an imbalance in brain chemistry' (Royal College of Psychiatrists 2004). The APA suggests that antipsychotic medications 'help bring biochemical imbalances closer to normal' (American Psychiatric Association 1996).

Even when they acknowledge that there is no evidence for a 'chemical imbalance' many psychiatrists believe that the term is still justified and appropriate, thereby demonstrating a deep underlying commitment to the idea. Wayne Goodman, a prominent United States psychiatrist commenting on an article highlighting the fact that there was no established link between serotonin abnormality and depression, still maintained that the term chemical imbalance was a 'reasonable shorthand for expressing that this is a chemically or brain based problem and that medications help to normalise function' (quoted in Meek 2006).

The pharmaceutical industry employs similar language in its promotional material. An early advertisement for Prozac suggests that 'Like arthritis or diabetes, depression is a physical illness' (Valenstein 1988, reproduced on p. 181). A leaflet produced in 1996 by a consortium called 'America's Pharmaceutical Research Companies' neatly summarises the idea of the chemical imbalance and its relation to a disease-centred model of drug action:

> Today scientists know that many people suffering from mental illnesses have imbalances in the way their brains metabolise certain chemicals called neurotransmitters. Too much or too little of these chemicals may result in depression, anxiety or other emotional or physical disorders. This knowledge has allowed pharmaceutical company researchers to develop medicines that can alter the way in which the brain produces, stores and releases neurotransmitter chemicals, thereby alleviating the symptoms of some mental illnesses.
>
> (Valenstein 1988, cited on p. 182)

Philosophical considerations

This book concerns the creation of a myth, the myth of the disease-centred model of drug action, and how that myth could be accepted as a real description of the world. It therefore involves questions about the nature of knowledge and the relation between knowledge and power.

Karl Marx was one of the first philosophers to undermine the notion that knowledge is objective and neutral. His analyses of capitalism demonstrated that what was portrayed in one way by the capitalist class was experienced differently from the perspective of the working class. Thus for the owners of capital, the bourgeoisie, capital was an economic necessity and a generator of wealth. For the working class it was a means of exploiting their labour and transforming it into a source of profit for other people. In his early writings Marx used the term *ideology* to describe ideas that were stimulated by class interests and obscured the real nature of social relations: 'ruling ideas are nothing more than the ideal expression of the dominant material relationships' (Marx & Engels 1970, p. 64). By standing aloof from the interests of the ruling class, Marx was able to lay bare the workings of capitalism that had been obscured by a 'bourgeois consciousness' that needed to present the capitalist system as benign and necessary (Marx 1990, p. 175).

Twentieth-century philosophers of science, such as Thomas Kuhn and Paul Feyerabend have also challenged the notion of objective knowledge and revealed the extent to which empirical data is shaped by prior conceptions and interests. This critique was extended by some of its proponents to the terrain of philosophical relativism, a position which maintains that there are no criteria for differentiating one account of the world from another or that there is no uniquely privileged 'truth' (Feyerabend 1975). But, for all its impact elsewhere, relativism has always been rejected by natural science, which simply could not operate on a relativist platform where no theory or fact can be wrong or inferior. It has therefore been able to largely ignore questions about the notion of objective knowledge.

Several philosophers have attempted to arrest the 'slide into relativism' and yet preserve the importance of recognising the influence of extrinsic factors on the production of knowledge (Parker 1992). Critical Realists, influenced by Marx, maintain that the nature of the external world imposes limits on the variety of ways open to us to represent that world. Human interests may skew knowledge away from a true representation of reality. Hence, identifying such interests is important to the process of establishing 'true' and useful forms of knowledge. Unmasking the interests and assumptions enmeshed in certain forms of knowledge is also important because it allows an open and honest debate about what sorts of values and interests scientific knowledge ought to promote (Goldenberg 2006).

The philosophy of Michel Foucault helps us to understand further this relation between interests and knowledge. Foucault was concerned with the way in which power is a precondition of the development of a body of knowledge and how knowledge could, in turn, function as power. In his lectures on 'Psychiatric Power' Foucault illustrated this thesis with reference to psychiatry. The 'medical authority' of the psychiatric profession, says Foucault, 'functions as power well before it functions as knowledge' (Foucault 2006, p. 3). It is the pre-established power of the profession, the authority it obtained over the process of the management of madness, that enabled the profession to define madness and distress in its own terms, in Foucault's words, enabling 'the great re-transcription of madness as mental illness' (Foucault 2006, p. 346). This form of knowledge reinforced the profession's claim to legitimacy. Foucault describes the 'interplay of a power relationship that gives rise to a knowledge, which in turn founds the rights of this power' (Foucault 2006, p. 346). Although Foucault did not address the role of other players in the formation of psychiatric knowledge, and was in fact wary of locating power in particular groups, preferring to describe power as a system or network, his analysis allows us to understand the symbiosis between the interests of certain groups and the formation of knowledge about psychiatric drugs.

In the spirit of Marx and Foucault I will, in the rest of this book, attempt to uncover the interests that have led to the development and success of the disease-centred model of drug action and its accompanying model of psychic distress. By reflecting on the motives that have generated this model I hope to be able to develop a deeper understanding of how psychiatric drugs work. I will attempt to demonstrate that research evidence, although it has been moulded to fit the disease-centred model, provides little justification for it. I outline an alternative 'drug-centred' approach that is consistent with a wide range of evidence, yields more information about what effects drugs have in different situations and forms a better basis from which to weigh up the pros and cons of drug treatment.

My thesis in this book is that the disease-centred model of drug action has been adopted, and recently widely publicised, not because the evidence for it is compelling, but because it helped promote the interests of certain powerful social groups, namely the psychiatric profession, the pharmaceutical industry and the modern state. Therefore, I offer the following study as an example of the way in which vested interests and the political environment can distort knowledge, in this case successfully deluding most of society for over half a century.

2
An Alternative Drug-Centred Model of Drug Action

The disease-centred model suggests that the important or 'therapeutic' effects of drugs are achieved by their effects on a particular disease process. By acting on the mechanisms of the disease, drugs move the human organism from an abnormal physiological state towards a more normal one. In contrast, the drug-centred model suggests that drugs themselves create abnormal bodily states. In the case of drugs that act on the brain or the nervous system, these states involve an alteration in subjective experience or consciousness. Psychiatric drugs are *psychoactive* drugs which, by their neurophysiological effects alter 'mental and emotional life and behaviour for the duration of the treatment' (Cohen & Jacobs 2007). When we consider drugs that are taken recreationally we have no trouble recognising this fact and we refer to the altered mental state drugs produce as 'intoxication'. But there is no fundamental distinction between drugs used for psychiatric purposes and other psychoactive drugs. They all act on the nervous system to produce a state of altered consciousness, a state that is distinct from the normal undrugged state. The only difference is that the state produced by recreational drugs is pleasurable whereas the effects produced by most psychiatric drugs are experienced as unpleasant. The characteristic features of the drug-induced state vary according to the chemical nature of the particular drug and its interaction with the brain and in subsequent chapters I will describe the features produced by ingesting some commonly prescribed psychiatric drugs.

Drug effects are always subject to individual variation. In other words, people vary in their biological response to drugs and in what they think of different drug-induced effects. The experience of taking a drug is also mediated by the context in which the drug is ingested, including the social circumstances and emotional state of the subject at the time. For example, someone forcibly injected with a benzodi-azepine drug[1] after being brought into hospital against their wishes, possibly by the police, is likely to have a different experience of the effects of this drug compared with a recreational user who chooses to take the same drug. In general, however the characteristic effects of a psychoactive drug are determined by its pharmacological properties, not by the presence of a disease. Therefore, according to the drug-centred model there is no absolute distinction between the response of a patient and that of anyone else.

The drug-centred model suggests that the therapeutic value of a drug is derived from the particular quality of the abnormal state it produces. Some drug-induced effects may be useful or desirable in certain social and interpersonal situations, including the situations that are brought to the attention of psychiatrists and called mental disorders. Deducing what therapeutic effects a drug might have therefore demands a detailed knowledge of the way it changes normal mental functioning which can then be matched up with the effects that the patient or others desire to achieve. But recognising that drugs produce altered states and do not return the body to normal indicates how drugs themselves constitute a source of stress, both physical and psychological. Although it may bring some temporary respite, a state of intoxication is unlikely to be con-ducive to leading a normal life. Individuals may end up having to strug-gle to counteract the effects of their drug treatment as well as their original problems. For this reason Peter Breggin, a psychiatrist and famous critic of psychiatric drugs, emphasises that psychiatric drugs impair brain function in the same way as physical intrusions on the brain, such as lobotomy. He calls them 'brain disabling' treatments stating that 'they exert their primary or intended effect by disabling nor-mal brain function' (Breggin 1993b, p. 72). Furthermore, according to Breggin, 'biopsychiatric treatments are deemed effective when the physi-cian and/or patient prefer a state of diminished brain function with its narrowed range of mental capacity or emotional expression' (Breggin 1997, p. 4). The implication that there are no justifiable uses of psychi-atric drugs may have limited the appeal of Breggin's ideas to psychiatric professionals and service users, but his work usefully highlights the general character of psychotropic drugs.

The case of alcohol illustrates how a drug-centred model can clarify the potential therapeutic uses of drugs for psychiatric or behavioural problems. Alcohol is a sedative drug that reduces nerve conductivity in the central nervous system. Ingestion of alcohol gives rise to character-istic physiological effects, such as dilation of blood vessels, smooth muscle relaxation and slowed reaction times. It produces various characteristic subjective experiences and behavioural effects that are dose dependent. At low doses it produces euphoria, some behavioural activation, social disinhibition and mild impairment of intellectual functioning. At higher doses it produces sedation and greater degrees of cognitive impairment. These effects have several consequences. They are responsible for the popularity of alcohol as a social lubricant and recreational substance and they can lead to aggressive and reckless behaviour in some circumstances. They can also help people to overcome behavioural inhibitions. Alcohol might therefore be deduced to have useful effects in social phobia, sometimes referred to as social anxiety disorder, not because the substance corrects an underlying physical abnormality but because some of the effects it produces might in themselves be useful for people experiencing difficulties in social situations. It has in fact long been officially recognised as an effective 'treatment' for social phobia.

Another example of a drug-centred explanation for drug effects is the effects of stimulant drugs on hyperactive children, now officially labelled as having 'attention deficit hyperactivity disorder' (ADHD). Mainstream psychiatry presents stimulants as a disease-specific treatment for this condition, although it cannot account for their mechanism of action. Stimulants are held to have a 'paradoxical' effect in children with attention deficit disorder, that is, their effects are believed to differ from their effects on normal people. However Peter Breggin, along with other critics and some mainstream commentators have long pointed out that the effects on children with attention deficit or hyperactivity are entirely predictable from our knowledge about the overall effects of stimulants on humans and animals (Breggin 2001; Grahame-Smith & Aronson 1992). At high doses stimulants such as amphetamine and methylphenidate (Ritalin) increase motor activity but at lower doses they only increase arousal and focused attention and activity, much like the weaker stimulants nicotine and caffeine. They do this by suppressing reactivity to the environment including social interaction, exploratory behaviour and emotional reactivity. In other words, they cause people to focus narrowly on a single activity and enable them to ignore other stimuli. At higher doses and with prolonged use this effect is magnified and expressed as obsessive and compulsive-type behaviours, and more extremely as stereotypies. These are rhythmic repetitive purposeless movements seen in both animals and humans when given high dose stimulants (they also form the basis of an animal model of psychosis discussed in Chapter 6). Thus, in the short-term low dose stimulants create a state of reduced responsiveness to environmental stimuli, increased passivity and compliance with set tasks, which may be desirable in hyperactive children, especially in a classroom, where focused attention is required. But this change involves a global reduction in responsiveness and initiative, which may undermine the benefits achieved. Whether the effect persists is another question, since the body rapidly adapts to counter the effects of drugs. Long-term benefits from stimulants have been difficult to demonstrate in controlled trials (Schachter et al. 2001).

Other examples of drug-centred thinking were provided by early proponents of modern psychopharmacology. Pierre Deniker, one of the psychiatrists who first used chlorpromazine, thought that its useful effects were attributable to the induction of an 'an experimental neurological disease' characterised by reduced movement (akinesia) and emotional indifference (Deniker 1960). It was these unique effects that Deniker and other early pioneers thought were responsible for the drug's therapeutic effects in schizophrenia and other cases of psychiatric disturbance (see Chapters 5 and 7 for further discussion of neuroleptic-drug effects). The utility of sedative drugs in anxiety also helps demonstrate the drug-centred model. The lessening of arousal and reduction of nerve conductivity produced by sedative drugs such as benzodiazepines, alcohol and barbiturates reduce anxious thoughts and ruminations, and dampen the heightened physiological arousal associated with these states. Some drug effects in general medicine can also be understood according to a drug-centred model such as the examples of antihistamines and their sedative effects and alcohol's effects on pain, which are described in Chapter 1. However in general, physical medicine prefers to use specific drugs where it can, since these are by definition more powerful.

The drug-centred model of drug action suggests that we can understand effects of drugs that are used therapeutically in essentially the same way as we understand the effects of recreational drugs. In the case of recreational use of drugs, it is effects such as euphoria, stimulation, indifference, disinhibition, psychedelic experiences and some types of sedation that are sought after. These effects are valued as pleasant in themselves, and also as ways of blocking out and anaesthetising people against painful memories and current difficulties. Drugs used in psychiatry have a similar range of effects, and several psychiatric drugs are also drugs of misuse. However these effects can be further discriminated. There are different types of sedation and stimulation, for example. Some drugs, such as benzodiazepines and opiates, produce sedation that is often appealing and others, such as neuroleptics, produce sedation that is generally experienced as unpleasant. Similarly, some drugs produce stimulant effects that are usually experienced as pleasurable, such as amphetamines and cocaine, whereas others produce stimulant effects that are intensely unpleasant such as the akathisia produced by neuroleptics.

As well as their immediate effects, drugs that are taken long term on a regular and frequent basis induce physical adaptations to the presence of the drug. These can be conceptualised as the body's defence against, or opposition to, the effects of a foreign substance (Breggin 1997; Jackson 2005). For example, long-term use of neuroleptic drugs that block dopamine receptors causes the body to develop increased numbers of these receptors, which also become more sensitive to dopamine (Muller & Seeman 1977, 1978). These adaptations have several consequences. Firstly, they may counteract the immediate effects of the drug so that to achieve these effects larger doses need to be used. This is the phenomenon known as 'tolerance'. Secondly, when the drug is stopped or reduced, especially if this is done suddenly, the bodily adaptations are suddenly unopposed by the presence of the drug. It is these unopposed adaptations that cause withdrawal symptoms and they may cause other problems such as precipitating an episode of psychiatric disorder (Baldessarini & Viguera 1995; Moncrieff 2006). These effects have profound implications for evidence about the efficacy and utility of long-term 'maintenance' treatment in psychiatric disorders as explained in the following section. Another important consequence of the body's adaptations to the presence of a drug is that these adaptations may themselves be harmful and sometimes irreversible, as in the case of tardive dyskinesia, which is thought to be due to overcompensating adaptations to dopamine-blocking drugs (Breggin 1997).

The disease-centred model presumes that drug treatment is a good thing because it helps correct a hypothetical underlying disease state and returns the body towards normal. Any unwanted effects of drugs are classified as 'side effects' and as such receive little attention. In contrast, the drug-centred model presents drug treatment in a much more ambivalent light. According to this model, drug effects cannot be parcelled off into therapeutic and adverse effects as if these were distinct. Instead drugs need to be seen as inducing 'global neurological syndromes' (Cohen 1997). The characteristics of these syndromes might be therapeutic in some ways but will almost certainly have negative implications too. The increased passivity and reduced initiative shown by a child on stimulants may be useful in a classroom but be a hindrance in a summer camp. The sedation produced by benzodiazepines may reduce tension but will also impair vigilance. Drug use is always a fine balancing act between the benefits that might be gained in some respects and the impairments that drug-induced effects almost always incorporate, especially in the long term. The drug-centred model also helps to alert us to the potential dangers of long-term drug use by stressing that drugs are foreign chemicals that interfere with normal biological functioning. Therefore, the body naturally tries to counteract their effects, sometimes leading to further harmful consequences.

Evaluating models of drug action

It is increasingly recognised that even the most rigorous methodology may not adequately control the influence of groups and individuals that stand to benefit from the results of medical research. The placebo-controlled randomised trial was devised to try and eliminate the effect of extraneous factors. It is designed to distinguish the effects of the general environment plus the natural history of the condition from the specific effects of a particular treatment. However these trials are based on the assumption that drugs act in a disease-centred way on the basis of a specific disease. The placebo or dummy tablet is employed to mimic the process of taking a drug because it is known that the positive expectations people have about the effects of taking treatment may, in themselves, improve the outcome of certain conditions. This is known as the 'placebo effect'. This effect is likely to be particularly influential in psychiatric disorders, especially depression and other 'neurotic' conditions, because of the subjective nature of symptoms and outcomes (Fisher & Greenberg 1993). However the placebo effect is only one aspect of what are called the 'non-specific' effects of treatment, so named to contrast with the specific or disease-centred effects. The drug-centred model suggests that in addition to placebo effects, drugs have non-specific *pharmacological* effects. In other words, they create drug-induced states that may impact on outcome without affecting the disease process. A standard placebo-controlled trial cannot distinguish between whether drugs exert disease-specific effects or whether they create a drug-induced state that suppresses the manifestations of mental disturbance or affects the way it is perceived. For example, various psychoactive drugs may appear to be beneficial in depression because they produce a state of intoxication that masks or supplants people's emotions, rather than having any specific effects on mood.

In addition, these non-specific pharmacological effects may affect people's expectations and thus interact with the placebo effect. The fact that psychiatric drugs are active agents means that they have detectable physiological effects such as dry mouth and nausea that are usually referred to as side effects. In addition, because they are psychoactive drugs, they induce a state of intoxication that is often readily distinguishable from the normal undrugged state. These effects enable participants in placebo-controlled trials to identify whether they are allocated to the active drug or the placebo. Therefore, double-blind trials can become 'unblinded'. In other words, some subjects can identify what they are taking because of the different physiological experience of taking an active drug compared to an inert placebo. A review of trials, where people were asked to guess the type of tablet they had been allocated to, found that in most studies people were able to guess more accurately than would be predicted by chance (Fisher & Greenberg 1993). If people know or suspect they are taking the active drug they may have a greater hope of recovery than people taking placebo. In other words, people on active drugs may show an 'amplified' placebo response (Thomson 1982). Conversely there may be a reduced placebo effect in people who suspect they have been allocated to the placebo due to negative expectations. Thus, people taking placebo in RCTs may fare even worse than similar people who are not offered drug treatment in ordinary life (Kaptchuk 2001).

Researchers can also often distinguish between people who are taking the active drug and people taking placebo, because they interview participants during the course of trials and during these interviews they ask about side effects as well as assess the state of the mental condition (Fisher & Greenberg 1993). In one trial they were even found to be able to distinguish between two different active drugs, imipramine and a benzodiazepine, alprazolam (Margraf et al. 1991). If researchers can guess the identity of people's treatment, their assessments of outcome may be influenced by their expectation that drugs are superior to placebo. A study that examined this possibility in a trial with people with chronic schizophrenia found that assessors rated people they believed to be on chlorpromazine as more improved than those they believed to be on placebo, to a degree that was highly statistically significant ($p < .007$), whereas in fact there was no difference between the two drugs ($p = .4$) (Engelhardt et al. 1969). Therefore, it is likely that many so-called double-blind trials are unblinded to some degree and that the effects of expectations are not eliminated by the use of a standard placebo.

A further problem with modern clinical drug trials is that people are usually dropped from the study once they relapse or if they stop the study drug for any reason. Therefore, there is no information about the ultimate outcome of these participants. In addition, the analysis is potentially invalidated because the remaining groups may differ from each other in ways that may affect treatment response. They are no longer the groups that were selected by randomisation and the analysis is not the 'intention to treat' analysis[2] that is recommended to prevent bias. Many trials nowadays claim to get round this problem by estimating the outcome for people who leave the trial early, usually taking their last recorded assessment as their final outcome. However it is not stressed enough that this is an estimate and not an actual measure of their final state. In addition, we know that positive studies are more likely to be published than negative ones, a phenomenon known as publication bias, and within published studies measures that show positive effects are reported and negative ones sometimes ignored (Melander et al. 2003; Stern & Simes 1997). Therefore, published data is likely to be inaccurately skewed towards showing beneficial effects of treatment.

Another major methodological issue in psychiatric drug trials, which is generally ignored, is the effect of drug discontinuation. Trials rarely start with people who are not taking any prescribed drugs to begin with. Trials of long-term or 'maintenance' treatment, in particular, take a group of people who have been mentally stable on drug treatment for some time, sometimes many years, and then randomise them into two groups. One group continues to take the treatment as before or is changed onto the study drug. The other group has their drug treatment withdrawn and replaced by the placebo. Studies of this sort generally find that the patients withdrawn to placebo have higher rates of problems. The conventional interpretation is that they have relapsed into their previous state of mental disorder due to the removal of the prophylactic effect of drug treatment. Hence these trials are believed to provide evidence that long-term drug treatment is beneficial in preventing the recurrence of mental disorders. However it is now widely recognised that the process of withdrawal from psychotropic drugs in itself causes a number of problems. Firstly, withdrawal syndromes occur with all classes of psychiatric drugs. These syndromes often include symptoms such as insomnia and agitation that may be mistaken for a relapse of a psychiatric condition. Secondly, several case studies suggest that discontinuation of neuroleptic drugs may occasionally provoke an iatrogenic episode of psychosis (Moncrieff 2006). These episodes appear to have their own distinct characteristics, and are more similar to stimulant-induced psychosis than to typical schizophrenia. Some cases have been reported in people who have no history of psychiatric disorder and were taking neuroleptic-type drugs for other indications (Lu et al. 2002). Therefore, it seems that these episodes may be unrelated to the original mental disorder and may comprise part of the spectrum of withdrawal effects of this type of drug. The fact that they occur most frequently after withdrawal of drugs with short half-lives,[3] such as clozapine, is in keeping with this explanation as such drugs are well known to cause the most severe withdrawal syndromes. This phenomenon has been referred to as 'supersensitivity psychosis' (Chouinard & Jones 1980) because it was suggested to be due to supersensitivity of dopamine receptors, but this mechanism has not been demonstrated. Thirdly, there is evidence that withdrawal of some psychiatric drugs makes people more vulnerable to a relapse of their underlying condition than they would have been if they had never started drug treatment in the first place (Baldessarini & Viguera 1995; Viguera et al. 1997). There is good evidence for this with lithium and some evidence for neuroleptics. It has been suggested to be due to 'pharmacological stress', which is the idea that the body's adaptations to a drug may act as a physiological stressor which precipitates relapse when the drug is withdrawn. However psychological mechanisms may also be relevant. Finally, the psychological effects of withdrawing from long-term medication are likely to be significant but they have received little attention. People who have been on medication for a long time are often intensely anxious about stopping it. In people with depression this anxiety may either be mistaken for relapse or it may actually make them depressed. Professionals are also often anxious when long-term medication is reduced or withdrawn and this may bias their ratings of outcome in clinical trials. Negative attitudes of staff and carers may also be communicated to patients.

All these problems may beset people who are withdrawn to placebo in randomised trials of long-term treatment, especially since withdrawal is usually fairly rapid. Gradual discontinuation appears to be less problematic in most studies, which may be because the physical adaptations to drug treatment have time to readjust to the absence of the drug (Viguera et al. 1997). Therefore, the superior performance of groups who continue drug treatment in maintenance trials could simply reflect the lack of withdrawal-related effects in these people and does not necessarily indicate that the drug has a true prophylactic effect.

Discontinuation problems may also operate in studies of treatment for acute problems like an episode of depression or psychosis of recent onset. Since patients are usually taking some sort of drug before the study starts, the placebo group is not a group of people who have no treatment; it is a group who have had drug treatment withdrawn. Participants in such trials have usually been on drugs for shorter periods than in long-term maintenance studies, hence the body has less time to develop adaptations and discontinuation problems may be less significant. However animal studies show that adaptations such as changes in dopamine receptors in response to neuroleptics occur within a week (Burt, Creese, & Snyder 1977; Muller & Seeman 1978).

Since standard clinical trials cannot distinguish between a drug's action on a disease process and the consequences of the abnormal state a drug induces, other sorts of evidence set out below are necessary to discriminate between the disease-centred and the drug-centred model. In the following chapters I will examine these types of evidence for different classes of drugs:

1. **Pathophysiology of the disorder:** The major justification of a disease-centred model is if the action of a drug can be understood according to the pathophysiology of a disease process, which is well established independently of the known actions of the drug. There are myriad examples in general medicine; the action of antibiotics can be ascertained from knowledge about the biology of bacteria, the action of anti-anginal drugs from the mechanisms (coronary artery spasm) underlying the symptoms of angina, the action of asthma drugs, such as salbutamol, by understanding the mechanisms of bronchospasm. However there is no established specific physical basis to psychiatric disorders. Biochemical theories about the origins of psychiatric disorders, such as the dopamine hypothesis of schizophrenia and the monoamine theory of depression, were themselves derived from the selected actions of drugs that were already thought to be specific. Therefore these theories *assume* that drugs act in a disease-centred fashion and do not, in themselves, provide any evidence that this is so. Reliable evidence, independent of drug effects, that particular biochemical states gave rise to particular psychiatric conditions is required to provide evidence of the disease-centred action of drugs.

2. **Rating scales:** In order for evidence from randomised trials to support a disease-centred model, it is necessary to be sure that rating scales used in these trials measure the manifestations of a disease process and not just drug-induced effects. However no psychiatric scales fulfil these criteria, since the disease processes have not been identified. Rating scales in all psychiatric conditions consist of collections of common complaints and observed behaviours, which are designated as 'symptoms' and many of these are not specific to any particular condition. Measurement scales for psychosis and depression, for example, include items on sleeping difficulties, agitation, tension, hostility and uncooperative behaviour. All these problems are likely

to respond to non-specific sedative effects associated with many commonly used types of psychiatric drug. In contrast, some items used to evaluate depression such as motor retardation, emotional withdrawal and depressed mood may respond to drugs which exert stimulant effects. Therefore changes in psychiatric rating scales scores may simply reflect drug-induced effects and do not necessarily provide any evidence for a disease-centred drug action. Evidence that particular drugs targeted more specific symptoms like delusions and hallucinations would be stronger evidence that there was an action on the underlying mechanism of the disorder.

3. **Animal models:** Animal research is generally assumed to identify compounds that have specific effects on particular psychiatric disorders by using animal models of psychiatric disorders. There are serious questions about whether animal behaviour can provide an adequate and meaningful model of human emotional states, but putting this question aside for a moment, evidence that these models selected supposedly specific drugs and not others might support a disease-centred model of drug action. Evidence on animal models and anti-depressants is reviewed further in Chapter 9. Some animal models have been developed to select drugs with a particular pharmacological profile, such as the stimulant-induced stereotypy model which selects dopamine blockers, as we shall see in Chapter 6. However these models simply determine what sort of pharmacological action a drug has and do not provide evidence about the specificity of action of drugs for particular behavioural states. These models only support a disease-centred model of drug action on the assumption that the mechanism identified by the animal model is the mechanism underlying the psychiatric disorder. This takes us back to the issue covered in point (1) of whether or not the pathology of the condition has been established.

4. **Comparisons with non-specific drugs:** According to the disease-centred model of drug action, drugs that are thought to have a disease-centred action should have superior effects to drugs that have only non-specific psychological or pharmacological effects. For example sedative drugs like benzodiazepines, which are not considered to act on the biological basis of depression or psychosis, could be compared with drugs that are regarded as having these specific effects. Surprisingly few such studies have been conducted. However demonstrating that non-specific drugs are inferior does not necessarily demonstrate that the supposedly specific drugs have a disease-centred action. It may merely indicate that the drug-induced effects

of one type of drug are superior in some situations to the drug-induced effects of other sorts of drugs. For example, neuroleptic drugs may be superior to other sedatives in psychosis, not because they act to reverse a disease process, but because of the particular characteristics of the state they produce. However in general, a finding that a supposedly disease-specific drug was not superior to drugs that were not considered specific would argue against a disease-centred model of its action.

5. **Healthy volunteer studies:** According to the disease-centred model, the therapeutic effects of drugs will only be expressed in an abnormal nervous system (Hyman & Nestler 1996). Therefore, studies of drug effects in human volunteers, that is, people without a history of psychiatric problems, will not be particularly useful in understanding how drugs affect patients. However a drug-centred model by contrast suggests that a drug's basic physiological and subjective effects will be the same in patients and volunteers, except insofar as effects of drugs show variation between individuals and are dependent on context.

6. **Improved outcome:** According to the drug-centred model, drugs would generally have no impact on the course of a psychiatric condition, even if their effects were useful. In contrast, the disease-centred model predicts that, by helping to reverse abnormal pathology, drugs would be expected to alter the outcome of a psychiatric disorder, at least for as long as they were taken. Therefore, if the outcome of psychiatric disorders could be shown to have improved significantly as a result of the use of a supposedly disease-specific treatment that might provide some encouraging evidence to support the disease-centred model. In contrast, if widespread use of supposedly specific drugs cannot be shown to have improved outcome, the case for it is weakened.

The drug-centred model should be the default position in psychopharmacology research. Since we know that psychiatric drugs have psychoactive effects, the consequences of these effects must be discounted before it can be concluded that a drug exerts its effects on the underlying disease process. In order to support the disease-centred model we must have evidence that a disease-specific action is necessary to explain results of research over and above the effects of the drugged state. A lack of evidence supporting the disease-centred model implies that the drug-centred model is sufficient to account for observed effects.

3
Physical Treatments and the Disease-Centred Model

In the late 19th and early 20th-century attitudes to psychiatric disorder became increasingly pessimistic. As the asylums filled up with an expanding population of chronic cases, the idea that had inspired the asylum-building programme of the 19th century, that a period of respite in a well-ordered asylum would cure people, appeared discredited. Ideas about hereditary became popular with the rise of the eugenics movement, and psychiatric disorders came to be seen as primarily inherited and therefore incurable. In this climate the morale of institutional psychiatry was low and methods of treatment were given little attention. A memoir of this period describes psychiatry as 'somnolent, if not actually asleep' and characterised by 'despairing therapeutic nihilism compounded by enforced inactivity' (Rollin 1990). Experiments with various physical procedures were recorded in published literature (Scull 1994), but none came to be widely accepted.

Psychiatric journals of the time were mostly concerned with the classification and causation of mental disorders, including ideas about hereditary and chronic infection, and from the 1920s there was an interest in hormonal disturbance as a cause of madness (Moncrieff & Crawford 2001). There were few papers about treatments. Textbooks contained only short discussions of treatment. Even when more optimistic attitudes were displayed, they usually emphasised the naturally remitting nature of some psychiatric conditions and the importance of general supportive and social measures, such as fresh air, massage, sunlight, rest and an 'atmosphere of hopefulness' (Hutton 1940). These attitudes were summed up by authors of the foremost British textbook

Donald Henderson and Robert Gillespie in the following passage on the treatment of schizophrenia:

> The peace and quiet of a mental hospital, the orderliness and discipline, the tolerant and understanding attitude of those in charge, and the simplification of life, may at once produce a most gratifying change.
> (Henderson & Gillespie 1927, p. 330)

Some psychiatrists even urged that intervention should be minimised. In his textbook of *Clinical Psychiatry*, Morris Braude suggests that 'except in very unusual cases manic patients abate their fury sooner or later and hence may call for little interference' (Braude 1937).

In the late 1920s the idea that inducing malaria might cure or benefit people suffering from General Paralysis of the Insane (a state of cognitive decline and neurological disorder caused by syphilis infection) was suggested and 'malarial therapy' started to be used in asylums. This consisted of infecting people with the malarial parasite. The rationale was that the high temperatures caused by the malaria infection would kill off the organism that caused syphilis. It remains uncertain whether this technique had any physical effect, but it helped to boost the morale of the asylum system (Braslow 1997). It also ushered in a new attitude to psychiatric disorders. The identification of General Paralysis as a manifestation of infection with the syphilis protozoa, and its possible treatment with malarial therapy opened up the possibility that some, and maybe many, psychiatric conditions might be curable, or at least treatable. It also gave the staff of asylums something to do, which involved a manipulation of the body, and allowed them to feel that they worked in a genuinely medical environment. From the early 1930s onwards insulin coma therapy, chemical and then electrically induced shock therapy and lobotomy were introduced into psychiatry and all became standard and accepted forms of treatment.

These treatments ushered in a major change of attitude to the nature of treatment in psychiatric conditions. By 1940 almost half of the papers published in the *British Journal of Psychiatry* concerned treatments, most of which described insulin coma therapy and chemically induced shock therapy. From the 1940s onwards textbook sections on 'treatment' got longer and gradually devoted more attention to a range of physical procedures including insulin coma therapy, electroconvulsive therapy (ECT), lobotomy and continuous narcosis, the practice of inducing prolonged sleep with large doses of barbiturates. Case notes of patients record ECT treatments, insulin coma therapy and discussions about referral for brain surgery (Moncrieff 1999). Psychiatry finally appeared to be confident that it had truly effective treatment procedures at its disposal.

Insulin coma therapy[1]

The introduction of insulin coma therapy is a seminal event in the history of modern psychiatry. Even though the aetiological theories behind its use were vague, insulin treatment is important because it was believed to act on the underlying pathological basis of the condition of schizophrenia. It rapidly became popular, its use spreading throughout Europe and North America. By 1940, it was being used in every major psychiatric institution in Germany (Ehrhardt 1966) and in most British and American asylums to treat schizophrenia (Valenstein 1988, p. 18). It was, therefore, the first treatment in widespread use that was considered to be a specific treatment for a particular mental disorder.

Insulin coma therapy was dreamt up by a Viennese psychiatrist called Manfred Sakel, in the early 1930s. In 1922 insulin was isolated and identified as a treatment for diabetes. This, and other advances in endocrinology, helped to stimulate great interest in the role of hormones in all sorts of conditions, and Sakel started experimenting with the use of insulin in morphine addicts to help them cope with withdrawal symptoms. After observing its calming effects, he went on to try it in acutely psychotic schizophrenic patients. In these patients he used injections of insulin to induce deep hypoglycaemic comas and fits. Sakel claimed that a course consisting of daily or almost daily comas over a period of two months produced impressive results, with 70% of patients being completely cured (Sakel 1937).

Two American psychiatrists involved in the use of insulin coma therapy recently provided a detailed description of what it had involved. A deep coma was induced by injection of insulin which lasted for around two hours. During this time most patients became calm, but some became excited and required restraining. Many patients soiled themselves and most were drenched in sweat. Signs of severe neurological impairment were present such as loss of reflexes and muscle spasm. Occasionally the patient had epileptic fits. Patients were left in the coma for about two hours and then woken up suddenly with an injection of glucose. Afterwards they would be calm but would show loss of memory and neurological abnormalities such as weakness and aphasia (loss of speech). Some became emotionally labile, showing fatuous laughing and crying (Fink & Karliner 2007). Insulin coma therapy was therefore a dramatic procedure and it carried a high mortality – about 5% of patients died in one large survey and higher numbers in smaller studies reported in the literature (Ebaugh 1943).

Evidence from journals, textbooks and patient case notes confirms that the use of insulin coma therapy was generally restricted to people diagnosed with schizophrenia (Moncrieff 1999). The socially inclined Henderson and Gillespie were sceptical about whether its effects were specific or not:

> insulin is capable of shortening the course of schizophrenic illness. What is not yet certain is whether it does more than this i.e. whether it cures or improves permanently cases which would otherwise not have been cured or improved.
>
> (Henderson & Gillespie 1944, p. 404)

However more biologically enthusiastic psychiatrists were less hesitant. Authors of another major British textbook admitted that 'a therapy which fails in two fifths of cases cannot very well be specific', but were still confident that 'hypoglycaemic treatment obviously touches the physical basis of schizophrenia more closely than all earlier modes of physical attack' (Mayer-Gross, Slater, & Roth 1954, p. 286). Attempts were made to explain its actions in terms of its effects on electrical circuits in the brain, an explanation that had become fashionable since the invention of the electroencephalograph (EEG), which measured brain waves, and was also applied to ECT (Fink & Karliner 2007; Paterson 1963). In 1966, a German textbook emphatically stated:

> The introduction of insulin coma treatment by Sakel was from a historical point of view the decisive step from a purely symptomatic to a curative therapy of the 'endogenous' psychoses.
>
> (Ehrhardt 1966, p. 838)

Insulin therapy was adopted with great enthusiasm and excitement. In 1937, cure rates of 70–90% were announced in Europe (Whitaker 2002, p. 86) and in 1938 investigators in the United States published results that claimed that two-thirds of patients benefited with most of these being discharged (Malzberg 1938). In 1939 one American psychiatrist proclaimed that 'the value of insulin treatment is now definitely established. Every institution that has given it a fair trial has found it to be effective' (Ross & Malzberg 1939). Insulin therapy was also celebrated as a great advance in American magazines and newspapers of the 1930s as unearthed by author Robert Whitaker. The *New York Times*, for example, described how patients had been 'returned from hopeless insanity by insulin' and explained the mechanism of action in these terms: after the deep comas the 'short circuits of the brain vanish and the normal circuits are once more restored and bring back with them sanity and reality' (*New York Times* 1937) (cited in Whitaker, p. 86). Evidence from case notes and correspondence show it was practised or endorsed by well-known social psychiatrists including British psychiatrist Aubrey Lewis (Moncrieff 1999) and the American Adolf Meyer (Grob 1983). Thus with insulin treatment, psychiatrists finally believed they had found a curative treatment for one of their most enduring psychiatric conditions and they were successful in persuading at least a section of the wider public that this was true.

ECT

In 1935 the Hungarian psychiatrist Ladislas von Meduna announced the benefits of using chemicals, firstly camphor and then the synthetic drug metrazol, to induce epileptic fits in psychiatric patients. The justification for this was a long-standing belief, whose origins are obscure, that schizophrenia and epilepsy are antagonistic to each other. Like insulin coma therapy, metrazol treatment rapidly spread throughout Europe and North America, with extravagant claims about its efficacy. In 1937 a 70% complete remission rate was claimed in a series of 1000 patients treated with cardiazol-induced convulsions, plus further partial or 'social' remissions (Kennedy 1937). In 1938 an Italian psychiatrist Ugo Cerlett began to use electricity to induce the convulsions and so ECT was born. Chemical and electroconvulsive therapies were used widely in European and American asylums in the mid-20th century, generally regardless of diagnosis. They were much easier to apply than insulin coma therapy – indeed von Meduna specifically emphasised how 'the best evidence for the simplicity of the procedure is the fact that 60–80 patients can be treated in one morning with the aid of only one assisting physician and at most two to three nurses' (von Meduna 1938, p. 46). Chemical and electrical shock therapies were therefore administered to a greater proportion of patients.

Descriptions of psychiatric hospitals of the mid-20th century record how ECT occupied a central place in the hospital routine (Braslow 1997; Rollin 1990). ECT 'clinics' were held several times a week, and inpatient wards were structured around preparing patients for these clinics. A British psychiatrist remembers how many patients, mostly diagnosed with schizophrenia, had 'maintenance' ECT consisting of one shock treatment a week for years on end resulting in many patients experiencing hundreds of episodes of ECT in a lifetime (Rollin 1990).

Like insulin coma therapy, chemical and electrical shock therapies were introduced for the treatment of schizophrenia and high rates of success were claimed in some reports. One early paper claimed that ECT produced complete remission in 67% cases of recent onset of schizophrenia and up to 43% of cases of longer duration (Kalinowsky & Worthing 1943), although other reports found disappointing results (Pollock 1939). Some authors recommended that its best effects were found in 'acute excitement, paranoidal or aggressive patients' (Bennett 1945) or that it could be used as a sedative for patients who were 'grossly uncooperative, assaultative or refused food' (Sharp, Gabriel, & Impastato 1953). Although people diagnosed as having schizophrenia continued to form the bulk of the patients to whom ECT was administered (Braslow 1997), gradually a consensus started to emerge that its best effects were limited to cases of depression or depression and mania. Many claimed that its best effects were obtained in 'involutional melancholia', a severe depression in older people, usually accompanied by agitation and sometimes delusions.

As with insulin coma therapy, explanations of its action were speculative and varied, but emphasised that ECT acted on an abnormal biological process that gave rise to depression. Like insulin coma therapy, one hypothesis concerned the ability of ECT to interrupt abnormal electrical circuits, replacing them by 'another form of homeostasis, that of normality' (Paterson 1963). Another proposal was that it acted by stimulating an underactive pituitary gland which was suggested as the origin of depression (Sadler 1953). Other authors, who admitted that its mechanism of action was uncertain, nevertheless appeared to regard it as a disease-specific treatment. For example, for involutional melancholia it was described as a 'specific and adequate means to relieve this common illness' (Moss, Thigpen, & Robinson 1953, p. 896).

Therefore by the 1940s psychiatry could present itself as having two specific treatments for its two biggest problems, 'manic depression' and 'schizophrenia', the two conditions defined by the Kraepelinian dichotomy, which had dominated psychiatry since the beginning of the 20th century.[2] In 1941, the Director of Institutions in California could write:

> While insulin shock therapy is applicable mainly in cases of schizophrenia in their comparatively early stages, electro-shock therapy is applicable to manic depressive psychoses and to involutional

melancholia. Thus these most common groups of mental disorders will soon be fully provided for.

(Rosanoff 1941, cited in Braslow, p. 101)

Other activities and physical therapies

Leading up to the 1930s and beyond it is evident that there was an 'orgy of experimentation' within psychiatry (Scull 1994, p. 8). Historian Andrew Scull lists some of the more outlandish interventions that were tried: surgical removal of teeth, tonsils, colons and uteri based on the theory that psychiatric disorders were the result of chronic hidden infection, inducing meningitis in people with schizophrenia by injecting horse serum, presumably patterned on the rationale for fever therapy in neurosyphilis, use of nitrogen and carbon dioxide to produce comas and convulsions, injections of cyanide and induction of extreme hypothermia. All these procedures were reported in reputable psychiatric journals of the time. As well procedures as insulin, there was interest in several hormones as treatments for schizophrenia. Thyroid hormone was regularly prescribed and case notes show that it was considered to be a specific treatment for schizophrenia. Its use was based on a theory that schizophrenia was due to thyroid deficiency, which was briefly fashionable (Jenner 1997; Mayer-Gross, Slater, & Roth 1954). Several journal articles from the 1930s to 1940s also discussed the theory that schizophrenia was caused by deficiencies or abnormalities of sex hormones and possibilities for treatment with sex hormones (Hemphill & Reiss 1945).

Lobotomy or leucotomy was introduced in the 1940s and had a profound influence on psychiatric thought. The numerous articles on its use in scientific journals and the fact that its 'inventor' was awarded the Nobel Prize testify to the excitement it inspired. Officially, indications for surgery were based on symptoms and many diagnostic groups were suggested to benefit:

> The general aim of the operation is to modify the disordered behaviour of many psychotic and neurotic patients whose illness has been of a prolonged type. The tendency is to select patients on a symptomatic than on a nosological basis.
>
> (Henderson & Gillespie 1944)

Another author suggested that it was most appropriately used 'to quiet a chronically disturbed and aggressively destructive patient' (Sadler 1953).

In this sense lobotomy was not a specific therapy. However Joel Braslow found that in the California state asylum it was performed predominantly on people diagnosed with schizophrenia and became associated with this diagnosis to such an extent that it was regarded as a 'specific therapy aimed at a specific disease' (Braslow 1997, pp. 141–2). Most descriptions of lobotomy tended to avoid the question of how it might produce its effects, in particular whether it was thought to be reversing a disease state or producing an abnormal brain state itself. More critical commentators, However suggested that 'lobotomy only exchanges one defect for another and even more permanent one' (Sadler 1953). For current purposes the importance of labotomy lies in the fact that psychiatric disorders were being treated by brain surgery, which confirmed the idea that they originated from brain pathology. It also conveyed the impression that psychiatry was a scientific enterprise engaging the most advanced technologies of medicine.

Despite the fact that in retrospect these physical therapies are generally felt to represent a 'therapeutic debacle', (Rollin 1990, p. 111) they had some positive consequences for the environment of the asylum. By their very nature they introduced much apparently therapeutic activity into asylums, which therefore became more convincingly like 'mental hospitals'. They caused new buildings to be constructed and equipped, such as insulin clinics, ECT clinics and asylum laboratories. They created jobs for people – ECT nurses, anaesthetists, asylum pathologists and neurosurgeons to perform the lobotomy operations (Anonymous 1990). And with most of the inmates trooping off several times a week for their ECT or insulin treatments, they helped create an impression that asylums were a hive of genuine medical activity. In this way they helped to boost morale in a previously run-down system. Henry Rollin describes how accompanying this wave of 'therapeutic optimism ... and in some degree occasioned by it, the ethos of mental hospitals underwent a dramatic metamorphosis' (Rollin 1990, p. 111). The furnishings and decoration of hospital interiors were updated so that they became physically more comfortable and homely, and locked doors and windows were unlocked. In all, they became more like hospitals or nursing homes and less like prisons.

Do insulin coma therapy and ECT work?

Insulin coma therapy

In 1953 a junior doctor, Harold Bourne, published a paper in the Lancet medical journal called 'The insulin myth' (Bourne 1953). In this paper he suggested that insulin treatment had no effect on schizophrenia at all, but that people believed it was effective because of its dramatic nature.

He pointed out that it had never been systematically evaluated, and that there were no studies that had attempted to control for these dramatic effects. A Medical Research Council funded randomised trial conducted in the United Kingdom in the 1950s appeared to support his conclusion when it found insulin coma produced no better outcome than a barbiturate-induced sleep used as a control procedure (Ackner, Harris, & Oldham 1957).

However there is another possible explanation for why insulin coma therapy was thought to be effective. Critics have suggested that insulin coma therapy affected people's behaviour by virtue of causing brain damage due to prolonged hypoglycaemia and anoxia caused during the comas and convulsions (Frank 1978; Whitaker 2002). Fink & Karliner's (2007) description of the process and its results lends support to this idea. They recorded how patients showed evidence of neurological impairment both during and after the comas and a labile emotional state typical of brain injury victims. Another psychiatrist described their condition as comparable to 'the behaviour of hanged persons after resuscitation, the sick after avalanches ... condition which comes on after head injuries, during the progress of uraemic coma, after carbon monoxide intoxication and other types of poisoning' (Palisa 1938). An approving psychiatrist of the time described how patients who received multiple comas appeared demented for days afterwards (Sadler 1953). In the 1950s it was recognised from animal and post-mortem studies that the procedure was associated with extensive and irreversible brain-cell destruction, whose severity was related to the number of treatments received (Kalinowsky & Hoch 1950; Sadler 1953). Sakel himself suggested that brain-cell death was the mechanism of action, but claimed that the treatment selectively killed or silenced 'those brain cells which are already diseased beyond repair.' He compared insulin treatment to 'fine microscopic surgery... the cure is affected (because it) starves out the diseased cells and permits the dormant ones to come into action in their stead.' (Sakel 1958, p. 334).

Whether insulin coma therapy merely worked through a placebo effect, that is, its dramatic nature convinced people, including the patient that he or she had improved, or whether it had real pacifying effects as a consequence of causing brain damage is uncertain. Both explanations seem plausible. Either way it is now generally believed that it was not an effective or specific treatment for schizophrenia.

ECT

ECT is still an accepted part of psychiatric practice, although its use is currently waning. It has become the most controversial of current psychiatric treatments and it evokes deep antipathy from many psychiatric service users who have experienced it. The efficacy of ECT in depression in the short term is still regarded as well established but it is acknowledged that it has no long-term effect. In other words, a few weeks after the ECT has taken place, people are no better than they would have been if they had never had it. A meta-analysis published in the Lancet in 2003 reviewed the evidence from studies that randomised patients to have either the real ECT, including the induced convulsion, or a 'sham' procedure consisting of a general anaesthetic only, without the fit. Although this review concluded that ECT was 'an effective short-term treatment for depression' (UK ECT review group 2003), one of these seven trials found no benefit of ECT at all compared with sham ECT (Lambourn & Gill 1978) and another found only minimal benefit (Johnstone et al. 1980). In this study the difference between the real ECT group and the sham group was a matter of about six points on the frequently used Hamilton Rating Scale for Depression after four weeks of treatment (estimated from the graph provided) and other rating scales used in the study did not show substantial and statistically significant differences between the real and sham procedures.

However the superiority of ECT over sham ECT like placebo-controlled drug trials, does not confirm that ECT has a disease-specific action. Alternative explanations can be derived from an understanding of the abnormal state that ECT produces, analogous to the drug-centred model of drug action.

Firstly, it is well known that ECT produces a syndrome of cognitive impairment consisting of disorientation, impaired attention and memory dysfunction that occurs immediately after experiencing ECT and is similar to the effects of an ordinary epileptic fit. A study in elderly people showed that they experienced a 3-point decrement in their Mini Mental State Score (a test of cognitive function used to assess people with dementia) during ECT (Rubin et al. 1993). Another characteristic of ECT is that it produces a sedating and calming effect, again similar to the aftermath of an ordinary epileptic fit. These effects were widely recognised in the early days of ECT use in the old asylums.

A state of disturbed behaviour similar to mania and sometimes with frank psychotic features has also been noted to occur occasionally following ECT. Peter Breggin has likened this syndrome to the effects of having a closed head injury (Breggin 1993b) and it is also reminiscent of other brain diseases such as the late stage of multiple sclerosis. The commonest features are the sudden development of a fatuous and over-familiar manner, spontaneous and unprovoked laughter and sexual disinhibition (Devanand et al. 1988). It is sometimes, but not always, accompanied by obvious cognitive deterioration, including disorientation. It usually improves rapidly with cessation of ECT. More unusually, ECT may provoke a state of frank delirium with neurological signs including agnosia, confabulation, aphasia and apraxia (Fink 1979). When ECT is given intensively and frequently, all subjects develop an extreme state in which they show 'complete confusion, and utter apathy' and are 'mute, incontinent and unable to take food without assistance' (Weil 1950). We know of these effects because there was a temporary fashion for therapies that involved intensive ECT in the 1940s and 1950s.

There has been intense controversy about whether ECT can induce lasting brain damage, with the psychiatric establishment adamantly denying this. In particular numerous early animal studies that showed evidence of brain damage have been criticised and their findings dismissed because they used an electrical stimulus of much greater intensity than used in normal ECT (Devanand et al. 1994). However some brain-imaging studies suggest that people who have had ECT have evidence of atrophy of brain matter and increased size of brain ventricles compared with brains of people who have not had ECT (UK ECT review group 2003). It seems logical enough that if an electrically induced fit can induce observable brain damage if prolonged and intense enough, ECT may produce milder levels of damage that may fall short of easy detection. Permanent memory problems may be further evidence of this. Psychiatrists have usually disputed the existence of long-term memory loss after ECT, pointing to studies, such as the Northwick Park study, where psychometric measures administered months after finishing ECT have not shown any adverse effects (Johnstone et al. 1980). They also suggest that memory complaints are attributable to depression rather than ECT (Coleman et al. 1996). However some studies do reveal persistent amnesia two months after cessation of ECT (Lisanby et al. 2000; Sobin et al. 1995). Subjectively many people perceive or experience lasting memory problems after ECT. In a recent survey of studies of patients' views of ECT up to 79% reported some memory problems following ECT, with 29–55% reporting persistent or permanent memory loss (Rose et al. 2003).

The state produced by ECT offers several explanations for the apparent therapeutic effects of ECT. Firstly, the acute cognitive effects may temporarily override underlying emotional states and reduce people's ability to express their emotions. The fact that the beneficial effects of ECT do not persist beyond the period of treatment would support this idea (Ross 2006). In addition, there is a correlation between the supposed efficacy of ECT and its cognitive effects. Thus unilateral ECT (placing the electrodes on the right side of the brain) is generally found to be less effective than bilateral ECT and causes a lower degree of cognitive impairment (Sackeim et al. 1993). Similarly, higher doses of unilateral and bilateral ECT were associated with higher response rates and longer periods of disorientation in one trial (Sackeim et al. 1993). The impairment of cognitive function is also likely to impair the ability to form the complex and exaggerated thoughts that form the basis of depressive delusions, which may account for the common perception that ECT is particularly effective in delusional depression. Interestingly, this possibility was entertained by some psychiatrists during the heyday of ECT. In the 1962 edition of their textbook Henderson and Gillespie attributed the effects of ECT to the 'disruption by the fit and the subsequent period of amnesia of recently acquired morbid patterns of behaviour and reaction' (Henderson & Gillespie 1962, p. 335). American authors similarly suggested that ECT produced 'a state of altered brain function in which many the patient can deny his problems' (Weinstein, Linn, & Kahn 1952). Since then there is little reference to this idea outside the critical psychiatric literature, which is remarkable since the acute cognitive effects of ECT are widely acknowledged. The fact that this obvious possible explanation for the effects of ECT has been forgotten is one of many examples we will see that testifies to the desire to construe psychiatric interventions as specific therapies.

Secondly, the sedative and calming effects of ECT may produce improvement especially in people with agitated depressions. As discussed in more detail later, depression-rating scales contain many items that would respond to sedative effects of drugs or ECT such as sleep difficulties, agitation and various manifestations of anxiety. Some older accounts suggest that it was indeed people with 'agitated depression' who responded best to ECT (Paterson 1963 p. 87).

Thirdly, the organic behavioural state produced by ECT, with its euphoria and disinhibition, may be mistaken for improvement. Often it is misdiagnosed as mania even in people who have no history of manic depression. It is credible that ECT may precipitate mania in people with a vulnerability, but this has not been definitively demonstrated (Devanand et al. 1988).

Fourthly, ECT may work psychologically. Although the sham ECT trials control for the effect of having a procedure involving an anaesthetic, the control procedure cannot replicate the acute cognitive effects of ECT. Hence, patients may know which treatment they are receiving, especially if they have had ECT before. Patients who believe that ECT worked for them in the past, which is likely to be most patients consenting to have ECT a second or third time, may be disappointed if they believe they are not getting the real ECT. Therefore patients randomised to the sham ECT group may do worse than expected due to poor expectations of outcome. Conversely, patients who get the real ECT may do better than the sham group as a result of suspecting they are receiving the real thing. In this respect it is interesting to note that in some of the trials which showed ECT to have the most marked superiority to sham ECT, a large proportion of patients had had previous ECT. In a trial carried out in Leicester, England, for example, 60% had had previous ECT (Brandon et al. 1984). In contrast, in the Northwick Park Study, which found only minimal differences between real and sham ECT, only 21% of patients had had previous ECT (Johnstone et al. 1980). Finally, ECT may operate by providing a psychological 'shock' which frightens the patient out of their depressive preoccupations, at least momentarily. This was also suggested as important in the early days of ECT (Henderson & Gillespie 1962). ECT is often a terrifying experience for patients, especially if forced on them against their wishes. An investigation of patients' responses to ECT found that many react with 'strong and enduring feelings of terror, shame, humiliation, failure, worthlessness and betrayal, and a sense of having been abused and assaulted' (Johnstone 2003).

These explanations offer a more compelling account of the effects of ECT than the idea that it is a specific treatment for depression. In addition, there is no currently accepted coherent theory about what it does to the brain that might help in depression. Its effects on increasing permeability of the blood-brain barrier and changes in cerebral blood flow have been noted, as has its effects on the hypothalamic pituitary – adrenal axis and on brain dopamine, monoamine (serotonin and noradrenalin) and cholinergic receptors. However research results have been inconsistent and no credible explanation has emerged. The fact that ECT has effects in people with schizophrenia also contradicts a disease-centred view of its action. A Cochrane review of randomised trials of ECT in schizophrenia revealed that in the short term patients who received real ECT were judged to be more improved by study raters, and showed more improvement in their rating-scale scores, than those who received the sham procedure (Tharyan & Adams 2005). Again the effect was not sustained after the end of the treatment period. The effect was not due to improvement in depressive symptoms (Brandon et al. 1985). The difference between schizophrenia and depression is that ECT was generally found to be superior to antidepressants but not to neuroleptic drugs in schizophrenia. However this may relate to the effects of these groups of drugs in their respective diagnostic groups rather than the efficacy of ECT, as we shall see in later chapters. Interestingly one randomised study comparing ECT with insulin coma therapy found no difference between the two procedures (Baker, Game, & Thorpe 1958). This is consistent with the possibility that both these techniques produce a state of temporary brain impairment that is misinterpreted as clinical improvement.

Why and when the idea emerged that ECT was specifically effective for depression is not clear. It is clearly stated in the 1940s (Jessner & Ryan 1943) but the idea that ECT is also effective in schizophrenia did not fade until the 1960s, possibly as a consequence of the widespread acceptance of the neuroleptic drugs by this stage. It may be that because ECT can cause an organic state frequently characterised by euphoria, it has been viewed as reversing the underlying biological basis of depression which is assumed to be the opposite to that of mania. Also, the acknowledged temporary nature of the effects of ECT may not have seemed worthwhile in people with chronic schizophrenic states as patients slipped back into their usual state. Since depression is usually a naturally remitting condition, people usually improve somewhat naturally by the time the effects of ECT wear off. Because insulin coma therapy was restricted to people with schizophrenia, where recovery is less common, it may have been more difficult to present it as a successful treatment. If insulin coma therapy had been employed in depression, it is possible it may have persisted for longer.

Whatever the reality of the action and effects of ECT, psychiatrists of the 1940s and 1950s believed that they had two specific treatments for the main disorders that they dealt with: insulin coma therapy for schizophrenia and ECT for depression or mood disorders in general. History has decided that insulin coma therapy was not an effective treatment, although it may have had some behaviourally calming effect through inducing brain damage in the same way that lobotomy did. The jury is still out on ECT. Its use has survived much longer, despite widespread opposition from some psychiatric survivors and the fact that it is widely acknowledged that its effects are not persistent. Its effects can also be explained by the acute cognitive impairment it causes, sometimes amounting to a brain injury-like state that may be mistaken for recovery from depression. Other mechanisms may also have a role. However in the face of opposition from an increasingly powerful and respected patient movement, and maybe also due to the demise of the asylum where it was born, it looks as if ECT will gradually drop out of use as insulin coma therapy did in the 1950s. The question of whether it really is or was a useful and specific treatment for depression will probably be quietly forgotten, as was the question of what effects insulin coma therapy really had in schizophrenia.

The importance of ECT, insulin coma therapy and the other physical treatments for understanding the current state of psychiatry is that they helped to encourage a confidence that mental illness could be cured with physical means. By the mid-20th century psychiatrists finally really believed they could resolve the problems experienced by people under their care by acting on what they presumed was the bodily basis of the problem. This was the context into which a new generation of psychotropic drugs arrived in the 1950s.

4

The Arrival of the New Drugs and the Influence of Interest Groups

Drug treatment prior to the 1950s

You might be forgiven for thinking that drugs were scarcely used in psychiatry prior to 1950s. Official literature such as textbooks barely mentioned them. When drugs were briefly mentioned, such as for the purposes of promoting sleep and managing manic excitement, they were recommended reluctantly with injunctions like 'they should be used as sparingly as possible' (Henderson & Gillespie 1927, p. 154) or 'it is well to withhold the use of drugs as long as possible' (Braude 1937, p. 16). Psychiatric journals contained only a small handful of papers on drugs for epilepsy and hormones (Moncrieff & Crawford 2001).

However despite official reticence, in practice psychotropic drugs were 'doled out by the bucketful', in the words of Henry Rollin, a psychiatrist reflecting on his experiences of psychiatry prior to the 1950s (Rollin 1990). Alec Jenner, another retired psychiatrist described to me how psychiatric hospitals of the time were permeated with the characteristic sickly sweet smell of paraldehyde, a commonly used sedative drug (Jenner 1997). Although drugs were not mentioned in the clinical notes or letters sections of the patient case notes I examined, prescription charts revealed that sedative drugs such as barbiturates, paraldehyde and bromides were commonly prescribed as well as stimulants. Inpatients were frequently prescribed several different drugs simultaneously and outpatients were also frequently prescribed drugs, mostly barbiturates and stimulants.

So, contrary to official descriptions, drugs were widely and routinely used in psychiatric practice prior to the 1950s. However unlike the physical treatments, which excited such excitement, they aroused little clinical or academic interest, and were not even considered worthy of mention in patient case notes. Where there was any attempt to classify the early drugs it was clear that they were generally regarded as acting in a drug centred rather than disease-specific manner. In Sargant and Slater's 1944 textbook of *Physical Methods of Treatment in Psychiatry*, drugs were classified into 'sedatives' and 'stimulants'. Sedatives, particularly the barbiturates, were further subdivided according to their speed of action and removal from the body. Phenobarbitone was recommended explicitly as a 'basic sedative and not *pro re nata*' (Sargant & Slater 1944, p. 87). The only exception to this drug-centred view was the use of stimulants in children with hyperactivity, a condition that Sargant and Slater believed 'may yield to the drug in what appears a specific way' (p. 96). Official reticence about the old drugs conveys the impression that they were a source of embarrassment, regarded as inducing only crude effects. Joel Braslow suggests that they were considered to be 'chemical restraints' and that they 'occupied the same non-therapeutic space as' as methods of physical restraint (Braslow 1997, pp. 37–38).

Attitudes to the new drugs

In contrast to views about the old drugs, the new generation of drugs introduced into psychiatry from the 1950s onwards were greeted with immense enthusiasm, verging on zeal. One contemporary observer noted disapprovingly that the atmosphere at conferences on the new drugs was akin to religious revivalist meetings (Bowes 1956). The period is still regarded as one of the most important moments in the history of psychiatry, even as 'one of the most important episodes in the history of medicine itself' (Ayd, quoted in Swazey 1974, p. 8), and is commonly referred to as the Psychopharmacological Revolution. From this time on, textbooks started to cover drug treatments in detail and proclaimed their transformative effects (Mayer-Gross, Slater, & Roth 1960, p. 300; Henderson & Gillespie 1962, p. 247).

Henry Rollin describes how the use of chlorpromazine 'tore through the civilised world like a whirlwind' (Rollin 1990, p. 113). Figures on its use in French hospitals support this statement (see Figure 4.1). In 1952 only 428 kg of chlorpromazine were used. By 1953, 7,5157 kg were used, rising to over a million by 1957 (Swazey 1974, p. 137). In the United States, Thorazine, the brand name of chlorpromazine, boosted Smith Kline & French's sales volume by over a third within a year of its launch (Swazey 1974, p. 162). Examining patient case notes confirmed the widespread use of these drugs. In contrast to the older drugs, the new drugs were explicitly discussed in clinical notes and letters.

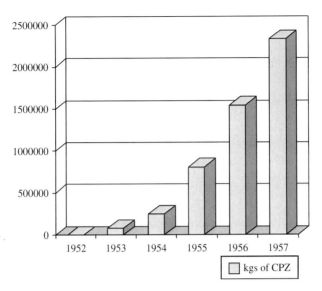

Figure 4.1 Kilogrammes of chlorpromazine used in French hospitals 1952–7 (Swazey 1974)

A vast research enterprise was rapidly spawned to investigate all aspects of drug action and related areas of biological psychiatry (Healy 1996). American Congress backed the new drugs by allocating extensive funds to research in mental health. By the mid-1950s, the U S National Institute for Mental Health (NIMH) had more money than it had research proposals to spend it on (Lehmann 1996). Numerous articles about drug treatment started to appear in psychiatric and medical journals. In the *British Journal of Psychiatry* one article out of 43 reported on drug treatment in 1945, and similar small numbers before this. By 1955, 15 out of 68 papers reported research into drug treatment and in 1960, 42 papers, almost a third of those published (145), concerned drug treatment (Moncrieff 1999).

Despite this evidence of the rapidity of the adoption of the new drugs and their influence on psychiatry, many of their advocates complained that there was resistance to using them. Pierre Deniker, one of the French psychiatrists who had first used chlorpromazine with psychiatric patients, complained in an interview in 1971 that this work had roused little interest (quoted in Swazey 1974, p. 138). Subsequently other prominent psychopharmacologists and historians of the period have reiterated this view (Healy 1996; Swazey 1974). Historian Judith Swazey's account of the introduction of chlorpromazine asserts that there was a general reluctance to accept it, despite presenting, on the same page, apparently contradictory data on the spread of chlorpromazine in French hospitals (Swazey 1974). Similarly, Francis Boyer, the president of Smith Kline & French and head of the Thorazine marketing task force complained of 'resistance to large scale hospital use of chlorpromazine' in some States (cited in Swazey 1974, p. 204). Undoubtedly there were psychiatrists who were suspicious of drug treatment and reluctant to use it. However the exaggeration of this response, and the downplaying of the enthusiasm with which many greeted the new drugs, paints a picture of a few heroic pioneers and an enlightened drug company helping to persuade a heathen profession to see the light. This attitude, not only portrays these individuals and the company in a good light, but also suggests that it was the benefits of the drug which persuaded the profession to change its ways. If, in contrast, it was admitted that the psychiatric profession was a sitting duck for a new medical type of treatment, the intrinsic benefits of the drug might seem more questionable.

Influence of physical treatments on attitudes to the new drugs

The enthusiasm surrounding the new drugs in psychiatry is reminiscent of attitudes to the physical treatments, especially ECT and insulin coma therapy. In fact, ideas about the physical treatments appeared to transfer smoothly onto the new drug treatments. Maudsley hospital psychiatrist and researcher Michael Shepherd described how psychiatric advocates of insulin coma therapy 'like a large shoal of fish ... simply switched direction to follow the lights of the more fashionable pharmacotherapy of schizophrenia' (Shepherd 1994, p. 93). One of the ideas that transferred was the specificity of action. When the new psychiatric drugs were first being developed there was no widely accepted precedent for the idea that a drug could act on the biological basis of a mental disorder. But, as described in Chapter 3, physical interventions such as electric shocks and insulin-induced comas were becoming identified as specific treatments that targeted some underlying pathology. With the introduction of chlorpromazine these ideas gravitated towards the new drug treatments as well. Because these physical methods were widely believed to be effective, and specifically effective in different conditions, psychiatry had become confident that manipulation of the body could reverse the biological abnormalities that gave rise to mental disorders. The new drugs were the natural inheritors of these beliefs.

The idea that treating the body can cure the mind is a longstanding one, and formed the implicit basis of the many physical treatments that were tried out in psychiatry in the 20th century (Scull 1994). The general acceptance of the efficacy and specificity of insulin coma therapy and ECT appeared to confirm the validity of this view. Many of the early pioneers of drug treatment had been advocates of the physical treatments. Hans Lehmann, who introduced chlorpromazine to Canada, compared its effects favourably to lobotomy (Lehmann 1955) and felt that it achieved 'about the same results' as insulin and shock treatments in schizophrenia (quoted in Swazey 1974, p. 157). Roland Kuhn, the Swiss 'discoverer' of imipramine, had worked with Jacob Klaesi, a psychiatrist in Berne, who had introduced barbiturate induced sleep therapy and was known as an enthusiast for physical treatments (Healy 1997). In an interview in 1970 Kuhn himself recalled 'our conviction that it must be possible to find a drug effective in endogenous depressions. This conviction arose from the literature study as well as from a great deal of experience we had acquired in the shock treatment of these depressions' (Kuhn 1970, quoted in Lehmann & Kline 1983, p. 234). Hans Lehman also explained that he and colleagues had been trying to find drugs 'to substitute for ECT' in depression (Lehmann 1996, p. 212). Many of the early pioneers of the new drugs, including the French psychiatrists Delay and Deniker and British researchers Elkes and Elkes were firm believers in a somatic or biological approach to treatment of psychiatric conditions and had been experimenting with other sorts of drugs before they used chlorpromazine (Swazey 1974).

Theories of drug action in medicine

Historians Edmund Pellegrino and Charles Rosenberg have described the history of the modern idea of a disease and of specific treatments. In contrast to the older 'humeral' notion of disease as a general state of bodily imbalance, the modern scientific view emerged during the late 19th and early 20th century. According to this latter view a disease was a collection of distinct symptoms caused by a biological mechanism, which could be identified in anatomical or physiological terms (Rosenberg 1977). Developments in microbiology crystallised this view with the discovery of the causative agents of several infectious diseases. The idea that substances might have specific actions on disease processes was clearly articulated at the end of the 19th century by Paul Erhlich with his idea of the 'magic bullet'. At first these ideas were greeted by scepticism among medical practitioners and their patients and much medical practice continued along humeral lines. However over the first decades of the 20th century confidence in science and scientific medicine grew. There was an acceptance of the disease theory of medicine and therapeutics among professionals and the public even before many effective medical treatments were available. Medicine became strongly associated with specialism and 'cure by specific therapy' became the 'only really proper sphere for the physician' (Pellegrino 1979, p. 255). In this period there was an almost unquestioning belief that science was for the good, that it would usher in a 'more humane, healthy and enlightened society' (Rosenberg 1986, p. 14), untempered by subsequent experience of atomic warfare and environmental degradation.

The new ideas brought with them a change in the nature and status of the medical profession and its relation to science. With the humeral model doctors prescribed drugs, or procedures such as bleeding, to induce bodily effects that were hoped to restore the body's balance and stimulate recovery. Drugs had to have noticeable physiological effects in order for people to believe they were doing their job. Rosenberg (1977) describes how mercury was particularly popular in the early 19th century because of the range of its effects; from diarrhoea to full-blown mercury toxicity depending on the dose taken. Prior to modern conceptions of disease and treatment, drug taking and prescribing were part of a 'fundamental cultural ritual' based on the shared humeral model of bodily health and disease. In this context patients and doctors had a more equal relationship than today. People took home remedies to produce purging and frequented quacks as well as regular physicians, but all treatments were based on the same principles.

By contrast, modern ideas about disease and its treatment require a technical knowledge that, by its nature, must be concentrated in the hands of specialists. The treatment of disease no longer requires an overt physiological effect, but consists in reversing or ameliorating the hidden biological process that gives rise to the symptoms. Thus it involves a detailed understanding of the specific mechanisms of disease based on a knowledge of the inner workings of the body that is not available to the layman. The medical profession was granted 'enormous social power' (Rosenberg 1986, p. 25) by this new orientation to treatment. In return doctors were expected to deliver more potent therapies.

Therefore, from the late 19th century the whole of medicine was seeking disease-specific treatments, a process that resulted in some very effective disease-specific drugs being developed starting with antibacterials like sulphonamides and hormones including thyroxine and insulin. Thus in developing disease-specific models of treatment, psychiatry was following a general trend within medicine. However in contrast to other areas of medicine, where this orientation offers a powerful and credible model, in the rest of this book we will see that there is little evidence to support the idea that psychiatric drugs work in this way. Therefore, we need to ask why it was that the disease-centred model of drug action became established in psychiatry, especially given that prior to the 1950s most drugs used were understood to act according to a drug-centred view. What motives extrinsic to the scientific data might have driven the adoption of a disease-specific view of the action of the new psychiatric drugs?

The psychiatric profession and the new drugs

There are two prevalent views of the nature of psychiatry in the 20th century. The first suggests that psychiatry has always been concerned to justify its place as a branch of medicine and therefore exhibits a continuous concern with biological explanations of mental conditions and physical methods of treatment. Biological theories and treatments played a central part in the professional struggles of 19th century psychiatrists or 'alienists' (Jacyna 1982) and, as we have seen, historians have documented the importance of physical interventions in the first half of the 20th century (Braslow 1997; Grob 1983; Scull 1994). According to this view psychoanalysis and moral treatment of the 19th century were anomalies in an otherwise consistent biological orientation (Scull 1994). The other view is that 20th-century psychiatry was dominated by psychoanalysis and social psychiatry (Wilson 1993). Often this view is put forward by those who decry this state of affairs, suggesting that during this period psychiatry was deflected from its proper biological and scientific orientation (Sabshin 1990; Shorter 1997).

Both views have some truth in them. The psychiatric profession has nurtured a long-standing concern to demonstrate its medical and scientific credentials. In the 19th century medical professionals had to struggle to justify their role in the management of madness and had to compete with successful examples of laymen fulfilling this role, such as at the famous York Retreat (Scull 1993). In the United Kingdom, it was only with the 1845 Lunacy Act that psychiatrists were awarded exclusive rights to run asylums. The emergent profession attempted to strengthen its position by asserting the physical basis of psychiatric disorders and their similarity with other medical conditions (Jacyna 1982). In 1858 an editorial in the *Journal of Mental Science* declared that 'Insanity is a purely a disease of the brain. The physician is now the responsible guardian of the lunatic and must ever remain so' (cited in Rogers and Pilgrim, 2001, p. 46). Similarly in the 20th century, the contents of the *British Journal of Psychiatry* revealed a continuous emphasis on biological explanations and approaches to mental disorder with little coverage of social or psychoanalytical approaches to mental disorder (Moncrieff & Crawford 2001). The *American Journal of Psychiatry* shows the same picture. Despite the supposed popularity of psychoanalysis and social psychiatry in the United States, only 7% of papers in available issues in 1940 covered these topics, 9% in 1950 and 7% in 1960. Again the overwhelming majority of the papers throughout reflected biological theories of psychiatry, such as genetics, electroencephalograph (EEG) recordings, treatment of epilepsy and the physical treatment procedures.

By the early 20th century, its role in the asylum system secured, psychiatry started to bemoan its second-class status in relation to the rest of medicine and sought greater parity with other medical specialties. In the United Kingdom in the early years of the 20th century psychiatrists were generally paid less than other doctors and were not highly regarded by the public or their medical colleagues. The profession attracted the least able medical students, people with disciplinary records and doctors from the colonies (Jenner 1997). Before they became part of the nursing profession, the attendants who staffed the asylums were of low status, had little if any education and received no training (Hannigan 2007). From the early years of the 20th century there is evidence that the leading figures of the psychiatric profession were trying to change this situation. In 1915 the president of the Medic-Psychological Association of Britain (now the Royal College of Psychiatrists) acknowledged the unpopularity of psychiatry as a medical career, calling it the 'Cinderella of medicine' and deplored the inadequate salary of most asylum doctors (Bond 1915). To address this situation he called for 'greater scientific training' and stressed the need for integration with general medicine, including a 'more satisfactory position for psychiatry in the medical curriculum' (Bond 1915, p. 8). In 1945 similar concerns were expressed in the Association's presidential address given by psychiatrist Lt Col. Petrie. Petrie also called for longer and tougher training, which he specifically hoped would attract more young neurologists and neuropathologists into psychiatry (Petrie 1945). There were similar concerns in the United States. In 1960 the president of the American Psychiatric Association called for 'adequate recognition by and closer affiliation with other professional and citizen organisations, particularly the general medical profession' (Malamud 1960, p. 3).

The physical treatments of the 20th century, especially ECT and insulin coma therapy, were greeted as potent symbols of psychiatry's status as a branch of medicine. Authors of a manual called *Shock Treatment in Psychiatry* argued that with ECT 'the psychiatrist takes on, in the patients mind, the characteristics of a "real doctor" in that he is able to apply and utilise a physical method of treatment' (Jessner & Ryan 1943). Subsequently the new drugs took on this role. They were credited with making 'the mental hospital a medical institution in the minds of the public' (Overholser 1956) and producing a 'profound intensification of medical orientation' (California State Senate 1956). They were also used as an argument for increasing psychiatrist numbers (California State Senate 1956). In 1970, Pierre Deniker reflected that one of the main contributions of the new drugs was to stimulate a 'more medically and scientifically oriented psychiatry' (Deniker 1970b).

Psychiatry had another concern during the 20th century, which was to disengage itself from the asylum. The large county mental hospitals built in the 19th century had become overcrowded with patients with chronic and severe conditions and they were perceived as a source of stigma and embarrassment for the psychiatric profession as well as their patients. The 1915 presidential address already identified the asylum as the cause of the unpopularity of psychiatry, and recommended the establishment of 'psychiatric clinics' in general hospitals (Bond 1915). During the 20th century the whole of medicine was developing a greater focus on milder conditions and their overlap with normality (Armstrong 1983). The rise of social medicine, health promotion and screening are some expressions of this trend as was psychiatry's increasing preoccupation with neurosis, outpatient practice, community psychiatry and the psychological health of the general population. However it was impossible to attract people with milder conditions to have cumbersome and dangerous procedures such as ECT and insulin coma therapy and these could not be conducted in an office-based practice. Psychoanalysis and psychotherapy were more suitable, which may partly explain their increasing popularity in this period. So was drug treatment, and drugs had the added advantage of seeming to be a proper medical treatment.

Although it can be overstated, the view that 20th psychiatry was strongly influenced by psychoanalysis is not altogether wrong. Mid-20th-century psychiatry was a curious mixture of the biological and the psychodynamic. Many psychoanalytical concepts and principles were accepted and psychotherapy was widely practised within mental hospitals as well as without. But for the most part it sat alongside physical approaches to treatment without there being much sense of contradiction or difficulty. Many psychiatric advocates of psychotherapy were also strong supporters of the new physical treatments (Linn 1955). Even Adolf Meyer, the great American social psychiatrist, approved of the introduction of insulin coma therapy (Grob 1983).

Some psychiatrists perceived difficulties with this situation and by the 1970s there was talk of a 'crisis in psychiatry', especially in America. This crisis was partly precipitated by the attacks of the antipsychiatry movement on the basis of biological psychiatry. But many prominent psychiatrists felt that psychiatry was vulnerable because the influence of psychoanalysis and social psychiatry meant that its theoretical underpinnings were vague and humanistic rather than what was regarded as truly scientific. Therefore, the psychiatric reaction to this perceived crisis was a deliberate attempt to remedicalise American psychiatry that culminated in the publication of the third version of the Diagnostic and Statistical Manual (DSM III) in 1980. DSM III replaced qualitative descriptions of psychiatric conditions informed by psychoanalytic concepts, with lists of symptoms and criteria for fulfilling different diagnoses. Superficially this produced a classification system that appeared to be more precise and more objective. It purged psychoanalysis from the conceptual basis of psychiatry and renewed the emphasis on biomedical science (Wilson 1993). There was also an economic impetus to this change in the United States. In the 1970s medical insurance agencies started to cut back on the amount of psychiatric treatment they would reimburse and it became more important for psychiatrists to be able to quantify and justify what they did (Wilson 1993).

The introduction of the new drugs, and especially their presumed specificity in different conditions was particularly important to the defense against antipsychiatry and to the development of DSM. The drugs justified the idea that madness and distress could be divided into discrete entities each with a characteristic aetiology and specific treatment. In 1973 the results of the 'Rosenhan experiment' were published, in which normal volunteers who got themselves admitted to mental hospitals were diagnosed as having suspected schizophrenia (Rosenhan 1973). This experiment appeared to call into question the ability of psychiatrists to identify genuine madness as well as the purpose and validity of psychiatric diagnosis. In a response to Rosenhan's challenge, leading American psychiatrist Robert Spitzer, the engineer of DSM III, defended psychiatric diagnosis by referring to the specificity of treatment. He argued that evidence for the 'superiority of the major tranquillisers (neuroleptics) in schizophrenia, of electro convulsive therapy in psychotic depression and more recently of lithium carbonate for the treatment of mania' justified the application of a medical process of diagnosis (Spitzer 1975). Martin Roth, a prominent British psychiatrist, also defended psychiatry from its antipsychiatry critics by referring to the 'beneficial effects of physical treatments' (Roth 1973, p. 377).

For many reasons therefore drugs had an obvious attraction to the psychiatric profession in the period of the 1950s to the 1970s. They were an intervention on the body and as drug treatment grew in importance in other areas of medicine they confirmed the desired parallels between psychiatry and physical medicine. This confirmation was needed to lift psychiatry out of the doldrums of the large asylum era and the easy administration of drugs made them perfectly suited to out-patient practice. They were also used as a weapon in the defence of psychiatry against its antipsychiatry critics. But for these endeavours to be successful, drugs needed to be presented as a specific treatment, not merely as a means of doping the patient into silence or submission.

Political attitudes to the new drugs

The modern state has been seeking a technical solution to the problem of madness since at least the end of the 18th century. In England, medical expertise was first legally endorsed in the 'Private Madhouses Act' of 1774, which required that patients admitted to private asylums be examined and certified insane by a doctor. However with its liberal political ideology, the 19th-century state was ambivalent towards the professions and saw its task partly as protecting the public from wrongful incarceration by unscrupulous private psychiatrists. Clive Unsworth's book the *Politics of Mental Health Legislation* describes the change in orientation of government policy at the beginning of the 20th century (Unsworth 1987). The liberal ideology of the 19th century was replaced by a belief that the state had a right and duty to intervene in social affairs. What had been perceived as individual moral weakness, such as crime and delinquency, was redefined as social problems that required state intervention and a technical solution. The idea that social problems could be prevented was also accepted. In order to achieve these aims the state formed an alliance with professional groups who were perceived to have the necessary technical expertise. It was at this point that the state unequivocally embraced a predominatly medical approach to the problems posed by the mad and the distressed. This attitude can be seen in government reports of the early 20th century, such as the Macmillan Report that underpinned the 1930 Mental Treatment Act. The report declared boldly that 'there is no clear demarcation between mental and physical illness' (Royal Commission 1926). It called for more laboratory facilities for research and recommended increased protection for doctors from suit against wrongful detention (Butler 1985). The Commission was preoccupied with ways to facilitate early treatment and believed that the long-standing involvement of a magistrate in the procedure of compulsory admission to mental hospital prevented this because of the stigma of association with the courts. The Commission expressed the belief that the involvement of an agent of the law was an unnecessary encumbrance that stood in the way of efficient medical treatment. At times, the Commission appeared to be more enthusiastic about the potential therapeutic powers of psychiatry than the psychiatrists they interviewed (Unsworth 1987).

Although, in the end, the 1930 Mental Treatment Act stopped short of abolishing the role of the magistrate, the concerns of the Macmillan Commission demonstrate that a commitment to a technical medical approach to the management of madness was present in government prior to the introduction of any psychiatric treatments that were generally thought to be effective.

The Percy Commission, reporting in 1957 was also confident that psychiatric conditions are medical problems and that medical treatments can resolve or eliminate them. 'Disorders of the mind are illnesses which need medical treatment' (Royal Commission 1957, p. 3), the report stated and it made numerous references to the similarity of mental and physical conditions. The report expressed great faith in the new treatments in psychiatry, which it referred to repeatedly. 'Great progress has been made during the present century in developing methods of treatment for many forms of mental disorder', it stated (p. 3), which have 'made the prospects of cure and recovery far better than they were 50 or even 20 years ago' (p. 75). It acknowledged that treatment 'is still at an early stage and much remains to be discovered' (p. 26), but denied that the mentally ill have any particular need for legal protection from ill treatment (pp. 38–39). The Percy Commission report formed the basis of the England and Wales 1959 Mental Health Act, which finally removed the process of involuntary incarceration from scrutiny by the legal process of abolishing the role of the magistrate. The power of commitment was, therefore, placed fully in the hands of professionals, those of doctors and social workers.

The other political objective of 20th-century mental health policy was deinstitutionalisation. The asylums, which had formed the 19th century's segregational response to madness, were costly to run and costs were increasing as the old Victorian buildings started to need extensive renewal (Scull 1977). Also, the isolation of the asylum system did not fit well with a belief that madness is a medical condition similar in kind to other physical conditions, whose management could be entrusted to qualified medical professionals. In the United Kingdom, the Macmillan Commission stated its approval of the development of outpatient and community services in the 1920s and by the late 1940s, a community-care survey was commissioned by the Ministry of Health (Titmuss 1968). The Percy Commission and the subsequent 1959 Mental Health Act stressed the importance of community care. In the United States expansion of community resources was seen as a solution to the overcrowding and appalling conditions in the public asylums. From the 1950s states started to fund outpatient services and by the 1960s the Kennedy administration was firmly committed to community psychiatry.

The desire to see the new drugs as a panacea is apparent in the selective representation of data on their relation to mental hospital occupancy rates. In the United States, studies by Henry Brill and Robert Patten from New York were widely quoted to support the conclusion that the new tranquillisers were responsible for increasing discharge rates from mental hospitals (Brill & Patton, 1957, 1958, 1962). A better-designed study conducted in Michigan, which concluded that the drugs were not responsible, was not publicised (Gronfein 1985). Data on the increasing rate of discharge of schizophrenic patients between 1914 and 1948, prior to the introduction of the new drugs, produced by the National Institute of Mental Health were also ignored (Grob 1994, cited p. 256). Numerous other data since then do not support a link between the use of the new drugs and decline in mental hospital numbers. Psychiatrist Michael Shepherd showed that inpatient numbers in the United Kingdom had started declining prior to the introduction of the new drugs (Shepherd et al, 1961). In the United States rates of discharge increased more before the introduction of neuroleptics than after (Gronfein 1985). In Norway inpatient numbers did not change with introduction of the drugs (Odegaard 1964) and in France they increased for a further 20 years after the new drugs came into use (Sedgwick 1982). These studies and others (Aviram, Syme, & Cohen 1976; Lerman 1982; Scull 1977) suggest that it was changing social policy and conditions rather than drugs that drove the reductions in asylum populations. However regardless of the reality of the drugs impact on patients, the political interest in the new drugs and the belief in their efficacy probably in itself hastened the process of deinstitutionalisation (Gronfein 1985). In 1963 US President John Kennedy confidently declared that the new drugs made 'it possible for most of the mentally ill to be successfully and quickly treated in their own communities and returned to a useful place in society' (*New York Times* 1963). He called for a 'bold new approach' based on 'new knowledge and new drugs' (Kennedy 1963).

The new drugs were also claimed to have quieted hospital wards. An official report declared that the new tranquillisers had 'delivered the greatest blow for patient freedom in terms of non restraint' (Joint Commission on Mental Illness and Mental Health 1961). But attributing this change to drug treatment was also fallacious. Efforts to transform the custodial regimes in asylums to more therapeutic ones were already afoot before the arrival of chlorpromazine. In the United States media exposés of the appalling conditions in mental hospitals in the 1940s led to political moves to improve conditions by increasing funding and staffing levels (Grob 1994). Hospital morale was also improved by the introduction of the physical therapies, which gave staff the impression that they were administering medical treatment. The new social therapies, such as milieu therapy, were also thought to be important (Greenblatt et al., 1955). The atmosphere of therapeutic optimism improved staff morale and introduced a less custodial attitude to patients. Psychiatrist Henry Rollin remembers how hospitals were refurbished and wards unlocked for the first time. The 'prison like atmosphere was largely eradicated', he notes (Rollin 1990, p. 111).

Thus the new drugs helped to fulfil political objectives as well as professional ones. Not only had Western governments long been trying to create a technical fix for the enduring and complex problem of how to manage psychiatric deviance, but by the 1950s they had financial incentives to reduce custodial care and find treatments that could be administered in the community. The new drugs provided the emergent political will for community care with the appearance of a scientific rationale.

The pharmaceutical industry and the new drugs

The pharmaceutical industry played a significant part in establishing the role of the new psychiatric drugs in the 1950s and 1960s. For doing so it is sometimes credited with helping transform psychiatry into a modern 'medical specialism' (Ban 1996). The large-scale marketing campaigns that helped to establish the use of the early neuroleptic and antidepressant drugs are documented in subsequent chapters, as well as the industry's role in propagating the modern view of depression as a common condition treatable with drugs.

The industry also helped to disseminate and reinforce the view that the new drugs were disease-specific treatments. Advertisements for antidepressants in the *British Medical Journal* and the *American Journal of Psychiatry* stress their specificity. Illustration 4.1 shows an early advertisement for Tofranil (imipramine), for example, asserting that it is a "specific" treatment for depression.

Niamid (nialamide, a monoamine oxidase inhibitor (MAOI)-type antidepressant), marketed by a branch of Pfizer, was described as a 'specific treatment' for 'depressive illness' (Niamid advertisement 1962). Laroxyl (amitriptyline) was heralded as a 'potent antidepressant' by one of its makers, Roche (Laroxyl advertisement 1962) and was described as being a 'specific treatment for depression and anxiety' by another manufacturer (Saroten advertisement 1962). Nardil (phenelzine) was claimed to be a 'true antidepressant which acts selectively on the brain' (Nardil advertisement 1961) in a British advert and a 'corrective' that 'helps remove the depression rather than masking the symptoms' (Nardil advertisement 1960) in an American advert. Adverts for the early neuroleptic Stelazine used the term 'antipsychotic' from 1960 in the *American Journal of Psychiatry* to stress the specificity of action. 'Stelazine', it is claimed 'exerts little or no sedative effect; rather Stelazine calms hyperactive patients chiefly because of its rapid effect against the psychotic process' (Stelazine advertisement 1960). The advert also notes that 'a striking response to Stelazine is the rapid reduction or elimination of delusions and hallucinations'. An advertisement for Largactil (chlorpromazine) in the *British Medical Journal* in 1961 was accompanied by a reproduction of a picture by Picasso of distorted machinery and a small caption picture of a brain (see Illustration 4.2). The implication is that the brain of someone with schizophrenia is like malfunctioning machinery that needs to be repaired with drugs.

However the industry's attitude to treatment specificity in this period was ambivalent. On the one hand the idea that drugs act directly on the biological basis of a disorder lends credibility and respectability to drug treatment, but on the other hand, it may limit its application. The idea that psychotropic drugs can induce effects that may be useful in a variety of situations is likely to create a larger market than the idea that they cure a specific psychiatric disease.

Therefore some advertisements emphasised the sedative action of tricyclic antidepressants. Amitriptyline, for example, was frequently recommended for its sedative action. It was described in one advert as having 'intrinsic tranquillising properties' and 'additional sedative action which relieves insomnia, agitation and anxiety'(Tryptizol advertisement 1964). Drinamyl, the combination of amphetamine and a barbiturate

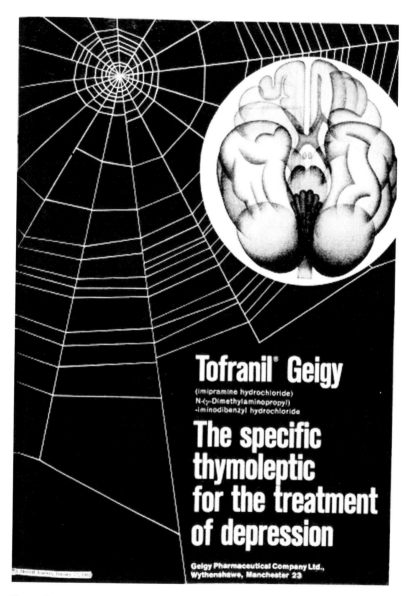

Illustration 4.1　Tofranil advertisement (reproduced with kind permission of Novartis)

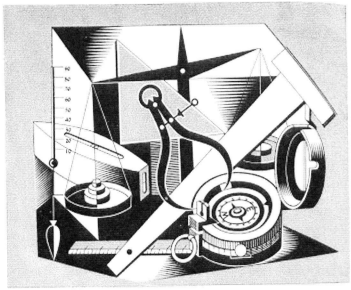

'*Largactil*' (CHLORPROMAZINE HYDROCHLORIDE)

the standard by which all other drugs
with a similar type of action are assessed

"Even if the other drugs do prove successful,
it is probable that some patients will respond better to
chlorpromazine than anything else, and because of this
it is likely to be of use to several practitioners for at
least some time to come."

Chlorpromazine and Reserpine—"the Rôle of the
General Practitioner," *Practitioner*, 1961, 18, 1961.

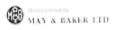

Distributed by
MAY & BAKER LTD

Illustration 4.2   Largactil advertisement (reproduced with kind permission of
Sanofi-Aventis)

marketed by Smith Kline & French, was described in one advertisement as 'the standard treatment for mental and emotional distress in everyday life' (Drinamyl advertisement 1962), although the same compound was promoted as having a 'proved antidepressant effect' in an American advertisement (Drinamyl advertisement 1960). Roche described the 'typical indications' for Parstellin, a combination of a neuroleptic and a monoamine oxidase inhibitor antidepressant, as 'emotional fatigue, menopausal symptoms, and many psychosomatic disorders' (Parstellin advertisement 1962). Many drugs were still advertised for their sedative or stimulating properties. In the 1960s several neuroleptics were marketed as everyday tranquillisers including Stelazine (trifluoperazine), Trilafon (perphenazine), Permitil (fluphenazine) and Melleril (thioridazine), which was described as 'a tranquilliser pure and simple' (Melleril advertisement 1962) and there were numerous adverts for benzodiazepines such as Librium. In 1964 an advertisement recommended Largactil for the 'querulousness of old age' (Largactil advertisement 1964). Ritalin was promoted as an 'antilethargic' for the period 'after childbirth, in convalescence, mild depression, oversedation, the menopause and in many old patients' (Ritalin advertisement 1964). However stimulants were also referred to as 'antidepressants' in adverts in the 1960s (Dexedrine advertisement 1960).

The action of neuroleptics on psychosis was also described explicitly in drug-centred terms in some advertisements as late as the 1960s. Trilafon, or perphenazine, a drug still used in the United States was advertised as producing 'symptomatic control of overactivity in psychopathological states' and inducing 'rapid response and early alteration of undesirable behaviour', minimising 'the problem of sedation and lethargy' (Trilafon advertisement 1960). Prolixen (fluphenazine) was described as an 'exceptionally effective behaviour modifier' (Prolixen advertisement 1960). The way in which this emphasis on drug-induced effects facilitated a wider market is clear as many adverts emphasised the numerous indications for their neuroleptic tranquillisers. An advert for Thorazine (chlorpromazine) claimed it controlled 'agitation – a symptom that cuts across diagnostic categories' (Thorazine advertisement 1960).

Recent promotion of the disease-centred model

The promotion of drugs for their drug-induced effects has become less respectable over recent years, especially in the wake of the scandal over benzodiazepine dependence. Although the benzodiazepines are associated with the treatment of anxiety and attempts have been made to articulate a disease-centred account of their action involving the neurotransmitter called GABA, the smell of non-specificity hovers around them. They are used recreationally by drug misusers because of their euphoriant effects, as well as being employed in diverse situations in medicine and psychiatry for their sedative and muscle-relaxant action. In the mid-1980s it became clear that they are physically and psychologically addictive in a similar fashion to alcohol or opiates and the massive scale of their use also became apparent. The subsequent scandal brought the idea of a non-specific drug for emotional problems into public disrepute. David Healy has suggested the industry's response was to transform the 'everyday nerves' that were the market for benzo-diazepines into 'depression' in the late 1980s and 1990s. In countries such as Japan, where there was no backlash against the benzodi-azepines, their sales remained high and there was no need to promote the idea of depression or the new antidepressants (Healy 2004).

Since this time the industry started to promote particular 'diseases' or diagnoses and allowed drug marketing to follow from the promotion of the condition. As well as depression, drug companies have organised campaigns to promote a number of entities such as panic disorder, social anxiety disorder, premenstrual dysphoric disorder, compulsive buying disorder and intermittent explosive disorder (Koerner 2002; Moynihan, Heath, & Henry 2002). It is not clear that conceptualising these difficulties as medical conditions is either meaningful or useful. Company funded research into the recently publicised 'conditions' of compulsive buying disorder and intermittent explosive disorder is being conducted at prestigious American universities and its results published in leading journals (Kessler et al. 2006; Koran et al. 2003). The industry has also funded campaigns to extend the medicalisation and drug treat-ment of childhood behaviour problems by promoting the diagnosis of attention deficit hyperactivity disorder (ADHD) and have successfully medicalised conditions such as substance abuse and bulimia that were not previously thought to be amenable to drug treatment.

Along with this emphasis on particular disorders, recent pharmaceu-tical industry literature for conditions like depression and psychosis refers increasingly commonly to imbalances in brain chemicals, echoing the statements of official psychiatric literature described in Chapter 1. On depression, Eli Lilly's website claims that 'a growing amount of evidence supports the view that people with depression have an imbal-ance of the brain's neurotransmitters ... many scientists believe that an imbalance in serotonin may be an important factor in the development and severity of depression' (Eli Lilly 2006a, accessed 10.02.2006). Wyeth, makers of the antidepressant Venlafaxine (brand name Effexor in the United Kingdom) suggest that it works by 'affecting the levels of two chemicals in the brain – serotonin and norepinephrine. Correcting the imbalance of these two chemicals may relieve symptoms of depression' (Wyeth 2006, accessed 21.09.2006). On schizophrenia, a Pfizer website states that 'imbalances of certain chemicals in the brain are thought to lead to the symptoms of the illness. Medicine plays a key role in balancing these chemicals' (Pfizer 2006) (accessed 06.02.2006). Eli Lilly claim that their drug Zyprexa (olanzapine) 'is believed to work by balancing the chemicals naturally found in the brain'(Eli Lilly 2006b). The word 'naturally' here suggests that these sorts of drugs are physically benign interventions, which merely restore the brain to a normal state, without exerting any additional effects.

Several publications now document the enormous and increasing influence of the pharmaceutical industry over the process of medical research and over the global health agenda (Angell 2004; Moncrieff 2003c; Moynihan & Cassels 2005). One of the most significant mechanisms of influence is the ability to market direct to consumers. In the United States and New Zealand, where direct-to-consumer advertising has been made legal, numerous television and radio adverts now promote prescription drugs. One recent survey found that one in five primary-care consultations was precipitated by someone seeing an advertisement (Gottlieb 2002). Even in countries without legal direct-to-consumer advertising, the Internet and 'disease awareness campaigns' provide an opportunity for drug companies to get a message to consumers. Many company sites now contain screening questionnaires, which present themselves as instruments that can detect the presence of a condition like bipolar disorder, social anxiety disorder or depression. If you score above a certain number of points on the questionnaire you are told you might have the condition in question and you are encouraged to see your General Practitioner. There is little check on the information companies are offering. Non-compliance with advertising regulations is common, with one in four adverts in the United States failing to meet the Food and Drug Administration's requirements (Aitken & Holt 2000) and even higher levels of non-compliance reported from New Zealand (Medawar 2001).

What we have witnessed over the last decade and a half is a powerful movement to promote the idea of the chemical imbalance led by the pharmaceutical industry, but with the psychiatric profession in tow. Previously, biological theories were only generally applied to severe psychiatric disorders and had little relevance to the general population. However social scientist Nicholas Rose has written of how these ideas have now seeped into public consciousness as never before and have started to change how people come to conceive of themselves. 'It seems' he says 'that individuals themselves are beginning to recode their moods and their ills in terms of the functioning of their brain chemicals' (Rose 2004, p. 28).

People corresponding on Internet websites demonstrate this development. One discussant on the 'Antidepressant Web', a website generally critical of psychiatric drugs and the pharmaceutical industry, stated: 'I truly believe that what I have is a biochemical imbalance centred around serotonin; whether it be lack of serotonin or receptors or an over-active re-uptake mechanism' (posted on 07/06/99). Another correspondent felt that 'coming from a family of mental imbalance, I knew it is everchanging and continual work to stay on top of the chemical wonder we call the brain' (posted on 13/10/02). Another referred to depression as a 'true brain disorder – treatable but not curable at this time' (posted on 26/04/04). Many participants endorsed the disease-centred view of drug action by talking of how antidepressants, in this case, 'worked' or 'helped' them in a general sense. Without a description of particular drug-induced effects, it appears that these people assumed that the drug had treated a disease or helped reverse an underlying biological process. One man effused about how antidepressants had changed his life and personality, 'it was the drug. It changed me – my brain's biochemistry. I've been on it for 6 years now and will continue because I love the new me' (posted on 07/06/1999) (Antidepressant Web 2006).

It appears that recent propaganda has been effective enough to persuade a large section of the population that their biochemistry is awry and that they need drug treatment to correct it. Thus the industry has been responsible for disseminating and popularising a disease-centred model of psychotropic drug action on a wider scale than ever before.

Conclusions

In this chapter I have described how enthusiastically the new drugs were received when they were introduced into psychiatry in the 1950s and 1960s and how they appeared to take over the mantle of interest that had been associated with the physical treatments. The whole of medicine in this era was searching for disease-specific treatments, and the psychiatric profession had additional professional motives to desire this sort of treatment. Western governments also supported a medical approach to the management of madness and distress, which stressed the similarity of general medicine and psychiatry. The pharmaceutical industry with its obvious motives to expand drug use, promoted drugs as a treatment for psychiatric conditions and lately have unambiguously promoted a disease-specific model of drug action and a chemical imbalance theory of the nature of mental disorders. Intense publicity from the combined forces of the pharmaceutical industry and the psychiatric profession has started to mould public attitudes to reflect professional and commercial ones.

So we have established that there were powerful interests behind the adoption of drugs as the principle form of psychiatric treatment and behind the transformation of views about drugs from chemical restraints to chemical cures. The question we now need to address is whether the evidence supports the idea that modern drugs are disease-specific treatments. Do psychiatric drugs deserve the prominence and respectability that they have now achieved? And if the evidence does not suggest that they act on disease processes, then how do they act? What are the characteristics of the psychological state they induce and how does this impact on normal mental functioning?

5
The Birth of the Idea of an 'Antipsychotic'

The neuroleptic drugs are psychiatry's most notorious drug treatment. They are the principle treatment for the most severe and symbolic of psychiatric conditions, such as schizophrenia or psychosis, but they are intensely disliked by many patients who therefore often have to be forced or pressurised to take them. They are also a focus of controversy due to claims about their brain damaging effects. They have been known under many names including major tranquillisers and phenothiazines, but are now mostly referred to as 'antipsychotics' a term that originated in North America. However to avoid the implications of disease specificity that this name implies I will mainly refer to them here as 'neuroleptics', a term that, as I explain below, better describes their characteristic actions.

These drugs are widely used within psychiatry and their use is increasing. The number of people using neuroleptic drugs in the United States increased from 2.2 million in 1997 to 3.4 million in 2004 and total expenditure on these drugs more than tripled over the same period (Stagnitti 2007). Psychiatric textbooks and guidelines recommend that they are effective for short-term treatment of an acute psychotic episode and should be used on a long-term basis to prevent recurrence or relapse. As well as patients with schizophrenia and psychosis, patients with many other diagnoses are prescribed neuroleptic drugs, usually alongside other types of psychotropic medication, including patients with anxiety, depression, mania, manic depression, personality disorder, etc.

Since the 1990s a range of new compounds have been introduced for the treatment of psychosis and schizophrenia. Although these compounds vary significantly in their pharmacological actions, they are collectively referred to as 'atypical antipsychotics' or second-generation antipsychotics. The property they are all supposed to share is a lower propensity to induce extrapyramidal side effects[1] than the first generation of such drugs, although they vary considerably in this regard. They have been heavily marketed by the pharmaceutical industry, with several becoming best-sellers, such as Eli Lilly's drug Zyprexa (olanzapine). They are widely recommended in current treatment guidelines and algorithms, although it is difficult to demonstrate that they are superior to the old drugs in terms of efficacy or adverse effects.

Over recent years it has been accepted that neuroleptic drugs should be started as early as possible in someone who is suspected of having a psychotic episode. 'Early intervention' teams have been set up in the United Kingdom and elsewhere, and numerous papers and conferences tout its benefits. The use of neuroleptics to prevent the onset of psychosis in so-called high risk individuals has also been advocated. The pharmaceutical industry has been active in this area, sponsoring academic symposia and journal supplements on early intervention (Lewis 2002; McGorry, Nordentoft, & Simonsen 2005) and funding the two trials of preventive drug treatment. A recent advertisement for risperidone depot injection features an adolescent girl walking near a playground, a doll dropped in her wake, with the caption 'Prescribe early, because what she loses she could lose forever' (*British Medical Journal* 2007; Risperidone Consta advertisement 2007).

When I started my psychiatric training in the United Kingdom in the early 1990s it was respectable practice to delay drug treatment for a time in someone with a suspected psychosis to make sure that they really did display psychotic features and to see if they improved without drug treatment. There was an air of caution about starting drug treatment and an acknowledgement of the negative effects this might have. It is becoming less easy for psychiatrists to practice in this way. It is now frequently suggested that drugs can prevent the progressive effects of an underlying brain disease and this idea is widely believed and presented as a fact, despite the fact that there is little evidence to support it. On the other hand, indications that the drugs themselves induce brain damage have been virtually ignored (see Chapter 8). Many psychiatrists are now convinced that not starting drug treatment early amounts to negligence.

Neuroleptic drugs are believed to be effective in schizophrenia and psychosis by interfering with the function of neurotransmitters in the brain. The most popular neurotransmitter candidate is dopamine, although others have been proposed sporadically. The drugs are thought to exert their main effect on the dopamine system by blocking transmission at D_2 (Dopamine 2) receptors (there are several known types of dopamine receptors), and thereby reducing the effects that dopamine has in the brain. It has been suggested that the correlation between clinical effects and D_2 receptor blockade is 'among the most clear-cut findings in psychopharmacology' (Healy 2002, p. 214). However the basis of this observation is that the *order* of the dose of a drug depends on the strength of its dopamine-blocking action. Drugs with particularly strong dopamine-blocking action, such as haloperidol are used at lower doses than drugs like chlorpromazine with weaker actions. But this is not evidence of a correlation with clinical improvement. It is simply an indication that the effects of dopamine blockade are difficult to tolerate above a certain level. In fact drugs with other profiles of action can produce clinical improvement such as non-neuroleptics and neuroleptics with relatively low dopamine-blocking potential, including clozapine.

A more consistent finding is that the blockading action at the D_2 receptor is responsible for the production of Parkinson's disease-like symptoms, often referred to as a type of extrapyramidal side effect. It is commonly held that 65% of D_2 receptors need to be blocked to produce a therapeutic effect and that overt Parkinson's-like symptoms appear at levels of 70–80% occupancy (Seeman & Kapur 2000).

The idea that the effects of antipsychotic drugs on the dopamine system represents an action on the basis of the disease of schizophrenia or psychosis, is derived from the dopamine theory of schizophrenia. This theory is one of the major 'chemical imbalance' theories of the nature and causation of mental disorders. It states basically that the symptoms of psychosis or schizophrenia are produced by an abnormality of the dopamine system, whether or not this is the ultimate cause of the condition. Drugs that act on the dopamine system can therefore help to correct at least part of this pathological process. However although nowadays the dopamine theory of psychosis and schizophrenia is central to the idea that antipsychotic drugs have a disease-centred action, it was the presumption that the drugs exerted a disease-specific action that was the initial inspiration for the dopamine theory. Therefore I will first describe how a disease-centred model of the actions of neuroleptic drugs developed before turning to the history of the dopamine theory of schizophrenia.

History of the disease model of antipsychotic drug action

In 1952 a French surgeon, Henri Laborit, used chlorpromazine to aid anaesthesia in surgical operations. His description of its effects led French psychiatrists Jean Delay and Pierre Deniker to wonder about its utility in psychiatric patients and they began to prescribe it to their patients in St Anne's psychiatric hospital in Paris. In these early days the effects of chlorpromazine were understood according to a drug-centred model and early names for this type of drug reflect this view. The French doctors who first used chlorpromazine called it a 'neuroleptic'. The word comes from the Greek meaning to 'take hold of the nervous system'. The term 'tranquilliser' was also frequently used to describe the effects of chlorpromazine and similar drugs and in Britain they were known as the 'major tranquillisers' for many years to distinguish them from the benzodiazepines, which were referred to as 'minor tranquillisers'. The term 'antipsychotic' with its clear disease-specific implications was not coined until the early 1960s. Its earliest appearance in an indexed scientific paper is 1962 (Mapp & Nodine 1962) and it was not frequently used until the 1970s and then mostly in North America.

Several authors have documented the way that this new type of drug was perceived to work in the early days after its introduction into medicine and psychiatry (Breggin 1993b; Cohen 1997; Gelman 1999; Valenstein 1988; Whitaker 2002). In 1952 Delay and Deniker noted that 'the apparent indifference or delay in response to external stimuli, the emotional and affective neutrality, the decrease in both initiative and preoccupation without alteration of conscious awareness or in intellectual faculties constitute the psychic syndrome due to treatment'. They also described how patients returned to normality when the drug was stopped: 'the patient, if he has been pale, regains his normal colour and activity and his normal "spirit"' (Delay & Deniker 1952, pp. 503–504).

Interestingly, Delay and Deniker first tried out chlorpromazine in patients with a range of psychiatric disturbances. Although some of their subjects had diagnoses of schizophrenia most were said to have 'excited or agitated' states or 'confusional' states. The term 'confusional' state is usually applied to a state of delirium caused by an organic condition such as a high fever, although it is not clear if this is the way Delay and Deniker were using the term. They concluded that the best effects of chlorpromazine were found in the excited, agitated and confusional states rather than in people with chronic schizophrenia (Delay & Deniker 1952).

Other psychiatrists noted early on how it produced 'a calming effect with a minimum of drowsiness and confusion' (Hoch, Lesse, & Malitz 1956), 'psychic indifference' (Anton-Stephens 1954) and a 'pathological tranquillity of mind' (Winkelman, Jr. 1957). Hans Lehmann, the first North American psychiatrist to use chlorpromazine described it as having the 'power to quiet severely excited patients without rendering them confused or otherwise inaccessible' and also recommended that it was most effective at controlling 'severe excitement' (Lehmann & Hanrahan 1954). Early on it was observed that the drugs produced effects similar to symptoms of Parkinson's disease, including reduced movement and facial expression and increased muscle tension. These observations were made more or less as soon as chlorpromazine started to be used (Steck 1954). Initially they were thought by many psychiatrists to be intimately related to the therapeutic action of the drugs. One wrote that 'the ability to induce an extrapyramidal action is a *sine qua non* of therapeutic effectiveness' (Denber 1959, p. 61). Another wrote: 'We busied ourselves to produce these states systematically through continuous treatment with Reserpine and Chlorpromazine ... Approximately half the patients [were] completely immobile. One could move them about like puppets' (Flugel 1956). This is a description of what was later called 'catalepsy', that is a state of extreme drug-induced Parkinson's disease, which is produced in animals when testing the side effect profile of potential antipsychotic drugs. As late as 1966, van Rossum, usually credited with the first articulation of the dopamine hypothesis of schizophrenia, stated, 'it seems as if extrapyramidal side effects are a prerequisite for neuroleptic action' (Rossum 1966, p. 492). Pierre Deniker likened the effects of the neuroleptics to encephalitis lethargica, an epidemic that had swept Europe between 1916 and 1926, leaving many of those affected with persistent Parkinson's disease-like symptoms (Deniker 1970a).

Several doctors who gave chlorpromazine to their patients in the 1950s compared its effects favourably to those of a frontal lobotomy. American Henry Winkelman, who was investigating chlorpromazine for Smith Kline & French in the United States, reported that 'the drug produced an effect similar to frontal lobotomy' making patients 'immobile', 'waxlike' and 'emotionally indifferent' (Winkelman, Jr. 1954). In a 1955 article Lehmann also speculated that it might prove to be 'a pharmacological substitute for lobotomy' (Lehmann 1955). Delay and Deniker are also said to have compared the effects of chlorpromazine to a frontal lobotomy (Swazey 1974, p. 155).

Although they were mostly enthusiastic about the potential therapeutic benefits of chlorpromazine, these early pioneers were at pains to point out that they did not believe that the drug acted on the disease process or had any specific effect on psychotic or schizophrenic symptoms. The authors of an early British study of chlorpromazine's effects in chronically psychotic long-term institutionalised patients concluded that 'in no case was the content of the psychosis changed. The schizophrenic and paraphrenic patients continued to be subject to delusions and hallucinations, though they were less troubled by them' (Elkes & Elkes 1954). In a succinct expression of the drug-centred model of drug action, psychiatrists at a symposium in 1955 concluded that chlorpromazine could be used 'to attain a neuropharmacologic effect, not to "cure" a disease' (Proceedings held under the auspices of Smith Kline & French laboratories 1955).

These beliefs about the effects of neuroleptic drugs quickly disappeared, however and the drugs rapidly metamorphosed into a 'miracle cure' for schizophrenia. These views start to appear very early on. Despite later comparing its effects to lobotomy, in 1954 Winkelman was already suggesting that 'chlorpromazine should not be considered merely a chemical restraint that has no real effect on the patient's illness' (Winkelman, Jr. 1954, p. 21). By 1958 a British book was hailing the new tranquillising drugs as being of a 'different order' from previous drug treatments, enabling psychiatrists to wipe out the 'symptoms of psychotic patients just as internists can use insulin for the elimination of the symptoms of diabetes' (Himmich 1958). Textbooks of the early 1960s hesitate about describing the effects of the new drugs as 'specific' but suggest that 'they appear to do more than tranquillise' (Henderson & Gillespie 1962). Another one suggests that 'the drugs penetrate much closer to the site of mechanism of the disease itself than any other procedure applied hitherto' (Mayer-Gross, Slater, & Roth 1960). Thus the disease-centred view of the action of the neuroleptic drugs appears to be already established by the time of the landmark National Institute of Mental Health (NIMH) study of their use in acute schizophrenia. This study reported in 1964 and, as well as apparently confirming the efficacy of these drugs in a large-scale RCT, it set the seal on a disease-centred view of their action. The study referred to the neuroleptic drugs as being '"antischizophrenic" in the broad sense' (The National Institute of Mental Health Psychopharmacology Service Center Collaborative Study Group 1964). In a conference held in 1962, they were described as 'astonishingly specific', able to produce 'change in the actual psychopathological mechanism' (Flugel 1966). By 1970 Peirre Deniker admitted that his early hypothesis about neuroleptics inducing a neurological disease was controversial and suggested, somewhat reluctantly, that it had been contradicted. He deferred to the disease-centred notion of neuroleptic drug action by referring to chlorpromazine as a 'drug that was found to act directly on a psychopathological process' (Deniker 1970b, p. 164).

Patient case notes also reveal that chlorpromazine and the new tranquillisers were regarded differently by psychiatrists and credited with a more direct therapeutic action than previous drugs had been. In contrast to older drugs, they were more often mentioned in the medical notes and were referred to in letters to General Practitioners when patients were discharged. The case of a male patient illustrates the point. He was treated with numerous shots of ECT and insulin coma therapy during his frequent admissions in the 1940s and 1950s, which were recorded in his medical notes and discharge summaries along with his progress. At the same time he received paraldehyde and barbiturate drugs, but this was only apparent from the medication charts and never mentioned in the notes. In an admission in 1958 he was treated with large doses of chlorpromazine. This was reported in his medical notes and a letter to his General Practitioner on discharge stated that 'he is leaving us today, *with his medication, of course ...*' [italics added].

The author Robert Whitaker records how this transformation was reflected in the popular press of the time in the United States. In an article in *Time* magazine entitled 'Wonder drug of 1954?', it is stated that 'there is no thought that chlorpromazine is any cure for mental illness, but it can have great value if it relaxes patients and makes them accessible to treatment' (Time 1954). Treatment here refers to psychotherapy. Stories in the *New York Times* in 1955 referred to chlor-promazine and similar drugs under development as 'one of the most significant advances in the history of psychiatric therapy', that will 'revolutionise the treatment of mental illness'. They were described as 'miracle' drugs, bringing 'peace of mind' and 'freedom from confusion' without the 'lethargy that follows the use of barbiturates' (cited in Whitaker 2002, pp. 152–153). Time magazine suggested that neuroleptic drugs represented an advance as significant as the 'germ killing sulphas discovered in the 1930s' (Time 1955).

With the metamorphosis of the neuroleptic drugs into 'antipsy-chotics', there was a conceptual separation between their therapeutic and adverse effects. Within professional circles early descriptions of their global effects were obliterated from the collective memory. Parkinson's symptoms and other neurological effects came to be regarded merely as incidental side effects not related to the mechanism of action. Effects that had been clearly described in the 1950s were presented subse-quently in the literature under a number of different names as if they had been newly discovered. In 1977 three eminent American psychia-trists rediscovered a 'side effect' of neuroleptics they called 'akinesia'. They described how this consisted of 'a lessening of spontaneity, paucity of gestures, diminished conversation and apathy' (Rifkin, Quitkin, & Klein 1975). In the 1970s other psychiatrists, notably Van

Putten, rediscovered drug-induced 'dysphoria', which was noted to be associated with neurological effects, especially akathisia[2] (Van Putten 1974, 1975). This was later labelled as 'akinetic depression' (Van Putten & May 1978). In the 1990s the term neuroleptic-induced deficit syndrome was coined to describe 'affective and cognitive impairment' (Lader 1994) and drug-induced dysphoria was revisited (Hollister 1992; King, Burke, & Lucas 1995).

A story was being woven of effective and specific drugs whose side effects were incidental and relatively minor. The numerous published accounts that contradicted this picture or suggested a different interpretation were ignored and forgotten. Only when the second-generation neuroleptics came onto the market, which were supposed to reduce the incidence of extrapyramidal side effects, was it admitted how endemic these 'side effects' were. Similarly, the therapeutic benefits of the drugs were only questioned when drug companies were trying to prove the superiority of newer drugs and when clozapine started to be marketed as a specific intervention for treatment-resistant cases.

The pharmaceutical industry and other influences

Chlorpromazine was introduced to the United States in a huge marketing campaign conducted by the company Smith Kline & French. The campaign was wide ranging and had a huge impact. A 'Thorazine'[3] task force was set up which operated from 1954 to 1960, whose activities have been described in a personal interview with the company president and task force convenor, Francis Boyer (reproduced in Swazey 1974). The campaign was launched on national television in a programme presented by Boyer himself, called 'The March of Medicine'. The task force targeted psychiatrists, asylum administrators and state politicians to persuade them of the benefits of increasing their spending on drugs, euphemistically referred to as 'intensive treatment'. It provided coaching for psychiatrists and hospital administrators to help them lobby state legislatures for more money for drugs. It helped design rating scales for evaluating drug effects. The task force compiled statistics to show that the use of chlorpromazine reduced violent incidents and damage to hospital property and reduced staff turnover within asylums. Education was provided for General Practitioners, private psychiatrists and general hospital medical staff. A large focus of the campaign was on 'aftercare', by which was meant the continued prescription of chlorpromazine after discharge from hospital. Boyer described how the importance of aftercare became apparent from the high relapse and readmission rate of discharged patients. Although he did not think that these patients were stopping their treatment after discharge he was concerned that they were being prescribed lower doses than they needed by nervous community practitioners. The task force supplied free Thorazine to several aftercare projects, and worked with state officials to produce aftercare protocols for regional clinics. Thus long before there were any evaluations of long-term treatment, patients were routinely being prescribed such treatment, with the pharmaceutical industry encouraging this approach.

A United States Senate enquiry chaired by Senator Estes Kefauver, published in 1961, revealed the extent of the industry's influence over the scientific portrayal of the new drugs. It alleged that many articles published in medical journals were 'ghost' written by the medical writers employed by pharmaceutical companies. Papers that were critical of drugs were rarely published because journals did not wish to jeopardise advertising revenue (U.S. Senate Subcommittee on Antitrust and Monopoly 1961). Much of the picture of chlorpromazine as a 'wonder drug' presented in the lay press in the 1950s was also concocted by the pharmaceutical industry (Whitaker 2002). The Senate enquiry revealed how newspapers and magazines were offered advertising revenue in return for printing favourable stories about the drugs and how journalists received high fees and other perks. A physician working for Pfizer admitted to the enquiry that 'much of what appears (in the lay press) has in essence been placed by the public relations staff of the pharmaceutical firms. A steady stream of magazine and newspaper articles are prepared for distribution to the lay press' (U.S. Senate Subcommittee on Antitrust and Monopoly 1961). These articles, described earlier, helped to shape a popular conception of the new drugs as miracle cures.

The psychiatric profession and Western governments also embraced and promoted the new tranquillisers, as described in Chapter 4, helping to transform them into exciting, disease-specific treatments. They were declared responsible for quieting psychiatric wards and emptying the mental hospitals and they were applauded for giving psychiatry a firm medical foundation. The neuroleptics came into psychiatry at a propitious time. They suited professional objectives to ally psychiatry closer to general medicine, and they facilitated political aims to run down the ageing and expensive asylums and find treatments that could be delivered in cheaper settings. They were also the perfect technical fix for the complex social problems posed by severe psychiatric disturbance.

The neuroleptics allowed the social control involved in the treatment of such disturbance to be presented as an unobtrusive and apparently thoroughly medical activity.

History of the dopamine theory of schizophrenia

The dopamine theory of the causation of schizophrenia is clearly central to the argument that neuroleptic or antipsychotic drugs have a disease-specific action. However the theory was not clearly articulated until the early 1970s. This is almost 10 years after the NIMH study declared that chlorpromazine and related drugs were 'anti-schizophrenic in the broad sense'. Although Van Rossum's paper of 1966 is often cited as the first expression of the dopamine theory of schizophrenia, in fact it only concerned the mode of action of neuroleptic drugs. In the paper Van Rossum states: 'The hypothesis is therefore put forward that dopamine receptor blockade is an important factor in the mode of action of neuroleptic drugs' (Rossum 1966, p. 492). In a book published the same year he speculates briefly that this discovery may have 'far going consequences for the pathophysiology of schizophrenia. Overstimulation of dopamine receptors could then be part of the aetiology' (Rossum 1966, p. 327). However despite the fact that it had not yet been clearly formulated, there are indications that the theory was already influential by the early 1970s. In 1974, for example, it was described as being 'shared by many investigators' and exerting 'a substantial influence on the design of experiments' (Matthysse 1974). Yet in the scientific literature the idea stayed at the level of brief speculation until the mid-1970s (Faurbye 1968; Kety 1972; Klawans, Jr., Goetz, & Westheimer 1972). For many researchers in the field, the dopamine hypothesis remained a hypothesis about antipsychotic drug action rather than the aetiology of schizophrenia (Snyder et al. 1970). As late as 1973, Steven Matthysse, in one of the first reviews of research pertaining to a possible dopamine theory of schizophrenia, argued that 'this simple hypothesis is by no means the only possible interpretation (of some research data). It is not even the most plausible' (Matthysse 1973). A year later he was more confident, stating that 'ideas connecting dopamine and schizophrenia have reached a certain maturity' (Matthysse 1974). By 1976 a comprehensive and substantial review concluded that 'the evidence for a role of dopamine in the pathophysiology of schizophrenia is compelling but not irrefutable' (Meltzer & Stahl 1976).

The fact that the theory was stimulated by observed actions of neuroleptic drugs on dopamine is clearly demonstrated in these early accounts. The dopamine theory was first postulated in the context of research into the dopamine-blocking actions of neuroleptics in cats (Rossum 1966). Later Meltzer and Stahl (1976) described neuroleptic drug action as 'one of the cornerstones of the dopamine hypothesis of schizophrenia' (p. 37). In 1988 it was noted that 'the dopamine hypothesis is still almost entirely based on pharmacologic evidence' (Carlsson 1988). In line with evidence that the drugs blocked dopamine receptors, the earliest incarnation of the dopamine hypothesis stated that schizophrenia was caused by overactivity of some dopaminergic neurons (Meltzer & Stahl 1976).

The notion of a neurochemical balance is also introduced in some of these early accounts. Matthysse (1973) suggests that 'It may be that a system inhibited by, or inhibiting dopamine neurons is deficient in schizophrenia, and the dopamine blocking actions of antipsychotic drugs *restores a balance*' (p. 204, italics added).

However it soon became apparent that there was little evidence of an intrinsic abnormality of dopamine activity in people diagnosed with schizophrenia, other than abnormalities induced by drug treatment with dopamine-blocking drugs. Other evidence also contradicted the hypothesis. But the dopamine theory of schizophrenia has proved remarkably tenacious. In 1991, Kenneth Davis and colleagues published a paper setting out a revised version of the dopamine theory of schizophrenia, designed to accommodate the theory to the problem that the common negative symptoms of schizophrenia[4] appear to be incompatible with what is known about dopamine's range of effects. Dopamine excess is associated with increased movement and mental activity and negative symptoms involve reduced activity. They suggested that schizophrenia was due to a simultaneous deficiency of dopamine activity in the frontal cortex of the brain (the area broadly responsible for complex thought, motivation, feeling and social behaviour) and an excess of dopaminergic activity in the subcortical (striatal) area. The dopamine deficiency caused the 'negative' symptoms of schizophrenia and the excess was responsible for positive symptoms (Davis et al. 1991). This theory is still influential (Abi-Dargham 2004), although how a single disease could produce the unusual situation of opposite biochemical changes in different brain areas has not been addressed. Other attempts to marry up the theory with contradictory evidence include the serotonin–dopamine version of the hypothesis, which was developed after it was noted that clozapine, thought to be a particularly effective antipsychotic drug, had substantial effects on the serotonin system and relatively weak effects on dopamine. This version suggested that the balance between the two neurotransmitters dopamine and serotonin was abnormal in schizophrenia and could be restored by drug treatment (Huttunen 1995).

A Canadian researcher, Shitij Kapur, has recently restated the dopamine hypothesis, suggesting that dopamine 'dysregulation' is the cause of psychotic symptoms rather than schizophrenia itself. Kapur's ideas have revived the popularity of the dopamine theory, which is now the subject of large international conferences and considerable research activity. Kapur proposes that 'before experiencing psychosis, patients develop an exaggerated release of dopamine' (Kapur 2003, p. 15). This 'dopaminergic dysregulation' is what he calls the 'aberrant neurochemistry' underlying psychotic experiences. He suggests that dopamine is responsible for the 'salience' of experiences. Excess dopamine leads to a state of 'aberrant salience', in which ordinary events are misinterpreted as meaningful and personally significant and become what we refer to as delusions and hallucinations. He then goes on to describe how the neuroleptic drugs counteract this abnormal process by reducing dopamine activity and thereby dampening the abnormal salience of phenomena characteristic of psychosis. Kapur emphasises that his theory does not explain the ultimate cause of schizophrenia, only 'how the symptoms of psychosis arise given certain neurochemical abnormalities' (Kapur 2003, p. 18). He also tries thoughtfully to accommodate psychological theories about the origins of some psychotic symptoms by suggesting that some symptoms such as delusions are cognitive responses to abnormal salience. The thesis about the ability of neuroleptic drugs to reduce salience is reminiscent of, and indeed derived from, early descriptions of the state of psychic indifference they produce and is consistent with a drug-centred view of the drugs' actions. However Kapur turns this drug-centred view into a disease-centred view by the proposed thesis that this action reverses an underlying 'neurochemical abnormality'. The therapeutic impact of antipsychotics are therefore explained, not in terms of how such effects might impact on psychotic symptoms, but in terms of their actions on an aberrant biological process.

A new zeitgeist

The story of how the new tranquillising drugs of the 1950s came to be seen as having a specifically 'antipsychotic' action demonstrates how desire won out over observation. David Cohen (1997) writes of a 'zeitgeist of psychotropic drug bias' (p. 203), which allowed evidence to be constructed and interpreted along lines that maximised the proposed therapeutic effects, minimised the significance of adverse effects and obscured the relation between the two. In this way the idea of a disease-specific treatment was superimposed on observations of drug-induced effects. A theory of the aetiology of schizophrenia and psychosis, the dopamine hypothesis, was constructed post hoc to provide a justification of this view. In the next chapter I will review the existing evidence on whether neuroleptic drugs do act in a disease-centred fashion, including evidence for the dopamine hypothesis of schizophrenia and psychosis.

6
Are Neuroleptics Effective and Specific? A Review of the Evidence

In this chapter I will look at the main body of research on which current beliefs about the nature and efficacy of the so-called antipsychotic or neuroleptic drugs are based. I will attempt to evaluate whether the data from this and other research supports a disease-based theory of neuroleptic drug action in disorders diagnosed as psychosis or schizophrenia.

Are neuroleptics better than placebo for short-term treatment?

There is no doubt that neuroleptic drugs have profound effects on the human body and brain. The question that we need to ask about their short-term use is whether they have any clinical advantage over placebo, *and* over other sorts of drugs that might be used in people with acute psychosis. By advantage we could mean a number of things. Firstly we could ask whether antipsychotic drugs speed up the natural process of recovery from psychosis, that is, do people get better quicker than they would without them? We know, for example, that for most people periods of psychosis are self-limiting. Secondly we could ask whether people who were prescribed these drugs achieve a fuller recovery when compared with people taking no treatment, placebo or other types of drug. Finally we might want to know whether these drugs help more people to recover than would do otherwise. One immediate problem with addressing these questions is that our information about the natural history of acute psychosis without modern drug treatment is limited. We do not actually know how many people might get better without drug treatment, how fast or how completely.

Studies of the effects of short-term treatment show that being on a neuroleptic is superior to being on an inert placebo on measures of symptoms and behaviour over a relatively short period. Since many episodes of acute psychosis are likely to last for months at least, and all such trials last a few weeks at most, there is little data with which to consider the overall advantages of drug treatment on the outcome of an acute episode. However these studies demonstrate that patients taking placebo also improve and in some trials the difference between the drugs and placebo is not large (Johnstone et al. 1978).

Longer-term follow-up of the results of acute treatment studies are rare. A one-year follow-up study of the earliest trial conducted by the NIMH in the United States found no evidence that patients who had been randomised to drug treatment fared better than those randomised to placebo. In fact the placebo group had a lower rate of hospital readmission during the year of follow-up, which was the only statistical difference between the two groups (Schooler et al. 1967). Similarly follow-up of another randomised trial with patients with first episode psychosis found that only 27% of the placebo group were rehospitalised compared with 62% of the patients initially randomised to chlorpromazine ($\chi^2=8.43$, $p<.01$) (Rappaport et al. 1978). The three-to-five-year follow-up of a large randomised trial comparing neuroleptics with psychotherapy, milieu therapy (consisting of admission to a well staffed hospital ward with no specific additional treatments) and ECT showed little difference between the groups. This was despite the fact that the short-term results showed clear differences in favour of drug treatment. The follow-up results were especially remarkable since the study excluded 'good prognosis' patients who were expected to do well without drugs (May et al. 1981). Between 15% and 44% of patients who were not allocated to antipsychotic drug treatment during the initial study phase managed to avoid the use of neuroleptic drugs for at least three years of follow-up. Therefore research suggests that neuroleptic drugs reduce the symptoms of psychosis or schizophrenia over the short term in some patients compared with the use of placebo, but there is little to suggest that this has any ultimate benefit.

The concept of 'treatment-resistant schizophrenia', which was developed to delineate a market for the relaunch of clozapine, has lead to public acknowledgment of the extent of non-response to treatment with other neuroleptic drugs. It is now widely admitted that at least 25% of patients do not show any significant clinical improvement with drug treatment. A recent comparison of two of the newer neuroleptic drugs, risperidone and olanzapine, found that 46% and 56% of patients, respectively, did not respond after four months of treatment (Robinson et al. 2006). In addition, the majority of inpatients with psychosis are treated with other sedative drugs in addition to neuroleptics, implying that the neuroleptics alone are insufficient to control their symptoms. In 1995, a survey found that 70% of patients on neuroleptics were taking other psychotropic medications, mostly benzodiazepines and "mood stabilisers" (Baldessarini, Kando, & Centorrino 1995). Therefore, it seems that antipsychotics are often unable to significantly improve the condition of someone who is acutely psychotic.

Are neuroleptics better than other drugs for short-term treatment?

The next important question is whether the short-term improvement produced by neuroleptics is better than that obtained with other sorts of drugs. Table 6.1 shows that studies have found that a variety of drugs have comparable effects to neuroleptics in the treatment of psychosis or schizophrenia. Two early randomised trials concluded that barbiturates were inferior to neuroleptics, but these may have been influenced by negative expectations of barbiturates, which were part of the old generation of disregarded drugs and are referred to in the studies as the 'control medication' (Casey et al. 1960, p. 98).

After the introduction of the benzodiazepine drugs in the 1960s, several studies were conducted evaluating their effects in schizophrenia. Since benzodiazepines were fairly new at the time, they did not suffer from the

Table 6.1   Studies comparing neuroleptics to other sedatives for short-term treatment of psychosis or schizophrenia

Drug group	Studies	Results
Barbiturates	2 randomised controlled trials (Casey et al. 1960a, 1960b)	Barbiturates inferior to chlorpromazine
Opiates	1 randomised controlled trial (Abse, Dahlstrom, & Tolley 1960)	Opium equivalent to chlorpromazine
Benzodiazepines	6 randomised controlled trials (Hankoff, Rudorfer, & Paley 1962; Hekimian & Friedhoff 1967; Maculans 1964; Merlis, Turner, & Krumholz 1962; Nishikawa et al. 1982; Smith 1961)	Benzodiazepines equivalent to neuroleptic in three studies, superior in two, inferior in one
Lithium	2 randomised controlled trials (Braden et al. 1982; Johnstone et al. 1988)	Lithium equivalent for moderately ill patients; inferior for overactive patients

same stigma as the barbiturates. Ratings of their effects might therefore be less susceptible to bias. Wolkowitz and Pickar (1991) reviewed 14 double-blind trials comparing benzodiazepines with placebo and neuroleptics for the treatment of psychosis or schizophrenia. The studies suffered from problems such as small sample sizes, short duration and mixed groups of chronic and acute patients. Six studies compared a benzodiazepine and placebo for patients with acute and chronic psychotic disorders; only the largest study found the benzodiazepine to be markedly superior to placebo at a statistically significant level. However in the six trials comparing benzodiazepines with neuroleptics, the outcomes were equivalent in three, the benzodiazepine was superior in two, chlorpromazine was superior in one, and in one trial the benzodiazepine was equivalent to haloperidol but inferior to chlorpromazine. Most interestingly, in seven of the ten studies where psychotic symptoms were evaluated, benzodiazepines reduced symptoms as much as neuroleptics or better than placebo. A recent study of the treatment of early signs of exacerbation in schizophrenia found that diazepam was superior to a neuroleptic (Carpenter, Jr. et al. 1999).

Trials of lithium in patients with acute psychosis (and not just mania) showed that lithium was inferior for the treatment of severely overactive patients, presumably because of its toxicity, but comparable to neuroleptics for the treatment of less overactive patients, regardless of diagnosis (Braden et al. 1982; Johnstone et al. 1988). A trial conducted in the 1960 comparing opium and chlorpromazine in acute schizophrenic patients showed equivalent improvement over three weeks with both drugs (Abse, Dahlstrom, & Tolley 1960).

The drug-centred model of drug action suggests that neuroleptics might be superior to other sedative drugs because of the nature of the neurological state they induce with its characteristic psychic indifference. Overall however there does not appear to be strong evidence that the effects of neuroleptic drugs are superior to the effects of other drugs with sedative effects, except possibly the barbiturates. There is little evidence even that they are superior for the core symptoms of psychosis such as delusions and hallucinations, since most comparative studies found benzodiazepines to have equal effects on these symptoms.

Are neuroleptics better than placebo for long-term treatment?

There is overwhelming consensus in psychiatric circles that continuous use of neuroleptic drugs by people with episodes of psychosis or schizophrenia reduces the risk of relapse or deterioration considerably.

Common estimates are that 80% of people relapse without drug treatment compared with 20–40% with drug treatment (Hogarty & Ulrich 1998). Guidelines recommend that people should remain on drug treatment for one to two years after an episode or relapse (National Institute for Clinical Excellence 2002), but in practice professionals are extremely reluctant to stop medication and people are likely to remain on drugs indefinitely unless they actively challenge medical advice and decide to stop the drugs themselves. A recent study found that people with long-term schizophrenia under the care of a General Practitioner had not had their psychotropic medication changed to any degree for decades in some cases, despite being clinically stable for long periods (Challoner 2006).

However the studies of maintenance therapy on which current recommendations are based are deeply flawed and cannot yield data on the efficacy of preventing relapse. This is due to the confounding effects of discontinuation-related problems. These studies start by selecting a group of people who are already taking drug treatment, and whose mental condition is currently stable. These people are then randomised either to continue drug treatment or to have the drug withdrawn and replaced by inert placebo tablets or injections. The placebo group are, therefore, vulnerable to all the adverse effects of having their drug treatment discontinued. The fact that it is usually done quite rapidly is likely to exaggerate these effects. Therefore, the fact that outcomes of patients allocated to placebo in long-term discontinuation trials appear to be inferior to those of people who stay on medication may merely reflect the difficulties of stopping long-term drug treatment. Somatic withdrawal symptoms may be mistaken for signs of relapse. The pharmacological stress placed on the body by withdrawal may induce a relapse and a small proportion of people may experience an episode of psychosis that is part of the withdrawal syndrome and may be nothing to do with their original condition (Moncrieff 2006). In addition, there are the likely effects of negative attitudes of staff, patients and others towards being on placebo. Most people who work in the mental health system believe that drug treatment is beneficial and that withdrawing it will inevitably lead to the recrudescence of the underlying problem. Given that people taking neuroleptics and placebo are likely to be easily distinguished on the basis of the many obvious effects of neuroleptics, such as extrapyramidal effects, it is possible that negative expectations further depress the outcome in the group withdrawn to placebo. Staff might overreact to minor withdrawal symptoms, for example, or focus on negative events that would normally be ignored in people they suspect have been withdrawn from drugs. One study revealed nursing staff's negative attitudes to reducing medication and concluded that staff attitudes were just as important as a patient's mental condition in determining drug treatment (Thomas, Katsabouris, & Bouras 1997).

A large review of 66 discontinuation studies published in 1995 found that overall, over an average period of 10 months follow-up, 16% of patients who continued drug treatment relapsed compared with 53% of patients who discontinued drug treatment (Gilbert et al. 1995). Further analysis of this set of studies revealed that the relapses after medication discontinuation were clustered around the point at which the drugs were stopped. Fifty per cent of those relapsing did so within three months of discontinuation (Baldessarini & Viguera 1995). In studies using randomised or matched controls, the risks of relapse after discontinuing medication appeared to converge over time with the risk of relapse while staying on medication. In other words, with increasing time after drug withdrawal the increased risk of relapse seemed to dissipate. Another meta-analysis of 28 discontinuation studies, mostly randomised controlled trials, confirmed these findings (Viguera et al. 1997). After abrupt discontinuation of drug treatment relapse risk was 50% within 30 weeks and by six months following drug discontinuation there were few further relapses. Overall 54% of patients relapsed in the first year after discontinuation compared with a further 2% in the following year.

There are at least two explanations for the clustering of relapses around drug withdrawal. The first is that somatic discontinuation symptoms are mistakenly labelled as relapse. The second is that the withdrawal process itself provokes significant psychopathology, either in the form of a withdrawal-related psychotic episode, or in the form of withdrawal-induced relapse of the underlying condition. Several studies included in Gilbert et al.'s review used broad criteria for relapse, such as small increases in rating scale scores that may easily have led to misdiagnosis of people experiencing somatic discontinuation symptoms. In addition, in many early studies relapse was not defined at all, but left to the discretion of the treating physician or investigator. In others it was simply defined as the 'need to resume treatment'.

If mild discontinuation symptoms can be mistaken for relapse, it would be predicted that studies that used hospitalisation as the relapse criterion would find smaller differences between drug treatment and placebo than other studies. The only study included in the Gilbert et al. (1995) meta-analysis to define relapse exclusively as hospitalisation found a difference of only 17% in relapse rates between people who continued to receive drugs and those withdrawn to placebo after two years (Carpenter, Jr. et al. 1990). This compares with an average difference in relapse rates of 37% at 10 months for all studies included in the analysis.

So there is an indication that some of the excess morbidity in the placebo group in randomised maintenance trials represents mild somatic withdrawal symptoms, or psychological symptoms relating to withdrawal, which are mistaken for signs of impending relapse. It is difficult to judge what proportion of severe relapses represent the re-emergence of the underlying illness in the absence of treatment, and what proportion may be episodes provoked by medication withdrawal. Studies among people with first episode psychosis may be instructive, since they are likely to have a shorter exposure to drug treatment than people with a long history of psychiatric disorder. This does not eliminate the possibility of drug withdrawal-induced psychosis and relapse since patients are likely to have been taking medication for some months at least, but it may mean these phenomena are less common. Mistaking withdrawal symptoms for relapse is still a potential problem.

Surprisingly there is only one placebo controlled trial conducted with people experiencing their first episode of psychosis. It took place at Northwick Park hospital in London and was published in 1986 (see Figure 6.1) (Crow et al. 1986). Relapse was defined as readmission to hospital or need for resumption of antipsychotic treatment. Follow-up

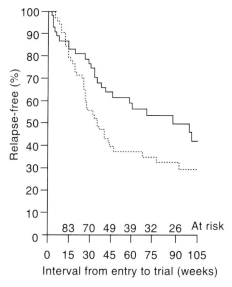

Figure 6.1   Northwick Park first episode study: Percentage of patients remaining relapse free on drug and placebo (reproduced with kind permission of the Royal College of Psychiatrists)

lasted two years. The results show a possible discontinuation effect, with the majority of placebo group patients relapsing in the first year and relatively few thereafter. In contrast, the drug-maintained patients continue to relapse throughout the second year.

Overall 46% of 54 patients on active medication were diagnosed as relapsed compared with 62% of 66 patients on placebo, giving a difference of 16%. Most patients defined as 'relapsed' were said to have psychotic symptoms, but not all. Since no breakdown is given by treatment group, it is difficult to judge whether some relapses on placebo might have been unrecognised drug-withdrawal symptoms.

Relapse rates in a more recent comparative study of haloperidol and risperidone for first episode psychosis were similar (Schooler et al. 2005). Forty-two per cent of the risperidone group and 55% of the haloperidol group were diagnosed as relapsed during the follow-up period of up to five years. However since rates of discontinuation were high (37% in the haloperidol group, 42% in the risperidone group), the proportion of patients who stayed in the study and had not relapsed at two years was only 28% of the haloperidol group and 44% of the risperidone group. Thirty-eight per cent of patients on placebo in the Northwick Park Study had not relapsed at the end of the two-year follow-up. Another large, government-funded trial, referred to as the CATIE study (Clinical Antipsychotic Trial of Intervention Effectiveness) consisted of a comparison of treatment with different neuroleptics in naturalistic conditions in people who were mostly stable and not treatment resistant. This study found that the median duration of 'successful' treatment[1] was only three months with olanzapine and one month with the other drugs (Lieberman et al. 2005a)!

Studies of long-term drug treatment in schizophrenia and psychosis emphasise relapse at the expense of other aspects of outcome such as social or occupational functioning or subjective effects. This is partly because relapse is considered to be an indisputable catastrophe, which trumps all other considerations. This helps to reinforce the disease-centred model, obscuring the impact of the global effects that drugs produce. The fact that almost all RCTs of maintenance treatment stop at the point of relapse confirms this way of seeing things, by generating a limited set of data. If patients were followed through relapses, firstly it would allow for discontinuation effects to dissipate and secondly it would enable a comparison of outcome in a number of different realms over a period of time.

Discontinuation effects also mean that in ordinary clinical practice people who take long-term medication and stop or reduce it for any reason (especially if this is done abruptly) may be more likely to relapse than they would be if they had never started on long-term treatment. In other words, long-term treatment may produce the very problems for which it is prescribed.

Neuroleptic drugs and long-term outcome of schizophrenia

Since the 1950s extravagant claims have been made about the impact of neuroleptic drugs on the outcome of schizophrenia. Modern textbooks of psychiatry still assert that the drugs were responsible for the decline in mental hospital populations, despite contrary evidence (Cookson 2005, p. 9). The authors of a meta-analysis of outcome studies over the 20th century, attribute the apparent improvement of outcome between the 1950s and 1980s to the introduction of the new drug treatment, among other things. However in the 1990s improvement rates declined to levels comparable with those found in the early part of the 20th century prior to the availability of modern drugs. Hence, the review provides no strong evidence that drug treatment has improved outcome (Hegarty et al. 1994).

Comparing outcome studies conducted at different times in this way is complicated by variations in diagnostic fashions and judgements of outcome. What is considered a good outcome in one era may not be considered so in another historical context. Similarly diagnostic fashions are known to have varied considerably over the 20th century. A study that retrospectively compared the outcome of patients admitted to psychiatric hospitals in 1947, just before the introduction of neuroleptic drugs with those admitted just after their introduction, in 1957, is useful in this respect (Bockoven & Solomon 1975). There was little difference in outcome between the two cohorts with 76% of the earlier cohort living in the community at five-year follow-up compared with 87% of the later cohort, despite the political impetus towards community care over the period. The authors of the study concluded that 'these drugs might not be indispensable' (p. 796).

A recent study of people admitted to hospital with a first episode of schizophrenia found that there were an average of two readmissions per person over an average of 3.6 years follow-up (Tiihonen et al. 2006). Another recent five-year follow-up of people with a first episode found that only 14% were deemed to fully recover (Robinson et al. 2004). Figures like these make it difficult to believe that the availability of neuroleptic drugs has much ameliorated the harsh and recurrent nature of this condition.

Not only is it difficult to prove that the long-term and widespread use of neuroleptic drugs has improved the outcome of schizophrenia but there are some hints that it may actually depress the outcome – that drug treatment may make people worse in the long term. It is well known that the outcome of schizophrenia, diagnosed by exactly the same criteria, is worse in the West than it is in the developing world (Jablensky et al. 1992; Leff et al. 1992). This is usually explained as demonstrating the detrimental effects of industrialised society, which is probably partly the case. However Robert Whitaker suggests that these studies provide evidence that drug treatment makes outcomes worse, since use of drugs is lower in the developing world (Whitaker 2002). In addition, as described earlier, follow-up studies of short-term treatment trials have either shown no difference between people initially randomised to placebo or non-drug treatment (May et al. 1981) or a better outcome in the placebo group (Rappaport et al. 1978; Schooler et al. 1967). In the Northwick Park maintenance study a subgroup of patients with good prognostic indicators had a better occupational outcome on placebo than on drugs (Johnstone et al. 1990). A recent follow-up study also found that people who took neuroleptic drugs for a shorter period had better social and vocational outcomes. However this association disappeared in the multiple regression analysis, suggesting it was attributable to other factors that predict outcome (Robinson et al. 2004). In addition, a number of studies have shown that a substantial proportion of people who experience a psychotic episode can recover without the use of neuroleptic drugs. These include the Soteria Project, set up in the United States by psychiatrist Loren Mosher, with the aim of reducing reliance on neuroleptic drugs. Published data showed that around 30% of patients allocated to the project had good outcomes without drugs (Bola & Mosher 2003). More recently a well-conducted study in Finland managed to treat 43% of patients with a first episode of psychosis successfully without neuroleptic drugs (Lehtinen et al. 2000).

Within cohorts of patients in Western settings, patients who consistently avoid the use of neuroleptic drugs do better than those who use them (Bola & Mosher 2003; Carone, Harrow, & Westermeyer 1991; Harrow et al. 2005; Lehtinen et al. 2000). In one long-term follow-up 40% of those people not taking any medication were classified as recovered after 15 years compared with only 5–17% of those who were taking neuroleptic drugs (Harrow et al. 2005). Use of neuroleptics was associated with a highly statistically significantly worse global adjustment and outcome ($p<.001$). In contrast, a recent follow-up study found higher readmission rates and mortality among people not taking neuroleptic drugs compared to those who were (Tiihonen et al. 2006). However in this analysis people classified as not taking neuroleptics included people who had just stopped them. Such people may be at risk of withdrawal-related problems, which may also include a heightened risk of suicide. Baldessarini and colleagues found a markedly increased risk of suicide after lithium discontinuation, for example (Baldessarini, Tondo, & Hennen 1999).

The association between the use of drugs and poorer outcome is partly attributable to the fact that people with more severe conditions are more likely to be prescribed long-term drug treatment. Or to put it another way, in the Western world, only those with the mildest of disorders who can function at a fairly high level are going to have a chance of evading the ubiquitous prescription pad. However no one has demonstrated that this is the entire explanation. Until then, the possibility that antipsychotic drugs are damaging to the long-term prospects of recovery has to be entertained. Morbidity associated with discontinuing the drugs and drug-induced neurological impairment, described further in the next chapter, provide possible mechanisms for this scenario.

Are the newer drugs better?

A meta-analysis of placebo-controlled studies of atypical or second-generation neuroleptics found only modest differences between the drugs and placebo. The difference in response rates was only 16% and even the authors comment that this seems small (Leucht et al. 2007). However even this figure may be exaggerated due to the many methodological failings of these trials. Most will have been confounded by discontinuation effects, since none of the studies involved only people with a first episode who had not previously been on drugs. Many studies were conducted with people who were previously stable, and then randomised them to have the new drug or placebo. All patients who had previously been on drug treatment and were put on placebo would therefore be susceptible to discontinuation effects. There was also no examination of the integrity of the double blind and it is likely that side effects lead to unblinding in many cases. Dropout rates were high, at 47% overall. The meta-analysis also demonstrates publication bias, with the funnel plot[2] showing clear evidence of the non-publication of more negative studies. The fact that known side effects of some of these drugs such as extrapyramidal effects and sedation were not detected also suggests that the trials were not reliable. They were all carried out by drug companies for purposes of getting the study drug licensed.

Drug company-sponsored studies suggest that the second generation of neuroleptic drugs are superior to older ones in terms of inducing lower levels of adverse effects, especially extrapyramidal effects and some claim to demonstrate better efficacy (Haro et al. 2005). This is not surprising in view of findings that most comparative studies find the sponsors' drug to be superior (Heres et al. 2006; Kelly, Jr. et al. 2006). Several meta-analyses of studies comparing old and new neuroleptics have now been conducted and they give conflicting results. Some suggest that the newer neuroleptics have a superior profile (Davis, Chen, & Glick 2003) and some show no difference between the new and the old drugs (Davis, Chen, & Glick 2003; Geddes et al. 2000). Government-funded studies have not found the new drugs to be superior. Three of these have now been conducted. A study of veteran patients in the United States using flexible doses of haloperidol combined with an anticholinergic drug to reduce extrapyramidal symptoms found no difference in efficacy between that and olanzapine and no difference in the incidence of extrapyramidal side effects (Rosenheck et al. 2003). Akathisia (unpleasant restlessness) was lower in the olanzapine group, but weight gain was higher. In the CATIE study, sponsored by the NIMH, there were no statistically significant differences in the main outcome between newer drugs versus an older drug, perphenazine, in this case. The main outcome was the proportion of patients who discontinued treatment, not the symptomatic or functional state of the patient. This is a curious outcome for an effectiveness study since it assumes that remaining on drug treatment is beneficial, but the benefits of drug treatment are precisely what the trial was designed to determine. The study found that a slightly higher proportion of patients stayed on olanzapine, although this was not statistically different from the proportions taking the other drugs. People taking olanzapine gained an average of 1 kg per month (Lieberman et al. 2005a). A United Kingdom-based study compared patients randomised to be prescribed a second-generation neuroleptic of the clinician's choice with an older drug of choice (Jones et al. 2006). There were no statistical differences between the groups in terms of symptoms, levels of functioning, quality of life, extrapyramidal side effects, akathisia, compliance and depression. If anything the differences slightly favoured patients randomised to the older drugs. The most commonly prescribed older drug was sulpiride, which is thought to have a relatively high threshold for inducing extrapyramidal effects and the most commonly prescribed second-generation drug was olanzapine. However the authors did not believe that their findings were attributable merely to the frequent prescription of sulpiride, and anyway they note the pharmacological heterogeneity of both groups of drugs.

Evidence for early intervention and preventive drug treatment

Initiatives for 'early intervention' in psychosis are founded upon the observation that people who have a longer evolution of symptoms before they come to psychiatric attention have a poorer outcome in the long term. This observation used to be interpreted as showing that a more severe and globally disabling form of schizophrenia was characterised by a gradual onset of symptoms, whereas an acute onset indicated a less-severe condition. For example, it is generally accepted that people who have a psychotic episode in response to environmental stress generally have a better prognosis. However possibly under the influence of the pharmaceutical industry, which has sponsored much of the research and discussion in this area, the interpretation of the situation has changed. It is now claimed that a longer evolution of symptoms is associated with poorer outcome because of the delay in the patient receiving treatment. A whole new term has been introduced, 'the duration of untreated psychosis' and the notion of the speed of onset as an indication of the inherent severity of the condition has been forgotten. A recent review of evidence concerning 'duration of untreated psychosis' does not even mention this previously common view (Marshall et al. 2005). The only trial published so far, which compared outcomes for patients in areas with Early Detection teams compared with areas without, found that there was no difference between the areas for severity of positive and general symptoms of schizophrenia, global functioning, quality of life, time to remission and the course of the psychosis. Only negative symptoms were better in patients in early intervention areas, but these symptoms are likely to be influenced more by a general increase in professional support than by a specific effect of earlier drug treatment (Larsen et al. 2006). Further research is clearly needed before any benefits of early treatment can be claimed. Despite this Early Intervention teams have already been established in the United Kingdom and other Western countries.

The idea that the occurrence of a psychotic episode can be prevented by treating individuals believed to be at high risk for developing psychosis is also currently fashionable. Two randomised drug trials have been conducted with young people, mostly those referred to child and adolescent services. Those judged to be at 'high risk' for developing psychosis by virtue of having a family history of psychosis or some vague transitory psychotic symptoms were entered into the studies. One study compared olanzapine with placebo (McGlashan et al. 2006) and the other compared a combination of risperidone and cognitive behaviour therapy with usual care (McGorry et al. 2002). Both studies found that the drug-treated group had lower rates of onset of acute psychosis during treatment. However the olanzapine study did not find a statistically significant difference, and in the risperidone study it was impossible to say whether it was the drug or other aspects of experimental treatment such as cognitive behaviour therapy that made the difference. In the risperidone study the evaluations were also not conducted double-blind. About a third of the non-drug-treated groups developed psychosis in both studies, but only 12% were classified as having schizophrenia in the one study that gave a diagnostic breakdown (McGorry et al. 2002). In the olanzapine study drug-treated participants gained 9 kg of weight during a year.

Preventive treatment has been criticised on ethical grounds because, even if it works, it involves treating people who will never develop psychosis in order to prevent some cases. The notion of the high-risk individual is also worryingly vague and could easily be expanded to include the majority of young people who attend psychiatric services. Combined with the popularity of the notion of early intervention, the idea of preventive treatment seems likely to decrease the prescribing threshold in child and adolescent services. Evidence suggests that this is exactly what is happening, with prescriptions of antipsychotics to this age group rising rapidly over recent years (Olfson et al. 2006). This should be a major cause of concern, given the vulnerability of the developing brain and evidence presented in the next chapter about the damage neuroleptic drugs can inflict.

The dopamine hypothesis of schizophrenia and psychosis

The dopamine hypothesis of schizophrenia and psychosis appears to justify a disease-centred view of the actions of neuroleptic drugs. However in a tautological loop, it was the action of neuroleptic drugs that gave rise to the dopamine theory in the first place, on the assumption that the drugs act on the biological basis of the condition. In turn the theory has come to be viewed as evidence that the drugs act in a disease-specific way. The action of neuroleptic drugs is still regarded as the strongest evidence for the dopamine theory of schizophrenia. However if their action is understood according to a drug-centred model, as inducing a characteristic neurological state, then it does not follow, as the theory assumes, that psychotic symptoms or the condition of schizophrenia are produced by the opposite biochemical state to that produced by drugs. As we shall see in the next chapter, neuroleptic drugs dampen down all spontaneous thought and action and their effects are not restricted to psychotic phenomena. Therefore, if we abandon the assumption that neuroleptic drugs act in a disease-centred manner, their effects provide no support for the dopamine theory of schizophrenia.

The other piece of evidence commonly said to have inspired the dopamine hypothesis is that chronic ingestion of stimulant drugs such as amphetamine, cocaine and L-dopa can produce psychotic symptoms in some individuals without a psychiatric history. These drugs increase dopamine activity and it has, therefore, been assumed that this is the mechanism responsible for inducing psychosis. However stimulants affect numerous other neurotransmitter systems. Amphetamine causes a substantial increase in noradrenalin release, for example. Extensive research in the 1970s did not demonstrate what particular aspect of their biochemical activity is responsible for psychosis (Meltzer 1976) and nor did it suggest whether any single neurotransmitter system could be pinpointed, given their complex effects. Dopamine may be involved but so may noradrenalin, other neurotransmitter systems or it may be due to complex interactions between different systems. Or the explanation may lie at another level, like the consequences of prolonged or extreme arousal. Cannabis, which is also well known to cause a psychotic syndrome on prolonged use, does not elevate dopamine levels substantially.

In addition, it has long been recognised that the features of stimulant-induced psychosis are not equivalent to those of schizophrenia (Snyder 1972). Characteristic schizophrenic symptoms such as 'thought disorder' (confused and rambling speech), delusions of control, delusional perception and an inappropriate or flattened mood are rarely seen in stimulant psychoses. In contrast, in amphetamine psychosis mood is usually one of extreme anxiety, sexual behaviour is heightened and visual hallucinations are more common than they are in acute schizophrenic psychosis (Snyder 1972). There is usually also increased motor activity, including sometimes repetitive meaningless, compulsive movements called stereotypies which are not characteristic of schizophrenia or idiopathic psychosis (Batki & Harris 2004). Dopamine is thought to be the main neurotransmitter involved in stimulant-induced hyperactivity and stereotypies, based on animal research that showed that stimulant-induced stereotypies are suppressed by dopamine-blocking drugs to a greater extent than other sorts of drugs (Pycock, Tarsy, & Marsden 1975). It has simply been assumed that because dopamine is involved in causing stimulant-induced hyperactivity and stereotypy, it must also be the cause of stimulant-induced psychosis. However there is actually no evidence to support this supposition. In addition, some research suggests that noradrenalin may also have a role in increasing locomotor activity (Borison & Diamond 1978; Herman 1970). However since hyperactivity and stereo-typies are very uncommon in people with untreated psychosis or schizophrenia, whatever causes them has no obvious relevance for the aetiology of these psychiatric disorders.

It has not been possible to show abnormalities in overall dopamine content of brains of people with schizophrenia. Total dopamine content can, incidentally, only be measured at post-mortem (Scott 2006), and overall such studies have not shown any differences between people with schizophrenia and those without (Reynolds & Czudek 1988). As one of the main researchers in the field put it, 'the dopamine content is found to be normal in the schizophrenic brain' (Seeman 1995). Research into levels of dopamine metabolites in the cerebrospinal fluid,[3] which initially claimed to find increased levels in people with schizophrenia, also proved to be inconclusive when people who had not been treated with drugs were investigated (Reynolds 1989; Tuckwell & Koziol 1993).

Findings of increased D_2-receptor density in the brains of people diagnosed with schizophrenia were first reported from post-mortem studies in the 1970s. At first these findings were regarded as evidence of a pre-existing dopamine abnormality in the brains of people with schizophrenia, 'we have now obtained direct evidence for some abnormalities for brain dopamine receptors in schizophrenia' (Lee et al. 1978). However the patients whose brains were examined had been taking antipsychotic drugs for long periods before they died. No one asked the obvious question of whether the observed effects were due to drug treatment, even though it had already been established that antipsychotic drugs increase brain concentrations of D_2 receptors in animal studies (Muller & Seeman 1977). Subsequent post-mortem studies found that the abnormalities of dopamine receptors were entirely attributable to the effects of drugs (Kornhuber et al. 1989; Mackay et al. 1982; Reynolds et al. 1981). In the 1980s it became possible to visualise dopamine receptors in the living brain, using positron emission tomography (PET). One early study of this kind claimed to find increased density of D_2 receptors in brains of 'neuroleptic naïve' patients with schizophrenia (Wong et al. 1986), but these findings were not confirmed in many subsequent studies (Farde et al. 1987; 1990; Nordstrom et al. 1995; Pilowsky et al. 1994). Studies of D_1 receptors have found them to be unchanged (Cross, Crow, & Owen 1981), decreased (Hess et al. 1987) or more recently increased (Abi-Dargham et al. 2002), although effects of previous drug treatment and age were not fully controlled for in the most recent report. Therefore research has not shown any consistent abnormalities in dopamine receptors in schizophrenia per se. It has demonstrated that neuroleptic drugs, which block the effects of dopamine at D_2 receptors, cause a compensatory increase in the number and density of these receptors in the brain. This finding has been confirmed for some of the new 'atypical' antipsychotics as well as older drugs in recent brain imaging studies (Silvestri et al. 2000).

Despite these findings, some literature still maintains that schizophrenia or psychosis is associated with dopamine receptor abnormalities. A meta-analysis of post-mortem and imaging studies of dopamine receptors failed to mention the confounding effects of drugs, even though the analysis revealed a substantial and statistically significant correlation between the medication status of subjects and D_2-receptor density compared with controls across studies ($r=0.63$, $p<.05$) (Zakzanis & Hansen 1998).

By the 1990s the lack of evidence of dopamine abnormality combined with data which were obviously contradictory, reduced the popularity and credibility of the dopamine hypothesis of schizophrenia. The existence of negative symptoms seemed incompatible with the idea that schizophrenia is caused by increased dopamine activity, although, as described in Chapter 5, attempts were made to reconcile the dopamine theory with this problem (Davis et al. 1991). The reintroduction of clozapine was also problematic since it appeared to have relatively weak action at D_2 receptors. In order to make its actions consistent with the dopamine hypothesis of schizophrenia, Clozapine is now suggested to have a strong but transient effect on dopamine receptors. However the fact that it does not cause Parkinsonian symptoms at moderate doses suggest that at most it must be a much weaker dopamine blocker than other neuroleptic drugs. Since it is generally considered to be more, not less, effective at reducing psychotic symptoms than other neuroleptic drugs, its action contradicts the dopamine hypothesis.

Since the mid-1990s a diverse and confusing collection of studies have been published which are now regarded as providing evidence that dopamine function is abnormal in acute psychosis. These studies have examined a variety of indirect measures of dopamine activity. Some have investigated the level of increase of dopamine after amphetamine ingestion (Abi-Dargham et al. 1998; Breier et al. 1997; Laruelle et al. 1996). These studies suggest that, as a group, people with psychosis have an enhanced release of dopamine compared with healthy controls, although there is substantial overlap in results – that is not all patients with psychosis had higher levels of dopamine release than controls. Most studies also showed a corresponding increase in psychotic symptoms in patients after amphetamine ingestion, a phenomenon that has been observed before. This suggests that people with psychosis respond more intensely to stimulant drugs than controls, but this may be a function of their psychological state. In other words, people with psychosis may respond more strongly because they are already aroused. It does not necessarily provide evidence of a pre-existing biological difference.

Another group of studies have measured the uptake of a radiolabelled dopamine precursor molecule, presumed to reflect the synthesis of dopamine in people with psychosis compared with healthy controls (Dao-Castellana et al. 1997; Elkashef et al. 2000; Hietala et al. 1995; Lindstrom et al. 1999; Reith et al. 1994). Results of these are inconsistent. Even the results of the 'positive' studies are incongruous with some finding increased uptake in the putamen but not the caudate nucleus (parts of the basal ganglia) (Hietala et al. 1995) and another finding increased uptake in the caudate but not the putamen (Reith et al. 1994). One study found no effect (Dao-Castellana et al. 1997) and the largest study so far found the opposite finding of reduced uptake in the ventral striatal area of the brain (Elkashef et al. 2000). Two studies examined indirect measures of dopamine-receptor occupancy. Although the authors of one concluded that their results showed 'direct evidence of increased stimulation of D_2 receptors by dopamine in schizophrenia' (Abi-Dargham et al. 2000, p. 8104), effects of prior drug treatment were evident from the results and were not completely controlled for.

All recent studies were small, and although efforts were made to identify and include patients who had not previously taken neuroleptic drugs, known as 'drug naïve' patients, all but one of the studies also included patients who had taken these drugs in the past, often for long periods. Therefore prior treatment with drugs known to affect the dopamine system may be, at least partially, responsible for the findings. However the biggest problem with all this research is the complete disregard for other possible explanations for increased dopamine activity. Dopamine release is known to be associated with numerous activities and situations that may differ between patients and healthy controls and may account for the difference in dopamine activity

independent of the presence of psychosis. Motor activity and attention have been shown to increase dopamine activity and dopamine is
involved in arousal (Berridge 2006). People with acute psychosis are
likely to be more aroused and agitated than healthy controls and this
may account for increased dopamine activity. None of the recent
dopamine–psychosis studies have examined these possible confounders. Nicotine increases dopamine release and people with psychiatric disorders are notoriously heavy smokers. Only one of the
recent studies attempted to control for the effects of smoking. It found
no evidence of an association between dopamine and smoking, but
the study was too small to detect anything but a very large effect
(Meyer-Lindenberg et al. 2002). Several studies in animals and humans
have found that dopamine is released in response to stress (Adler et al.
2000; Breier 1989; Finlay & Zigmond 1997; Frankenhaeuser et al.
1986; Pruessner et al. 2004; Rauste-von Wright & Frankenhaeuser
1989), although one study with humans using a mild stressor failed to
find an association (Montgomery, Mehta, & Grasby 2006). Since
patients with psychosis are likely to be in a state of high stress, and
research shows their stress hormones are elevated (Pariante et al. 2004;
Tandon et al. 1991), it may be that increased dopamine in people with
psychosis is a non-specific indication of a state of stress, rather than a specific correlate of psychosis per se. A meta-analytic review of the
amphetamine challenge studies was the only report to consider the
role of stress in the studies of dopamine in psychosis (Laruelle et al.
1999). It found a statistically significant level of increased anxiety in
people with psychosis compared with controls both before and during
the procedure.

Overall the evidence in support of the dopamine theory of psychosis
or schizophrenia is weak. Much early research was negative and findings that were thought to support the hypothesis turned out to be due
to the effects of drug treatment. Recent studies are inconsistent and
although some suggest enhanced dopamine activity in some situations,
such as following amphetamine ingestion, there has been no allowance
made for the numerous other factors that affect dopamine activity.
These factors are likely to influence dopamine levels in patients quite
independently of their psychotic symptoms. The persistence of the
dopamine hypothesis and its recent resurgence in popularity are testimony therefore not to the state of the evidence but more to the need
of the psychiatric profession to have medical models of the disorders it
is confronted by, particularly ones that provide a medical justification
for its treatments.

Is a disease-centred view of neuroleptic drug action justified?

Before moving on to a drug-centred analysis of the effects of neuroleptics, I will conclude this chapter by evaluating the evidence for a disease-centred view of their action according to the headings outlined in Chapter 2.

(1) *Is there a demonstrable pathological basis to psychosis/schizophrenia from which the action of 'antipsychotic' drugs can be understood?*

Decades of research have failed to produce clear and independent evidence of a dopamine abnormality in people with psychosis or schizophrenia that cannot be attributed to some other cause.

(2) *Do rating scales for acute psychosis or schizophrenia reliably measure the manifestations of a particular disease process?*

Rating scales used to measure effects of drugs in trials among people with schizophrenia or psychosis contain numerous items that are not confined to these situations or diagnoses and would be likely to respond to any drug with sedative effects. Thus the commonly used Brief Psychiatric Rating Scale (BPRS), which has a total of 18 items, contains items on 'tension', 'uncooperativeness,' 'excitement' and 'hostility'. Each item can score up to 7 points. Differences of 10 points on this scale are usually considered significant. This was the difference between patients treated with clozapine and patients treated with chlorpromazine in the seminal study heralding clozapine as an effective treatment for treatment-resistant schizophrenia, for example (Kane et al. 1988). Similarly of the seven items in the 'positive symptoms' section of the Positive and Negative Syndrome Scale (PANSS), two concern 'excitement' and 'hostility'. Thus decreases in symptom-rating scales after drug treatment do not necessarily indicate improvement in core psychotic symptoms, but may simply reflect sedating effects on various aspects of behavioural disturbance and overarousal. A difference of 10 points on the BPRS could easily reflect sedating effects on behavioural disturbance rather than any specific 'antipsychotic' effect. Use of the 'psychotic symptoms cluster' of the BPRS is a better measure of change in specific symptoms.

(3) *Do animal models of psychosis select antipsychotic drugs reliably?*

The principle animal model of psychosis has for many years been the hyperactivity and stereotypies induced by stimulant drugs. In animals and humans prolonged or high-dose stimulants, such as amphetamine, produces repetitive, compulsive movements that are referred to as 'stereotypies'. An example is gnawing movements in rats. Because stimulants can also produce psychosis in humans, it was assumed that a drug which could reduce their motor effects would also have antipsychotic properties. It was observed that dopamine-blocking drugs could reliably reduce stimulants' motor effects and did so more than other sedatives (Pycock, Tarsy, & Marsden 1975). Experiments with animals were also believed to show that dopamine rather than noradrenalin or serotonin was responsible for the effects (Ernst 1967). However the literature on this subject is extremely confusing. Some authors suggest the model detects the extrapyramidal activity of drugs rather than their antipsychotic actions (Pycock, Tarsy, & Marsden 1975), and others regard stereotypy as a model for tardive dyskinesia rather than psychosis (Klawans, Jr. & Rubovits 1972). Some research suggested that noradrenalin might also be implicated (Borison & Diamond 1978; Von Voigtlander & Moore 1973). A recent paper shows that noradrenalin and dopamine are involved in arousal and motor hyperactivity induced by amphetamine (Berridge 2006). Some studies demonstrate that non-neuroleptics like diazepam can also reduce stimulant-induced hyperactivity (Hsieh 1982; Thiebot et al. 1980).

However it is surely not surprising that dopamine-blocking drugs are particularly effective in reducing hyperactivity given their propensity to reduce movement and produce a Parkinson's type picture as described further in the next chapter. Therefore, the model seems to reflect drugs' extrapyramidal action and can be regarded as a screen for drugs with dopamine-blocking activity. In line with this idea, most research shows that second-generation neuroleptic drugs such as clozapine, which have weaker antidopaminergic effects, have relatively weak antistereotypic actions (Costall & Naylor 1976; Tschanz & Rebec 1988).

Therefore the effects of drugs on stimulant-induced stereotypies says nothing about the action of drugs on a disease process, but can be better understood as a reflection of particular drug-induced effects in line with a drug-centred model of drug action.

Numerous other animal models of psychosis have been proposed, but few others have been used routinely for drug screening. The model called the conditioned avoidance response is considered important, however. Smith and colleagues describe the test as follows:

> In a typical Conditioned Avoidance Response experiment, a rat is placed in a two compartment shuttle box and presented with a neutral

conditioned stimulus (CS) such as a light or tone, followed after a short delay by an aversive unconditioned stimulus (US), such as a foot shock. The animal may escape the US when it arrives by running from one compartment to the other. However after several presentations of the CS-US pair, the animal typically runs during the CS and before the onset of the US, thereby avoiding the US altogether. Animals treated with low (noncataleptic) doses of antipsychotic drugs fail to perform avoidance responses to the CS, even though their escape response is relatively unaffected.

(Smith et al. 2004, p. 1040)

As this description illustrates the conditioned avoidance response represents the ability of animals to connect to different stimuli. In other contexts, such as research on effects of toxins on the brain, a reduced conditioned avoidance response is taken to indicate an impairment of learning and memory. The initial rationale for using this as a test for antipsychotics was that drugs considered mainly sedative primarily decreased spontaneous motor activity in animals, whereas neuroleptics were thought to selectively suppress the conditioned avoidance response more than motor activity (Cook 1958). However reduction of the conditioned avoidance response is also achieved by many sedatives, albeit with concomitant reduction of motor activity (Arnt 1982; Dielenberg, Arnold, & McGregor 1999) and histamine (Tasaka et al. 1985). Anything that impairs cognitive function including numerous toxins and radioactivity also impair the conditioned avoidance response (Gao, Wang, & Zhou 1999; Shukakidze, Lazriev, & Mitagvariya 2003). Therefore, again, this model provides no evidence of disease specificity but appears, rather, to reflect the particular drug-induced effects of neuroleptics on learning, effects that are shared by other drugs and toxic processes.

(4) *Are drugs considered to have non-specific actions inferior?*

It is not clear that so-called antipsychotic drugs are superior to other types of drugs with sedative effects but different mechanisms of action. Lithium, benzodiazepines and opium have been shown to be comparable to neuroleptics in the treatment of psychotic states in some studies. The ability of the neuroleptic drugs to reduce the most characteristic symptoms of psychosis such as hallucinations, delusions and thought disorder have often been interpreted as evidence of their specifically antipsychotic or 'antischizophrenic' action (The National Institute of Mental Health Psychopharmacology Service Center Collaborative Study

Group 1964), although benzodiazepines have also been found to reduce these symptoms in most studies where this has been examined.

However showing that neuroleptic drugs were superior to other sedative drugs would not necessarily demonstrate a disease-centred action, since some of the effects induced by neuroleptics may be particularly useful in psychosis. The most obvious of these effects is the capacity of neuroleptic drugs to induce indifference, discussed in more detail in the next chapter. In this respect it is interesting to note that the only RCT of an opiate, another group of drugs that are noted to induce a state of indifference, albeit a rather different one, found that opium was as useful as chlorpromazine for the treatment of a psychotic state. However the data on benzodiazepines, a group of drugs not noted to produce emotional or psychic indifference, suggest that a sedative effect alone may be capable of ameliorating psychotic symptoms.

(5) *Do studies with healthy volunteers show different or absent effects?*

In the next chapter I describe research in which 'healthy volunteers' have taken neuroleptic drugs. This shows unambiguously that volunteers experience the same range of effects that are seen in patients.

(6) *Is the outcome of psychosis/schizophrenia improved by the use of antipsychotic drugs?*

Data on the course of schizophrenia have not been able to demonstrate that the introduction of neuroleptic drugs has improved outcome. They may even impair outcome due to harmful effects on the brain or due to the iatrogenic problems encountered when discontinuing psychiatric drugs.

Conclusions

Neuroleptic drugs clearly have different effects from inert placebo. These effects may be beneficial in the short term for some patients with psychotic episodes, in terms of reducing symptoms and getting out of hospital. However some patients with psychosis recover spontaneously, and it is uncertain roughly what proportion gain added benefit from neuroleptic treatment. It is also uncertain whether other sedative drugs might not have the same effects. It is impossible to say whether long-term treatment confers advantages over placebo in terms of relapse prevention because of the potential confounding influence of discontinuation effects in placebo-controlled trials which depress the outcome in the placebo group. Randomised maintenance trials have also not addressed whether long-term drug treatment affects other aspects of functioning such as social functioning, work performance and quality of life. It is often claimed that neuroleptic drugs have improved the outcome of schizophrenia but it is actually quite difficult to find evidence to support this position. Some evidence even points to the possibility that widespread and long-term drug treatment may make the outcome worse, especially for people who might have done well without drug treatment. Although the bulk of research on neuroleptic drugs has been conducted on the assumption that they act in a disease-centred way, the data produced by this research does not justify this position. A drug-centred model is better able to explain the nature of their effects in people with schizophrenia and psychosis. A drug-centred model also provides a platform from which to weigh up the pros and cons of using such drugs and helps us to judge what role they should have in psychiatric treatment.

7
What Do Neuroleptics Really Do? A Drug-Centred Account

In contrast to the disease-centred model, the drug-centred model of drug action provides a framework within which to explore the full range of a drug's actions. In this chapter I will examine the evidence for what sorts of effects neuroleptic drugs induce, concentrating on their effects on mental function and brain state over the short and long term. Instead of measuring these effects in terms of the symptoms of a presumed disease state, and regarding other effects as incidental and unimportant, I will, following a drug-centred model try and develop a picture of their global action. Then we can assess whether they have any utility for people suffering from psychiatric disorders, especially those diagnosed as having psychosis or schizophrenia.

Short-term effects of the older neuroleptics

The mental and behavioural effects of the older neuroleptic drugs and many of the newer ones can be understood as a state of mild and sometimes overt Parkinson's disease. All neuroleptic drugs are known to block D_2 receptors and it is well recognised that a certain level of blockade of these receptors produces observable symptoms that mimic Parkinson's disease. Although the obvious physical manifestations only occur at high levels of receptor occupancy, over 80%, it seems logical that lower levels of occupancy will produce milder and more subtle symptoms. Hence the 'therapeutic' effects of neuroleptics, that are supposed to occur at 40–60% occupancy of D_2 receptors, can be understood as mild symptoms of Parkinson's disease. Classical idiopathic Parkinson's disease is a disease of unknown cause that consists of a gradual degeneration of dopaminergic nerves in a part of the brain called the substantia nigra, one of a collection of nuclei called the basal ganglia. It is essentially a state of dopamine depletion and it is treated with the dopamine precursor, L-dopa. Common symptoms, as well as the classical tremor, include reduced spontaneous movement, difficulty initiating movement, slowness of movements, reduced facial expression, apathy, reduced emotional responsiveness and slowness of thinking. One of the key components of the disease appears to be an inhibition of the will to move and to think; a general slowing up or restriction of mental and physical activity. Other diseases that affect the basal ganglia of the brain also produce symptoms of Parkinson's disease, such as encephalitis lethargica, the early 20th-century epidemic, some of whose victims are vividly depicted in Oliver Sacks's *Awakenings* (Sacks 1999).

The basal ganglia are part of what is referred to as the brain's extrapyramidal system of motor control, so called to distinguish it from the pyramidal nerve tracts that control voluntary movement. The extrapyramidal system is most directly associated with involuntary aspects of movement such as muscle tone and posture. However it has extensive connections with other parts of the brain, especially the frontal cortex, the seat of personality and rationality. This 'functional network ... mediates volitional motor activity, saccadic eye movements, emotion, motivation, cognition and social behaviour' (Wonodi, Hong, & Thaker 2005, p. 340). Thus conditions that effect neurotransmission in the basal ganglia can be expected to have far-reaching functional consequences.

The motor and psychic effects of neuroleptics are similar to those of Parkinson's disease, except that the classical tremor is less common. As Ross Baldessarini, a well-respected psychopharmacologist observed, 'nearly all of the neuroleptic agents used in psychiatry can diminish spontaneous motor activity in every species of animal studied, including man' (Baldessarini 1985, p. 394). In the extreme case the drugs are known to cause the state referred to as 'catalepsy'. In this state animals become immobile and do not resist being moved passively into abnormal postures, but are not as drowsy as they would be with sedative type drugs such as barbiturates (Klawans, Jr. & Rubovits 1972). As with idiopathic Parkinson's disease, the psychological effects of drug-induced Parkinsonism are more subtle. Peter Breggin has summarised the mental effects of neuroleptics in drug-centred terms as a 'deactivation syndrome'. He describes this state further as 'a continuum of phenomena variously described as disinterest, indifference, diminished concern, blunting, lack of spontaneity, reduced emotional activity, reduced motivation or will, apathy and in the extreme, a rousable stupor' (Breggin 1993b, pp. 11–12). This profile of effects was recognised by the early pioneers of the neuroleptic tranquillisers in psychiatry, as described in Chapter 5.

They described these drugs' effects using the following phrases: 'psychic indifference', 'psychomotor indifference' (Deniker 1970a), an 'akinetic-avolitional syndrome' (Flugel 1959), 'motor retardation and emotional indifference' (Lehmann & Hanrahan 1954), 'reduced reactivity to external and internal stimuli', 'decreased spontaneous activity' and 'blunting of emotional arousal' (Lehmann 1975). An American textbook of the 1950s comments that 'if a patient responds well to the drug, he develops an attitude of indifference both to his surroundings and to his symptoms' (Noyes & Kolb 1958, p. 654). More recently Baldessarini described how under the influence of neuroleptic drugs, 'exploratory behaviour is diminished, and responses to a variety of stimuli are fewer, slower and smaller ...' (Baldessarini 1985, p. 394).

The psychological effects are well expressed by patients themselves, and by non-patients who have taken these drugs for research purposes. An article by Marjorie Wallace, founder of the British mental health charity SANE, who is usually enthusiastic about medication, summarises how people described the experience of taking neuroleptic drugs during calls to a telephone helpline (Wallace 1994). Wallace describes how 'most people with schizophrenia dislike taking the drugs they are prescribed ... which they often describe as making them feel like a zombie' (p. 34). - 'I feel as though I am walking with lead in my shoes' was one person's description of how the drugs made them feel. Another said: 'I feel emptied out, devoid of ideas'. 'Almost all of our callers report sensations of being separated from the outside world by a glass screen, that their senses are numbed, their willpower drained and their lives meaningless', Wallace continues, referring again to callers' feelings about medication (Wallace 1994, p. 35).

In 1970, two Israeli doctors reported the effects of a haloperidol injection in similar terms, and also described the unpleasant experience of akathisia:

> The effect was marked and very similar in both of us. Within ten minutes a marked slowing of thinking and movement developed, along with a profound inner restlessness. Neither subject could continue work, and each left for over 36 hours. Each subject complained of a lack of volition, a lack of physical and psychic energy. The subjects felt unable to read, telephone or perform household tasks of their own will, but could perform these tasks if demanded to do so. There was no sleepiness or sedation; on the contrary, both subjects complained of severe anxiety.
>
> (Belmaker & Wald 1977)

This description highlights the surprising co-existence of deactivation and anxiety. A characteristic and common effect of neuroleptics is the occurrence of a state of physical and mental restlessness and tension known as akathisia. It is thought to be due to their effects on the extrapyramidal system. Symptoms of restlessness occur in idiopathic Parkinson's disease, but are not as frequent as they appear to be in the drug-induced state. Many subjective accounts of neuroleptic drug effects stress the occurrence and intolerability of akathisia. In an interesting study carried out by David Healy and colleagues, using droperidol,[1] all 20 volunteers described severe akathisia consisting of motor restlessness as well as irritability, impatience or belligerence. In association with this effect, there was also the typical psychic indifference, 'a general feeling common to all subjects to some extent of disengagement – a feeling of uninvolvement with the tasks at hand. ... Mental effort appeared to be difficult, with all subjects reporting some problems with concentration. Apparently simple tasks, such as obtaining a sandwich from a sandwich machine, proved too difficult for some people' (Healy & Farquhar 1998, pp. 115–116). Most subjects also felt sedated and many slept as soon as they were able to. Eleven out of the 20 were dysphoric.

When the effects of neuroleptic drugs are described in these terms, it is easy to understand how they can produce an apparent improvement in people with psychosis who are preoccupied with their own internal world. The general reduction in mental activity and accompanying psychic indifference are likely to dull the import of delusional thoughts and hallucinatory experiences. Patients confirm this view. Those who find neuroleptic drugs helpful do not regard them as removing their abnormal experiences or 'symptoms', but suggest that the drugs help them to disengage from their symptoms and become less troubled by them (Mizrahi et al. 2005). The physical aspects of the deactivation state could also be predicted to be useful to reduce excitement and resistive or aggressive behaviours. But there is a negative side to these effects.

In line with this 'deactivating effect' the original neuroleptic drugs impair intellectual or cognitive function in volunteers in the short term and impair measures of performance and learning in animal studies. Numerous studies of normal volunteers show that after ingesting doses of neuroleptic drugs, there is a reduction in co-ordination, motor speed, increased reaction time, reduced alertness, impaired attention and impaired and slowed performance on intellectual tasks involving learning and memory (Fagan et al. 1991; Heninger, Dimascio, & Klerman 1965; McClelland, Cooper, & Pilgrim 1990; Peretti et al. 1997; Ramaekers et al. 1999; Rammsayer & Gallhofer 1995). Although there are differences in the degree of sedation associated with different types of neuroleptic, most evidence suggests they are all sedating to some degree and all have some detrimental effects on intellectual performance (McClelland, Cooper, & Pilgrim 1990). However the cognitive effects are not simply due to sedation or inhibition of movement and one study noted the similarity between the cognitive defects induced by the neuroleptic drug sulpiride and those of Parkinson's disease (Mehta et al. 1999). Animal studies consistently show impairment of motor performance, learning and memory with neuroleptic drugs (Gemperle, McAllister, & Olpe 2003; Rosengarten & Quartermain 2002; Skarsfeldt 1996). As described in the previous chapter, the drugs' ability to reduce the conditioned avoidance response in animals, a measure of the failure or impairment of learning from previous exposure to a stimulus, is so well recognised that it is suggested as a screening test for antipsychotic activity!

In contrast to these findings, it is generally believed that neuroleptics do not impair cognitive function in patients with schizophrenia. In fact it is frequently suggested that they improve it. These claims, which were first made in relation to the older neuroleptics (King 1990), are based on the observation that cognitive performance, which is impaired when people are acutely disturbed, not surprisingly improves as people recover. However this finding may also reflect the fact that research subjects learn how to do cognitive tests and so performance improves over time (Fagerlund et al. 2004). Few studies have prospectively compared drug-treated patients with unmedicated patients to control for these effects and those that have use a withdrawal design, thus comparing effects of medication with effects of medication withdrawal (e.g. Weickert et al. 2003). Studies of gradual dose reduction in patients on long-term drug treatment show some improvements in cognitive function, paralleled by decreased apathy or 'negative symptoms' (Kawai et al. 2006; Seidman et al. 1993).

Recently it has started to be acknowledged that older neuroleptics might impair cognitive function in patients (Kasper & Resinger 2003). The new atypical antipsychotics, in contrast, are being claimed to have 'cognitive enhancing effects', and numerous company-funded studies claim to show their superiority to the older drugs (Bilder et al. 2002; Harvey et al. 2005; Keefe et al. 2006; Woodward et al. 2005). As with response rates, claims vary depending on marketing imperatives. When newer drugs come along assertions about older drugs are revised in order to provide a favourable comparison for the newer drugs. Only with time, if at all, is it possible to disentangle the promotion from the science.

In the short term, therefore, the typical or older neuroleptic drugs cause a syndrome that can be described as 'deactivation', which can be thought of as a mild form of Parkinson's disease. It is characterised by reduced motor and mental activity and particularly by a state of psychic indifference and a paralysis of the will. There is accompanying akathisia, or subjective and inner restlessness and varying degrees of sedation. This state is unsurprisingly associated with impaired cognitive function in volunteers, although this effect is less obviously detected in patients.

Short-term effects of the new or 'atypical' neuroleptics

There is much less information about the global effects of the atypical neuroleptic drugs. Since they come from a variety of different chemical classes and have divergent pharmacological profiles, it is likely that their effects will vary. Some, such as risperidone and ziprasidone appear to be similar to typical antipsychotics in that they can induce overt extrapyramidal side effects (Parkinsonism) at usual clinical doses (Shirzadi & Ghaemi 2006; Scherk, Pajonk, & Leucht 2007). Others, notably clozapine, olanzapine and quetiapine still induce such effects but do so only at higher doses (Rochon et al. 2005). These drugs in particular are known as 'dirty drugs' in that they act on a large array of neurotransmitter receptors. They all have some affinity for D_2 receptors, although less than other commonly used neuroleptics. Olanzapine and clozapine, which have a similar and distinct pharmacological profile, affect a wide range of neurotransmitter systems, particularly the serotonin, noradrenalin, histamine and cholinergic systems. They have a particular propensity to cause metabolic disturbance (described below), which may or may not be related to their psychoactive effects.

There are no official published reports of volunteer experiences with atypical antipsychotics comparable to the reports of haloperidol and droperidol described above, but there is some useful information on the Internet. A website called 'askapatient.com', which enables patients to record their experience of medical drugs, contains numerous entries from people taking olanzapine. Although many record that they found the drug helpful in suppressing psychotic symptoms, mania, anxiety, suicidal thoughts and obsessional symptoms, most people describe profound sedative effects, and many found these incompatible with leading a normal life. Most correspondents noted an increase in appetite, and many described how eating became compulsive and how they craved the most fattening of foods. Many also described how taking olanzapine made them feel 'dopey', like a 'zombie', or as if they had a 'hangover.' One notes 'I was sleeping 14 hours a night and was so hang-over during the day I couldn't go about my normal routines – I couldn't even get myself dressed or go out to the store'. Many participants also remarked on how they felt their emotions had been suppressed by taking the drug, describing themselves as 'emotionally flat', 'numb' or 'robotic' (Askapatient.com 2007)

Recreational drug users note the same effects. Several comment on similarities between olanzapine and quetiapine and the benzodiazepine drugs, such as diazepam (Valium), because of the intense sedation. However none report the euphoria that characterises benzodiazepine effects. One correspondent reported protracted insomnia after stopping olanzapine, comparing it to benzodiazepine withdrawal (Sixseal.com 2007).

Most evaluations of the cognitive effects of atypical antipsychotics con-sist of studies comparing them favourably to the effects of the older neu-roleptic drugs (Scherer et al. 2004). In-house company volunteer studies and some others show only minor cognitive impairment with atypical antipsychotics compared with placebo (Legangneux et al. 2000; Rosenzweig et al. 2002), but others indicate reduced motor performance, attention and learning similar in nature to the older neuroleptics (King 1994; McClelland, Cooper, & Pilgrim 1990). A recent non-industry-funded study showed that risperidone worsened working memory in peo-ple with a first episode of psychosis. The decline with treatment was greater than the initial impairment in working memory found in people with psychosis compared with healthy controls. The deficit persisted throughout a one-year observation period (Reilly et al. 2006). This find-ing may indicate that the deficit in working memory found in many chronically medicated patients (Lee & Park 2005) may be due to drugs, at least in part. In contrast, a short-term study in patients found that risperi-done did not impair working memory but clozapine did so (McGurk et al. 2005). Numerous animal studies suggest that the atypical neuroleptics impair learning and memory (Levin & Christopher 2006; Rosengarten & Quartermain 2002; Skarsfeldt 1996; Terry, Jr. et al. 2002). One study with rats showed reduced reward-seeking behaviour, a possible parallel of emo-tional indifference, with a range of typical and atypical antipsychotics, including olanzapine, clozapine, risperidone, quetiapine and haloperidol (Varvel et al. 2002).

Overall the effects of atypical antipsychotics appear more difficult to characterise. Some are probably similar in nature to the older neuroleptics, but they tend to be used at lower doses that are less problematic in terms of effects on the extrapyramidal system. Some, such as olanzapine and clozapine, are strongly sedative, induce sleep and cause metabolic disruption including increased appetite, obesity and diabetes. They may have similarities to benzodiazepines. It is not yet clear whether all the new generation of neuroleptics produce the 'psychic indifference' characteristic of the older drugs. Initial reports suggest that they might, but it needs to be clarified whether this effect exists over and above their sedating effects.

Long-term effects – Do neuroleptics cause brain damage?

Although most people who are prescribed neuroleptic drugs are continued on them long term, the question of whether their acute effects persist, or whether tolerance develops,[2] as happens with drugs of abuse such as opiates and benzodiazepines, has been virtually ignored. Recently one animal study has examined effects of continued use of haloperidol and olanzapine on animal models of psychosis. It showed that both drugs progressively lost their efficacy in suppressing stimulant-induced locomotion and the conditioned avoidance response. An increased dose temporarily restored the response (Samaha et al. 2007). Increased D_2 receptor density and sensitivity were detected, providing a possible explanation for the changes. Therefore, animal research suggests that long-term use of neuroleptic drugs is associated with loss of their dopamine-blockading activity and clinical effects as the body adapts to their presence.

In addition, there is considerable evidence that the long-term ingestion of neuroleptic drugs has an adverse impact on the structure and function of the brain.

Brain imaging studies

Critics of psychiatric drugs, such as Peter Breggin have long been arguing that neuroleptic drugs damage the brain (Breggin 1993b, 1997). He argued that the reduced brain volume found in patients with schizophrenia was evidence of drug-induced damage, rather than the official explanation that it was attributable to the process of schizophrenia. Two new studies support Breggin's interpretation. In 2005 results of the largest ever brain-imaging study of people with first episode psychosis was published in the *American Journal of Psychiatry*. The study was funded by Eli Lilly the makers of the 'atypical' neuroleptic drug olanzapine (Zyprexa) and involved 161 patients who were randomised to treatment with haloperidol or olanzapine (Lieberman et al. 2005b). Magnetic resonance imaging (MRI) scans were conducted at the start of the randomised treatment and then periodically thereafter and compared with scans from a matched group of 58 controls. The results demonstrate that even after 12 weeks of haloperidol treatment there was a statistically significant reduction in the grey matter in the brain[3] compared with controls ($p = .005$). After one year the difference was even greater ($p = .003$). The results show that olanzapine-treated subjects also had a reduction of overall grey matter volume after one year ($p = .03$) with evidence of reductions in frontal, parietal and occipital lobes of the brain. The olanzapine-treated group also showed reduced volume of the caudate nucleus after one year compared with controls ($p=.003$) and compared with haloperidol-treated patients ($p=.02$). The text of the study glosses over the effects of olanzapine, reflecting the interests of the sponsors. In fact, the authors only briefly admit the possibility that the effects may have been due to the drugs, focusing instead on the possibility that olanzapine may prevent the decline in brain volume associated with schizophrenia better than haloperidol!

However a second shorter study confirms that these effects are most probably attributable to the drugs. A group of researchers at the Institute of Psychiatry in London studied a group of 84 patients with first episode psychosis after 8–9 weeks of neuroleptic drug treatment (Dazzan et al. 2005). They found that compared with patients who were psychotic but not taking neuroleptics, patients who were taking older or 'typical' antipsychotics had reduced volume of grey matter in several brain areas and enlargement of the basal ganglia. Both findings were significantly associated with neuroleptic dose. Correlation with dose is traditionally taken as strong evidence of a causal effect in medical epidemiology. Atypical antipsychotics were associated only with enlargement of the thalamus,[4] a finding that was also correlated with dose. The exposure period may have been too short at nine weeks to detect other changes in this group. The findings may also have been more marked if the comparison group was restricted to patients who had never had neuroleptics, since about half of the group had had previous exposure.

Traditionally the atrophy of the brain observed in people with schizophrenia has been attributed to the process of schizophrenia itself and has been regarded as confirmatory evidence that schizophrenia is a brain disease involving neurodegeneration. Research on brain structure barely mentions the possibility that drugs may produce or exaggerate brain changes even though most studies involve patients who have received many years of neuroleptic and other drug treatment. For example, a study published in the *British Journal of Psychiatry* in 2005 revealed substantial deficits of grey matter (nerve cell bodies) and white matter (nerve fibres) in brains of long-term patients diagnosed with schizophrenia compared with age-matched healthy controls. Multiple brain regions were affected including the frontal cortex, the cerebellum, the temporal cortex, the basal ganglia, the thalamus and parts of the parietal lobe (McDonald et al. 2005). Patients with bipolar disorder, in contrast, showed deficits in white matter only. Despite the fact that all patients with schizophrenia were taking antipsychotic drugs and had most probably been taking them for a considerable time, there is no mention of the possibility that drug exposure might have been responsible for the reduced grey matter. No attempt is made to examine correlations between drug exposure and brain volume in the statistical analysis, which would have been a relatively simple procedure. The only mention of drugs is a sentence in the discussion section of the paper, which refers to the possibility that psychotropic drug exposure might account for white matter deficits. Why it should account for white matter but not grey matter deficits is not indicated and I can think of no plausible explanation.

Despite the common indifference to the possibility that drugs may affect brain structure illustrated by this paper, several studies have looked at patients with a first episode of psychosis or schizophrenia, partly to try and minimise the confounding effects of drugs. None of these studies was entirely restricted to patients who had never taken psychiatric medication before and where it was examined, a statistically significant correlation between exposure to neuroleptics and reductions in grey matter volume was found (Cahn et al. 2002; DeLisi et al. 1991; Gur et al. 1998). A recent meta-analysis of some MRI studies of first episode patients compared with normal volunteers found reduced brain volume and enlarged brain ventricles (cavities) in patients with psychosis, but the authors emphasised that the overall differences were so small that they were 'close to the limit of detection by MRI methods' (Steen et al. 2006, p. 510). In the Discussion section of the published paper they did acknowledge the possibility that the effects might be a result of early antipsychotic drug treatment, but this was not mentioned in the Abstract, which suggested that the study demonstrated that schizophrenia was a 'neurodegenerative' or 'neurodevelopmental' process. Curiously, the paper did not cite the results of the Lilly-funded first episode study of brain structure, and nor did they include data from this study in the meta-analysis, even though the first author of that study, Jeffrey Lieberman, was also one of the authors of the meta-analysis. Another review that specifically examined MRI evidence of drug-induced effects did include the Lilly study but it emphasised the superiority of atypical over conventional antipsychotics and ignored the observed brain atrophy with olanzapine (Scherk & Falkai 2006). It is as if the psychiatric community cannot bear to acknowledge its own published findings. Not only does the evidence on brain shrinkage have damning implications for antipsychotic drug treatment, it also weakens one of the strongest pillars of the case that schizophrenia is a brain disease.

Tardive dyskinesia

One of the best-recognised adverse effects of the original generation of neuroleptic drugs is a condition called tardive dyskinesia. The name refers to the most obvious manifestation of the condition, which is abnormal, involuntary, repetitive movements, most commonly involving the face and mouth, but which can involve the limbs and trunk as well. These movements are not seen immediately after drug ingestion, but occur usually after several months or years of drug exposure. However as several commentators have pointed out, the condition is almost certainly not restricted to abnormal involuntary movements, but also includes some degree of cognitive impairment and may also involve characteristic behavioural abnormalities (Breggin 1993a; Cohen & Cohen 1993; Waddington et al. 1993). A review in 1993 found 29 studies that compared the cognitive function of patients who showed signs of Tardive Dyskinesia with patients who did not (Waddington et al. 1993). Twenty-three of these found that there was greater cognitive impairment in people with tardive dyskinesia and the association persisted in studies that controlled for age, use of anticholinergic medication[5] and other potential confounders. The authors of the review also reported their own data, which confirmed the association. These studies used a wide range of tests, and so it is difficult to characterise or localise the dysfunction. Several demonstrated memory impairments. Others showed executive dysfunction and impaired abstraction suggestive of damage to the frontal lobe of the brain. Another recent study found patients with tardive dyskinesia showed greater mental slowness than other patients (Eberhard, Lindstrom, & Levander 2006). The association of tardive dyskinesia and cognitive dysfunction has also been demonstrated in other groups of patients including patients with affective disorder (Wolf, Ryan, & Mosnaim 1983) and mental handicap (Youssef & Waddington 1988).

The usual interpretation of this data has been to assume that people with pre-existing brain damage are more susceptible to tardive dyskinesia. Although this is plausible, a more obvious explanation has been overlooked, at least in most psychiatric literature. This is the possibility

that long-term drug exposure causes a state of generalised brain impairment whose manifestations include not only abnormal movements but
varying degrees of cognitive dysfunction. Longitudinal studies might
help to disentangle these competing interpretations. I could find four
such studies. Two of these found that people who subsequently developed tardive dyskinesia had pre-existing cognitive impairment relative
to people who did not (Struve & Willner 1983; Wegner et al. 1985). The
other studies, including by far the largest and most recent study found
no association between prior cognitive level and subsequent development of tardive dyskinesia (Jeste et al. 1995; Waddington, Youssef, &
Kinsella 1990). The only study to look at changes over time found that
patients who developed tardive dyskinesia experienced a deterioration
of their cognitive function over the same period that the abnormal
movements emerged (Waddington, Youssef, & Kinsella 1990). In addition,
abnormal movements are likely to be a late manifestation of a generalised state of brain impairment induced by long-term drug exposure.
If this is the case then mild cognitive impairment is likely to be present
in the early stages before the development of the abnormal movements.
Therefore patients with damage sufficient to cause abnormal movements
will show highest levels of cognitive impairment, but mild cognitive
impairment may predate the onset of the dyskinesia (movement disorder).
A study that provides some support for this continuum hypothesis
consisted of a comparison of patients with schizophrenia and tardive
dyskinesia, drug-treated patients with schizophrenia without tardive
dyskinesia and drug-free schizophrenic controls (Tegler et al. 1988).
Cognitive functioning in this study was worst in the group with tardive
dyskinesia and best in the non-drug -treated group with the drug-
treated non-tardive dyskinesia group in the middle.

Several authors have suggested that there is also a behavioural concomitant to tardive dyskinesia, which has been called 'tardive dysmentia'
(Myslobodsky 1993; Wilson et al. 1983). Wilson et al. (1983) described
the characteristic features as 'unstable mood, loud speech, and inappro-
priately close approach to the examiner' (p. 18). Myslobodsky (1993) has
summarised the features as consisting of excessive emotional reactivity,
enhanced responsiveness to environmental stimuli and reduced awareness of abnormal movements if these are present. He also notes features
such as heightened tension, aggression and a background mood of mild
elation. These authors suggest that the syndrome is a consequence of
organic brain damage and point to similarities between the characteristics of 'tardive dysmentia' and behaviours associated with brain injury,
especially in the frontal or prefrontal region of the brain. The reduced

awareness of abnormal movements, sometimes referred to as anosognosia, is well recognised in tardive dyskinesia and reminiscent of the denial of disability that occurs in other severe brain conditions such as stroke (when it is usually associated with damage to the parietal non-dominant lobe) and generalised brain diseases such as neurosyphilis and Korsakoffs.

It is well established that neuroleptic drugs cause tardive dyskinesia. Although there is debate about whether there might also be other causes, recent studies confirm a strong association between use of neuroleptic drugs and tardive dyskinesia (Jeste et al. 1995). The precise neural mechanism is unknown. For a long time supersensitivity of D_2 receptors was postulated to be the cause, but it has been hard to demonstrate any differences in D_2 receptor upregulation in patients with and without tardive dyskinesia (Andersson et al. 1990; Crow et al. 1982). Research on structural brain abnormalities is also inconsistent (Wonodi, Hong, & Thaker 2005). A recent hypothesis concerns the ability of neuroleptics to cause nerve-cell death via the production of free radicals (Lohr, Kuczenski, & Niculescu 2003). Whatever the cause, it seems unlikely that a condition that originates in the brain, and is manifested in involuntary movements, would not also involve other aspects of brain function.

The prevalence of the movement disorder of tardive dyskinesia has long been a matter of dispute and depends on the type of population surveyed. Most estimates put the prevalence at 20–40% of patients on long-term neuroleptic drug treatment with higher estimates for elderly patients who are consistently shown to be more susceptible (American Psychiatric Association 1980). One large study found that 60% of a sample of middle aged and elderly patients developed tardive dyskinesia within three years (Jeste et al. 1995). Another found a figure of 53% in the same period, even with relatively low doses (mean CPZ equivalents 80 mg) (Woerner et al. 1998). Estimates that included people with drug-induced cognitive impairment without abnormal movements might, of course, be much higher.

There have been frequent claims that the atypical drugs cause lower rates of tardive dyskinesia, and even claims that they do not cause it at all. However although rates of tardive dyskinesia may be lower with some atpyicals than with older-generation drugs, they all appear to have some propensity to cause it, just as they all appear to be associated with Parkinsonian symptoms at high doses (Rochon et al. 2005). It is probably too early to form clear estimates of their tardive dyskinesia inducing potential. Drug company studies predictably show low rates of tardive dyskinesia, for example, a 1% rate of new cases within a year on risperidone (Gharabawi et al. 2005). A study of outpatients at a Veterans Affairs centre in New York found rates of 3% in risperidone-treated patients and 5% in olanzapine-treated patients over a one-to-two-year period (Schwartz et al. 2002). An Eli Lilly-funded study of olanzapine versus haloperidol found rates of 7% of new onset dyskinesia visible during at least one assessment in a mean follow-up of around eight months with 1% of patients developing persisting dyskinesia (Tollefson et al. 1997). A recent study of patients with borderline dyskinesia at entry found rates of progress to full tardive dyskinesia within six months of 45% for patients taking older drugs and 24% for patients on 'atypicals' (Dolder & Jeste 2003). Many of the patients in all these studies had been on older drugs prior to taking atypicals and so there may be carry over effects. However a number of case studies suggest that the new drugs can cause tardive dyskinesia in their own right in people without a history of prior neuroleptic use (Bhanji & Margolese 2004; Margolese et al. 2005).

Research on cognitive function in schizophrenia

It is well recognised that chronic institutionalised patients with schizophrenia have impaired cognitive function. It also appears that patients with early schizophrenia or psychosis may differ from other people in their mental characteristics. The literature on cognition and schizophrenia is extensive and confusing. Studies of unmedicated people with acute psychosis find attentional deficits and possibly impaired memory and learning (Hill et al. 2004; Saykin et al. 1994). The attentional deficits appear to be related to symptoms and resolve with improvements in mental state (Elvevag & Goldberg 2000). In addition, having a lower overall IQ has been found to predict the subsequent onset of schizophrenia or psychosis (Bilder et al. 2006; David et al. 1997; Reichenberg et al. 2005) and some studies suggest that people who develop psychosis show a decline in intellectual performance prior to the onset of overt symptoms (Bilder et al. 2006; Reichenberg et al. 2005). Evidence as to what aspects of intelligence are most implicated is inconsistent. For example, one study found that only poor performance on verbal tasks, and not other aspects of intellectual ability, was associated with greater risk of subsequent diagnosis of schizophrenia after controlling for the impact of general intelligence (David et al. 1997). In contrast, another found that only impairment in non-verbal reasoning skills conferred any extra risk of developing a schizophrenic type disorder (Reichenberg et al. 2006).

Although the research is difficult to interpret, many psychiatrists are convinced that schizophrenia is fundamentally a 'neurodevelopmental disorder characterised by cognitive deficits' (Bilder et al. 2006).

However there are other interpretations of existing evidence. Cognitive decline may be an early psychological manifestation of the experiences that constitute psychosis. Being preoccupied with the internal world of incipient psychosis is likely to interfere with someone's ability to perform certain cognitive tasks. Another explanation is that deficits in the ability to reason and communicate may predispose people to the development of psychosis. The possibilities are numerous and the nature of the relation is unlikely to be simple.

There has been little attempt to tease out the potential impact of long-term drug treatment on brain function from the wealth of research in this area. Studies with patients who have not been exposed to drugs are few and open to different interpretations. Since neuroleptics impair cognitive function in volunteers, it seems difficult to believe that they do not have similar effects in patients. However there are no studies that compare patients who have recovered from an episode of psychosis with drug treatment with those who have recovered without the use of neuroleptics, or with people who have been withdrawn from the drugs for a reasonable period. Only in such a situation, when the effects of the acute psychosis have abated, is it possible to ascertain the real impact of drugs on cognitive function in people with a history of psychiatric disorder.

However there is now clear evidence from MRI studies that both older and newer neuroleptic drugs cause atrophy of the brain within a year. In addition, long-term treatment is associated with the development of a condition, tardive dyskinesia, characterised not only by involuntary movements, which may be relatively trivial in themselves, but also by generalised cognitive decline and possibly by other behavioural indications of brain dysfunction. The implications of this scenario should not need spelling out. The long-term use of neuroleptic or antipsychotic drugs appears to damage the brain. Since we know that some cases of tardive dyskinesia are permanent, this damage may not always be reversible on stopping the drug. The evidence points to the possibility that the use of these drugs has created an epidemic of iatrogenic brain damage, as Peter Breggin and other voices in the wilderness have been suggesting for a long time.

A drug-centred approach to the use of neuroleptic drugs

There are good reasons to expect that neuroleptic drugs might have the ability to reduce the intensity of psychotic symptoms. The reports of their effects in patients and volunteers suggest they do this by producing a state of reduced physical and mental activity, including reduced emotional reactivity or indifference. This has been referred to as a state of 'deactivation' (Breggin 1993b). In low doses it is plausible that psychotic thought processes may be suppressed without the deactivation effects reaching levels that would be experienced as unpleasant or start to inhibit functioning. On the other hand, many patients find the effects of these drugs more unpleasant than their psychosis. Peter Wescott, whose account of his experience was published in the *British Medical Journal*, felt that long-term treatment with neuroleptic drugs had helped to prevent his psychosis from recurring, but wrote poignantly that 'my personality has been so stifled that sometimes I think that the richness of my pre-injection days – even with brief outbursts of madness – is preferable to the numbed cabbage I have now become'. He continued, 'in losing my periods of madness I have had to pay with my soul' (Wescott 1979). Unless someone's behaviour is seriously antisocial or criminal, they should be allowed to decide for themselves whether the effects of the drugs or the mental disorder are more intolerable. By promulgating the disease-centred model of drug action, the idea that drugs are correcting a biological defect, we deny patients this possibility.

Since the drug-induced effects of neuroleptics are striking and profound, it is likely that clinical trials based on the disease-centred paradigm will show them to be effective in a range of psychiatric conditions. Thus they have been shown to have beneficial effects on depression-rating scale scores, manifestations of obsessive compulsive disorder, anxiety, and behavioural disturbances associated with dementia, learning disability and personality disorder. Whether the deactivating effects are really useful in these conditions depends on the nature of the experience and its impact on people's lives. Where preoccupation with intrusive thoughts is problematic, the psychic indifference and reduced mental activity produced by neuroleptics may be useful. In cases where someone is aroused and overactive, the physical deactivation they produce can be used as a chemical restraint. On the other hand, in cases such as depression, the drug-induced state may interfere with the process of psychological adjustment and healing that needs to occur.

As well as their effects on the brain, neuroleptics commonly produce other potentially lethal effects. They are all toxic to the heart, inducing conduction defects and arrhythmias. Olanzapine and clozapine also interfere with normal metabolism, causing what is known as 'metabolic syndrome'. This syndrome has only recently been described and is defined as the occurrence of obesity, diabetes, hypertension and dyslipidaemia[6] (Shirzadi & Ghaemi 2006). The underlying cause of the syndrome is thought to be resistance to insulin. All these effects increase the risk of coronary heart disease and other cardiovascular disorders such as stroke. Numerous studies show that these drugs cause substantial weight gain. In recent trials participants taking olanzapine gained an average of 1 kg per month (Lieberman et al. 2005a; McGlashan et al. 2006). Although long-term psychiatric patients have high rates of diabetes anyway, due to lack of excercises, obesity and poor diet, clozapine and olanzapine increase the risk of diabetes further and more than the older generation of neuroleptic drugs (Sernyak et al. 2002). It may be that this effect is simply due to their effects on body weight, but some evidence suggests that they have an independent effect on glucose regulation (Newcomer et al. 2002). The long-term, independently funded CATIE study showed a substantial increase in blood glucose and glycosilated heamoglobin (a measure of long-term glucose control) in people on olanzapine compared with other neuroleptics (Lieberman et al. 2005a). The metabolic effects of these drugs are not infrequent and incidental. Clozapine caused a marked increase in weight of more than 10% of baseline weight in 58% of patients treated for one year (Sussman 2002). About 30–40% of patients treated with olanzapine show weight gain of 7% or more over periods of up to 18 months (Lieberman et al. 2005a; Nemeroff 1997). Therefore, metabolic impairment appears to be an integral part of the action of these drugs.

Eli Lilly, makers of olanzapine (Zyprexa) tried to play down this effect to doctors and patients as revealed in company documents leaked to the *New York Times* (Berenson 2006). The company has also sponsored publications publicising the idea that the increased risk of diabetes is inherent in severe mental illness, helping to divert attention from the probable link with their drug (Dinan 2004). Numerous studies have shown that long-term psychiatric patients die earlier than the general population and most of the excess mortality is due to cardiac disease and other 'natural causes' (Osby et al. 2000). Several studies have shown that neuroleptic drug use contributes to this excess mortality (Bralet et al. 2000; Joukamaa et al. 2006; Waddington, Youssef, & Kinsella 1998). Cardiovascular deaths and stroke are associated with the use of these drugs in a dose-dependent manner. People on higher doses have a greater risk of dying of these causes compared with people on lower doses or people with severe mental illness who do not take them at all (Osborn et al. 2007). Using more than one neuroleptic drug also appears to be particularly risky. One study, which controlled for the effects of some other factors likely to increase mortality including smoking, found that each additional neuroleptic drug prescribed increased the risk of dying compared with the general population by two-and-a-half times (Joukamaa et al. 2006a).

Therefore, a drug-centred approach to the use of neuroleptics would need to weigh up the possible benefits on psychotic symptoms with the serious adverse effects of these drugs. In the short term, it might be argued that the particular benefits on mental state outweigh the harm sustained, especially since adverse effects are more likely to be reversible with limited exposure. However other sedative drugs such as opiates and benzodiazepines may achieve similar effects. Notably, opiates also produce a state of emotional indifference, but obviously dependence and craving are a major concern. In the long-term however the balance of pros and cons is less likely to favour neuroleptic drug use. Their efficacy in preventing relapse is questionable because of the discontinuation design of long-term studies. Many of their harmful effects such as brain atrophy, neurological impairment, cardiac toxicity and metabolic disorders are common. It is difficult to believe that the damage neuroleptic drugs induce is a price worth paying for a reduced risk of recurrence, even if this could be more securely demonstrated.

The consensus that antipsychotics are disease-specific treatments seems more secure now than ever. Focusing as it does on the idea that the drugs act on the pathology of psychosis or schizophrenia, the disease-centred model has obscured the global effects of neuroleptic drugs. Indications of damaging effects on the brain are either ignored (tardive dysmentia, cognitive impairment associated with tardive dyskinesia), parcelled off as unfortunate but incidental side effects (tardive dyskinesia), or attributed to the mental condition itself (structural brain abnormalities and general cognitive impairment). The fact that this has been possible in the face of the considerable evidence about adverse effects on brain structure and function, is perhaps one of the strongest testimonies of the need to believe in the disease model of psychotropic drug action. This is especially important for the neuroleptic drugs. As expressed in their other name 'antipsychotics', these drugs embody the idea that psychiatrists have a specific treatment to offer for the most devastating and frightening of mental disorders. This is a central plank of psychiatry's claim that psychiatric problems can be approached in essentially the same way as physical illness. Without it the medical edifice might start to crumble.

8
The Construction of the 'Antidepressant'

Current use of antidepressants

The first drugs that were specifically referred to as antidepressants were introduced into psychiatry in the late 1950s. The concept of an 'antidepressant' is an inherently disease-centred notion, as expressed in the word itself. It consists of the idea that a drug can improve symptoms of depression, not just through drug-induced effects, but by reversing the process of depression, at least temporarily. Implicit in this idea is that depression is caused by physiological mechanisms that drugs can act upon. The monoamine hypothesis of depression was formulated to underpin these assumptions. It suggests that symptoms of depression are caused by a deficiency of brain monoamines, a group of neurotransmitters that include serotonin and noradrenalin,[1] which are incidentally also related to dopamine. According to this theory antidepressant drugs are thought to exert their therapeutic action by increasing brain monoamine levels.

By the 1960s antidepressants were in widespread use in psychiatry and General Practice. However prescribing levels remained fairly constant from the 1960s to the late 1980s and there was a general perception that the best effects of antidepressants were obtained in severe depression, sometimes referred to as endogenous depression – the heir of the idea of melancholia or involutional depression (see Chapter 3). Since the arrival of the selective serotonin reuptake inhibitor (SSRI) antidepressants, under the influence of massive drug company promotion, this situation has changed dramatically. There has been an explosion in prescribing rates and antidepressants are now prescribed to a much wider proportion of the population (see Figure 8.1).

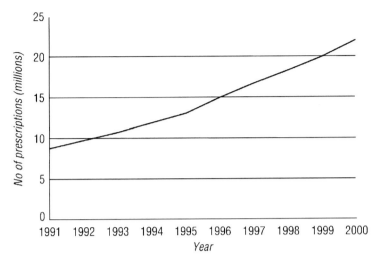

Figure 8.1 Trends in antidepressant prescriptions in the United Kingdom (1991–2000)

A community survey conducted in the United States in 2002 found that 11% of women and 5% of men were taking an antidepressant drug (Stagnitti 2005). Between 1997 and 2004 there was a 62% increase in the number of people taking them in the United States and the number of purchases made almost doubled (Stagnitti 2007). Use in children has also been increasing. There is now a widespread perception that taking pills for the downs of life's ups and downs is a perfectly ordinary activity. The popularisation of a biological view of depression has been one of the most significant changes of recent decades, leading to what Nikolas Rose has called 'the neurochemical re-shaping of personhood' (Rose 2004).

Antidepressant drugs are also prescribed to people with a variety of problems that are not labelled as depression including anxiety disorders, obsessive compulsive disorder, bulaemia, post-traumatic stress disorder, premenstrual syndrome, substance misuse, personality disorders, etc. Sometimes this use is justified on the grounds that the individual suffers from depression in addition to their other complaints. Increasingly, however antidepressants are becoming the primary recommended treatment for other disorders. The justification for their use is not usually made explicit, but implicitly it is based on a - disease-centred model of their action. Since no drug centred explanation is offered, such as what effects the drugs induce that might prove useful with the problems concerned, a message is conveyed that they act to reverse a biological disease process.

In the next chapter I will summarise the evidence for whether drugs currently referred to as antidepressants really do have specific effects on depression – that is do they act in a disease-centred manner? First I will trace the origin of the idea that certain drugs could improve depression by acting on its neurobiological basis – the idea that became known as the 'antidepressant'.

Treatment of depression prior to the 1950s

Although melancholia is a long-standing psychiatric diagnosis, in the first half of the 20th century only two syndromes involving depression were described in psychiatric textbooks, the depressive phase of manic-depressive psychosis and severe depression in old age known as 'involutional melancholia'. Both these syndromes were subsumed within the category of manic depression (Braude 1937; Henderson & Gillespie 1927). Descriptions of depressive conditions were brief and they were considered to be relatively rare and mostly confined to people who required admission to psychiatric hospital. Textbooks also covered neurotic disorders, such as anxiety and neurasthenia,[2] but these did not commonly include depression (Braude 1937; Henderson & Gillespie 1927; Mayer-Gross, Slater, & Roth 1954). It was not until the 1950s and 1960s that something resembling the modern concept of depression began to emerge. In 1962, for example, one of the major British psychiatric textbooks introduced a general disorder called 'depression', which was graded by severity (Henderson & Gillespie 1962).

Prior to the introduction of ECT, textbooks described the treatment of depression and mania as consisting of general measures such as bed rest, fresh air, occupational therapy and the use of prolonged baths (hydrotherapy) (Braude 1937; Henderson & Gillespie 1927). Some authors emphasised that 'there is no specific form of therapy' (Henderson & Gillespie 1927, p. 154). Evidence from patient case notes suggests that people with depression, along with everyone else in psychiatric hospitals, were given sedative drugs such as barbiturates and paraldehyde and some were also prescribed stimulants. The amphetamines were synthesised for the first time in the 1930s. Their physiological stimulant effects were remarkable for being quite different from effects of other drugs in common use. Some authors praised their effects and recommended their frequent use in depression (Sadler 1953) and patient case notes revealed that they were prescribed to both inpatients and outpatients with depression and neurotic disorders (Moncrieff 1999). They were advertised in the *American Journal of Psychiatry* in the 1940s for the treatment of depression. However they excited little official attention and were barely mentioned in major psychiatric textbooks or research papers (Moncrieff 1999). A well-known textbook of physical treatments described stimulants as having 'limited value in depression' because the euphoria they induce quickly wears off and 'the patient slips back' (Sargant & Slater 1944). The authors suggested that stimulants may have specific effects in children with hyperactivity, by implication denying that they might do so in depression. The lack of interest and negative perceptions of stimulants may have been due to the fact that no drugs were regarded as worthy of much scientific interest prior to the introduction of chlorpromazine. However their obvious effects in normal people coupled with rapid tolerance to their effects may have contributed to the view that their action was not disease specific.

By the 1940s ECT was in widespread use in psychiatric hospitals. Although it was still given to large numbers of patients with other diagnoses, mostly schizophrenia, it was already regarded as being most useful for the treatment of depression. ECT had prepared the ground for the antidepressants by suggesting that depression could be alleviated by physical means.

From stimulants to 'Psychic energisers'

The introduction of chlorpromazine transformed the way that drug treatment was regarded. Even before the disease-centred theory of its action crystallised, chlorpromazine was received with great enthusiasm. It was viewed as being superior to previous drug treatments and it inspired extensive research and publicity (Moncrieff 1999). It immediately stimulated a search for similar compounds and for possible drug treatments for depression (Lehmann & Kline 1983).

Although it is now little recognised, some of the first drugs that were later referred to as antidepressants were initially regarded as stimulants. David Healy has chronicled the simultaneous development of two different types of drug for depression (Healy 1997). In America, interest focused on two drugs used for the treatment of tuberculosis, namely iproniazid and isoniazid. Tuberculosis was still a prevalent condition in the mid-part of the 20th century and psychiatric hospitals had special wards for patients with the disease. In the mid-1950s research papers reveal that these drugs were well known to act as psychostimulants and produce serious psychiatric side effects similar in nature to those associated with amphetamine. In 1956, in a report of a small experiment in tuberculous patients, George Crane (later the man, who tirelessly publicised tardive dyskinesia caused by neuroleptics) described the effects of iproniazid in this way: 'The typical reaction to the drug consists of an increase in energy, appetite and resistance to fatigue. Mental aberrations are diversified and are in most cases, characterised by overactivity, insomnia, agitation and paranoid trends' (Crane 1956, p. 330). He likened it to amphetamine, but pointed out the difference that iproniazid appeared to stimulate appetite whereas amphetamine was a well-known appetite suppressant. Jean Delay, known for the first psychiatric use of chlorpromazine in France in 1952, also tried isoniazid in psychiatric patients around this time. He later described how the immediate subjective effects as 'a sensation approaching euphoric dynamism' (p. 52) and he noted the occurrence of 'psychomotor subexcitation', insomnia and anxiety (Delay & Buisson 1958). In 1958 Hans Lehmann, also involved in the introduction of chlorpromazine, described iproniazid as a 'drug with stimulant properties' (Lehmann, Cahn, & de Verteuil 1958).

However within a short space of time a change in the conception of the effects of these drugs can be detected. There came to be less emphasis on the nature of the effects the drugs produced and more stress on their effects on the patient's mental condition. Thus in a paper published in 1957, George Crane divided the effects of iproniazid into 'Therapeutic effects', which were presented first, and 'Toxic effects' including 'Psychological side effects' presented later. This is in contrast to the earlier paper in which an overall profile of the effects of the drug was presented. In the second paper the therapeutic response was described as 'marked psychological improvement' consisting of 'an increase in vitality, a feeling of well-being, and an almost unlimited resistance to fatigue'. There was no reference in this section to 'stimulant' effects or hyperactivity. However in the section on side effects it was briefly mentioned that three of the 20 subjects developed psychotic reactions and a further 15 had 'behavioural disorders' or 'overstimulation' (Crane 1957).

It was also in the year 1957 that the idea of the 'psychic energiser' was first elucidated by a group of American researchers, including psychiatrist Nathan Kline. Kline, who became an avid evangelist for the use of iproniazid and similar drugs in depressive states (Healy 1997), suggested that a 'psychic energiser' was a drug that stimulated the psyche without stimulating the body. In a paper describing the effects of iproniazid in depressed outpatients, Kline and colleagues contrasted 'psychic energisers' with 'general energisers' by which they meant stimulants, such as amphetamine. According to their theory stimulants effected motor function and arousal as well as psychological state, thus exerting a 'general rather than a specific action' (Loomer, Saunders, & Kline 1957, p. 130). The authors went on, 'it has heretofore been impossible to increase psychic energy without simultaneously increasing motor, alerting and cerebral activity – without resulting undesirable side effects when a certain level is reached'. 'But' they continued 'it is our conviction that the present preparation, iproniazid, acts more selectively than any of the others' (Loomer, Saunders, & Kline 1957, p. 130). They speculated that a purely or predominantly 'psychic energizer' would increase appetite, in contrast to the appetite suppressant effects of general stimulants, and through similar mechanisms would also increase sexual desire. Although the anti-tuberculous drugs were noted to increase appetite, which does distinguish them from classical stimulants, these observations were made in patients with tuberculosis, and may have been due to improvement of the disease, which is well known to suppress appetite.

The immediate uptake of iproniazid for use in people with depression illustrates the appetite that existed for a pharmacological treatment for this sort of problem. Kline himself later commented that 'probably no drug in history was so widely used so soon after the announcement of its application in the treatment of a specific disease'. Kline attributed this partly to the fact that iproniazid was already available because it was a recognised treatment for tuberculosis, but he also records the feeling of the time that there was an 'overwhelming need for an effective antidepressant medication' (Kline 1970, p. 202).

In the 1957 paper Kline and colleagues attributed the effects of psychic energisers to inhibition of the enzyme called monoamine oxidase. Since this enzyme is involved in the degradation of monoamines, inhibiting it was believed to lead to an increase in the availability of the monamines. However stimulants were also known to decrease the action of monoamine oxidase. Kline and colleagues acknowledged this, but did not offer any explanation for how the difference between general stimulants and psychic ones was mediated. Based on subsequent accounts written by Kline, David Healy describes how the concept of the psychic energizer also incorporated elements of psychoanalytical theory. None of this is evident in the 1957 paper however which is often claimed to be the first publication of antidepressant drug effects (Healy 1997). The importance of this paper for the evolution of the idea of the antidepressant is that the concept of the 'psychic energiser' is a clear step away from a drug-centred understanding of the actions of the antituberculous drugs in depression, drugs that later came to be classified as monoamine oxidase inhibitor antidepressants (MAOIs). The concept can be seen as an attempt to move the drug treatment of depression away from the focus of inducing general stimulant effects.

'Antidepressants'

The other drug tested around this time, which came to be regarded as an antidepressant, was imipramine. Unlike the tuberculostatic drugs, imipramine is not a stimulant. It is chemically similar to chlorpromazine and has sedating properties. Therefore, in contrast to stimulant drugs with their activating and euphoric effects, it was difficult to construct a drug-centred rationale for why it might be useful in depression. In other words, it was difficult to see that any of the physiological and subjective effects it induced would be useful in someone who was depressed, especially as there were many other known sedatives available to address insomnia and agitation. Therefore, its use could only be rationalised on the basis that it exerted its effects by acting on the pathological basis of a depressive illness. In this sense imipramine was the first 'antidepressant'.

Imipramine was first used by Swiss psychiatrist Roland Kuhn. According to subsequent accounts by Kuhn himself and Alan Broadhurst of Geigy, Kuhn tried out a compound called G 22355, later named imipramine, which was given to him by the drug company because of its likeness to chlorpromazine (Healy 1997). It was first given to a group of patients with chronic schizophrenia who were withdrawn from chlorpromazine and then started on the new drug. Many of the patients became agitated and some became euphoric. Although this makes little sense given the known pharmacological profile of imipramine, and in retrospect it seems more likely to have been due to the sudden withdrawal of chlorpromazine, the official story goes that imipramine made the patients manic or euphoric. Therefore, it was concluded that it might have beneficial effects in depressed patients. So in 1955 Kuhn started to give the drug to depressed patients. He published these results in a Swiss journal in 1957 and in the *American Journal of Psychiatry* in 1958. Neither of these papers contained any figures or quantitative data on levels of improvement in patients on imipramine, or any systematic comparison with patients having other sorts of treatment. The results consisted of Kuhn's personal impressions and opinions. In the American article he described imipramine as having 'markedly anti-depressive properties' (p. 459) and 'potent antidepressant action' (Kuhn 1958, p. 464).

Kuhn comes across as a passionate advocate of imipramine. He described dramatic transformations with the drug, reminiscent, as Healy observes, of the way Prozac was described three decades later (Healy 2002). He claimed that people who had been depressed for years were suddenly cured usually in two to three days, and that those patients and their relatives claimed 'they had not been so well for a long time' (Kuhn 1958, p. 460). He described how a homosexual man had been transformed to heterosexuality through treatment and another man had been cured of impotence. Kuhn dismissed imipramine's side effects as 'relatively slight' (Kuhn 1958, p. 460). For example, instead of noting its now well-known and potentially dangerous hypotensive effects, he suggested that it could improve hypertension. Only in passing did he mention that several instances of collapse had occurred among his patients, almost certainly due to hypotension (Kuhn 1958). He also suggested imipramine could cure constipation when this was associated with depression. Only later in the paper did he note the fact that imipramine appeared to induce constipation, which is now well recognised to be a common effect.

Although Kuhn admitted that imipramine's mode of action was uncertain, he was at pains to deny that imipramine had euphoriant effects. He did not explicitly propose a mechanism of action, but one can be inferred from certain remarks. Kuhn said that imipramine's effects were 'symptomatic', by which he meant that if the drug were discontinued 'the illness breaks out again, usually with undiminished severity' (Kuhn 1958, p. 460). He also believed that imipramine could induce mania in susceptible individuals, a belief that has persisted ever since in psychiatric folklore, despite the fact that controlled studies show no evidence that this occurs (Visser & van der Mast 2005). Therefore, Kuhn's report conveys the implicit idea that imipramine reverses the biochemical or physical substrate of endogenous depression. If the drug is stopped the abnormalities resurface and use of the drug may tip the patient into the opposite state of mania. Later on Kuhn expressed his views of imipramine's action more explicitly. In 1970, describing the discovery of imipramine, he stated that 'we have achieved a specific treatment of depressive states, not ideal but already going far in this direction. I emphasise "specific" because the drug largely or completely restores what the illness has impaired – namely the mental functions and capacity and what is of prime importance, the power to experience' (p. 214). In this account he acknowledged that the side effects of imipramine are greater than he had first reported, but he maintained that 'the neurovegetative and extra-pyramidal side effects are true side effects and clearly distinguishable from the specific antidepressive components' (Kuhn 1970, p. 214).

From the beginning Kuhn associated the benefits of imipramine particularly with endogenous, or what he sometimes called 'vital' depression. Endogenous depression replaced the idea of melancholia and referred to a state that was thought to originate from biological dys- function in contrast to 'reactive' or 'neurotic' depression that was thought to be a response to external events. Endogenous depression is held to be characterised by symptoms that indicate its biological origins, such as sleep and appetite disturbance. These are still referred to as 'bio- logical' symptoms of depression, although there is no basis for con- cluding that these have any more biological origin than any other features of a depressed state. Again Kuhn offered no data to support his assertion that imipramine was more effective in endogenous depression than other sorts of depression, only his overall impressions. Yet the claim that there is a particular type of depressive condition that responds to the drug also helps suggest a disease-specific notion of the effects of imipramine. It implies that the drugs' effects are not universal, but confined to people who are believed to have a truly biological condition.

In 1958, Hans Lehmann and colleagues published a paper describ- ing their experiences of using imipramine, which provides a transi- tion from a drug-centred to a disease-centred view of the drug treatment of depression. They described imipramine as having 'primarily inhibitory or depressing (in the physiological sense) action on the central nervous system' (Lehmann, Cahn, & de Verteuil 1958, p. 162). They also noted 'we are unable at this stage to express any opinion on the specificity of the pharmacological action of imipramine (G 22355). It is conceivable that similar results might have been obtained with other drugs' (Lehmann, Cahn, & de Verteuil 1958, p. 161). The authors then proceeded to formulate a physical theory of the aetiology of depression, providing a disease-specific rationale for the effects of imipramine in depressed states. Although their expla- nations involved the still fashionable theory of electrical circuits, interestingly they suggested the idea that depression represents a state of disturbed physiological equilibrium, which has echoes of the chemical imbalance metaphor employed so widely today. 'A thera- peutically effective drug (for depression) restores the disturbed equilibrium of excitatory gradients, either by direct influence on the disturbed focus or by acting on surrounding cerebral field.' (Lehmann, Cahn, & de Verteuil 1958, p. 162).

Dissemination of the concept of an 'antidepressant'

The evidence suggests that use of the term 'antidepressant' quickly caught on. Figure 8.2 shows the number of papers published using the term 'antidepressant' between 1957 and 1965, as retrieved from a search of *Medline*. By 1959 the term was being used routinely in over 100 papers. Where the meaning of the term was spelled out it was in vague terms suggesting some action on a disease process, reminiscent of the language of Kuhn. Thus antidepressant drugs were referred to as having a 'worthwhile effect upon depressive illness' (Ball & Kiloh 1959, p. 1054) or having 'value' or 'benefits' in the treatment of depression without any explication of what this effect might consist of (Ball & Kiloh 1959; Rees 1960). In 1961, leading American psychiatrist Frank Ayd confidently used the term antidepressant, explaining that antide-pressant drugs 'control or eradicate target symptoms such as depressed mood, psychomotor retardation, loss of interest' (Ayd, Jr. 1961a). Many papers repeated the assertion that imipramine's effects were strongest in endogenous depression. Often there was no reference to Kuhn's paper or to anything else, suggesting that the association between the benefits of imipramine and endogenous type depression was regarded as established beyond doubt (Ayd, Jr. 1961a; Dally & Rohde 1961).

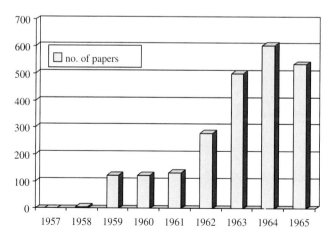

Figure 8.2   Papers using the term 'antidepressant' on *Medline* (1957–65)

However one early study already contradicted this proposed association (Rees, Brown, & Benaim 1961) and it has not been confirmed in subsequent overviews (Joyce & Paykel 1989).

As early as 1959 the idea that the new drugs for depression were disease-specific treatments was strongly and explicitly endorsed by prominent psychiatrists. At a major conference on depression held in Cambridge, England in 1959 Professor Erik Jacobsen expressed the belief that

> The MAOIs seem, in theory, to be closer to the ideal psychotropic drugs, with strong and clear-cut effects on pathological states and almost no effect on normals.
>
> (Jacobsen 1964, p. 210)

Jacobsen suggested that the effects of the MAOI antidepressants such as iproniazid were clearly distinguishable from effects of stimulant drugs. Like Kline and colleagues, he assumed that their effects in depression were due to monoamine oxidase inhibition, but did not explain how they could be differentiated from stimulants which were also known to act in this way.

At the same conference Pierre Deniker and his colleague declared that

> The action of imipramine, and to a lesser extent iproniazid, is not merely sedative and symptomatic, like that of the neuroleptics, but is curative.
>
> (Deniker & Lemperiere 1964, p. 230)

They proposed that it was possible to dispense with ECT for all but the most severe cases, and that it was in 'protracted involutional melancholia that imipramine gives results really superior to those of ECT' (p. 230). In contrast to Jacobsen, who was eager to detach antidepressants from stimulants, Deniker and Lamperiere (1964) made the remarkable assertion that imipramine as well as iproniazid 'behave as stimulants, and thus resemble amphetamine, even though their action is more complex' (p. 229). They suggested that imipramine induced insomnia, for example, and that it could be differentiated electrophysiologically from chlorpromazine. These statements are difficult to understand given that imipramine was already clearly described as having sedative properties and being closely related to chlorpromazine. Therefore, Deniker and Lamperiere's observations are still coloured by the idea that an antidepressant drug must induce a chemical stimulant effect. However they also demonstrate the desire for a coherent and single disease-based account of the action of drugs being used for depression.

At another psychopharmacology conference held in the United States in 1962, it was suggested that antidepressants 'strike almost specifically at the governing mechanisms of affectivity which are disturbed in manic depressive psychosis' (Flugel 1966, p. 495). Their specificity of action was again contrasted with stimulants:

> The earliest reports of the use of antidepressant medication seemed to indicate that the purpose of the medication was simply some special kind of stimulation which was useful in relieving lethargy and withdrawal. It was soon evident, however to good clinical observers, that the action of antidepressant substances was much more specific.
>
> (Goldman 1966, p. 526)

A similar sentiment was expressed in a later British textbook of psychopharmacology: 'Antidepressant drugs, like imipramine and the monoamine oxidase inhibitors differ from euphoriant drugs such as amphetamine in that they appear to act specifically against depressive symptoms' (Dally 1967, p. 10).

The ascendancy of the disease-centred model of antidepressant drugs is apparent in textbooks and formularies from the 1960s. As early as 1960 textbooks referred to iproniazid and imipramine as 'antidepressants' and explicitly distinguished them from stimulants (Mayer-Gross, Slater, & Roth 1960). The British National Formulary classification first included a category of 'antidepressants' in 1963 (British Medical Association and Pharmaceutical Society of Great Britain 1963), noting that 'the treatment and prognosis of mental depression has been considerably enhanced by the use of antidepressant drugs' (p. 85). The old category of 'stimulants' was abandoned in this edition and amphetamines and other stimulants were included in the category of antidepressants along with imipramine and 'monoamine oxidase inhibitors' such as iproniazid.

However some researchers challenged the view that antidepressants were disease-specific drugs. In 1964, a psychiatrist called E.H. Hare and his colleagues published a report of a controlled trial comparing 'Drinamyl' a widely used preparation containing barbiturates and amphetamine, with imipramine. They found no difference between the two treatments and concluded 'that imipramine has no specific antidepressive action' (Hare, McCance, & McCormick 1964, p. 819). Hare and colleagues also suggested that 'in so far as antidepressive drugs are effective in the treatment of depressive illness, this is in virtue of a sedative action' (p. 819) and recommended that they should be compared with other 'purely sedative' drugs (p. 820). In 1964, prominent American psychopharmacologists John Overall, Leo Hollister and colleagues set out to examine the 'specificity of drug classes' (p. 605) by comparing the effects of imipramine and an 'antipsychotic' drug thioridazine. They pointed out how imipramine and chlorpromazine 'share many pharmacodynamic effects, differing mainly in potency'. The study found no difference between imipramine and thioridazine in depressed patients (Overall et al. 1964). The authors concluded that they could not confirm 'the specificity of action ordinarily attributed to antipsychotic and antidepressant drugs' (p. 608). However these were already dissenting voices in a psychiatric climate that had overwhelmingly adopted the notion of the 'antidepressant' as a specific treatment for depression. Further expressions of scepticism were occasionally published subsequently but provoked little discussion (Thomson 1982).

History of the monoamine hypothesis of depression

The monoamine theory of depression is important because it provides a model for the idea that antidepressant drugs act on the biological basis of depressive symptoms. It forms the basis for the modern idea that depression arises from a chemical imbalance.

'Monoamines' is the term used to refer to the neurotransmitters noradrenalin and serotonin. In the mid-20th century there was widespread interest in medicine in the catecholamines noradrenalin and adrenalin. In 1928 an enzyme called monoamine oxidase was described that was involved in their metabolism and inactivation. In 1938 the actions of the stimulant ephedrine were linked to inhibition of this enzyme (Gaddum & Kwiatkowski 1938). In 1952 it was demonstrated that iproniazid inhibited monoamine oxidase (Zeller & Barsky 1952) and subsequently it became known as a 'monoamine oxidase inhibitor'. Its actions in various conditions including depression were attributed to this action. In the late 1950s there was a burst of interest in the use of iproniazid and other drugs referred to as MAOIs for a number of indications including angina, hypertension and cancer, as well as depression. Drug companies looked for other compounds with monoamine oxidase inhibiting action, and several were produced and tested in depression as well as other medical conditions. Although no clear disease theory of depression had been articulated in writing by this point, there was already an understanding, described by psychiatrist Nathan Kline in a memoir, that elevating monoamine levels with stimulants or MAOIs was necessary for its treatment (Lehmann & Kline 1983). Despite the fact that stimulants were later not considered to have disease-specific action, their ability to induce a state of euphoria and heightened activity inspired the idea that depression was due to the opposite biochemical state from that produced by stimulants.

When imipramine was suggested to be an 'antidepressant' it did not readily fit into this picture. In fact its actions were similar to chlorpromazine and reserpine. Reserpine, a drug used briefly as a neuroleptic, was thought to induce depression by reducing the availability of monoamines. In the early 1960s Julius Axelrod, who was investigating catecholamine (adrenalin and noradrenalin) metabolism, discovered that one action of some drugs was to block the reuptake of neurotransmitters into nerve cell bodies. In a paper published in 1961, it was reported that imipramine, chlorpromazine, reserpine, amphetamine, tyramine and cocaine inhibited reuptake of noradrenalin into heart, spleen and adrenal gland tissue and caused a brief five-minute increase in blood concentration of noradrenalin (Axelrod, Whitby, & Hertting 1961). Subsequently Axelrod and his colleagues demonstrated that the uptake of noradrenalin by brain tissue of rats was reduced by imipramine and amitriptyline but not chlorpromazine (Glowinski & Axelrod 1964). They concluded that this may be 'a mechanism for the antidepressant action' of the tricyclic drugs.

It has since been assumed that this is the therapeutic action of tricyclic antidepressants, which are sometimes referred to as monoamine reuptake inhibitors or MARIs. However the exact significance of this reuptake process is unknown, especially as the tricyclic antidepressants have numerous other actions and 'influence, directly or indirectly, almost all neurotransmitters, many neuropeptides and most hormones' (Khan 1999). Further studies of reuptake by heart muscle preparations showed that chlorpromazine was a stronger reuptake inhibitor than imipramine and not all the tricyclic antidepressants had this action (Lahti & Maickel 1971). In addition, it has not been possible to demonstrate that reuptake inhibition is actually correlated with increased availability or activity of noradrenalin or serotonin. In fact most evidence suggests that tricyclic drugs reduce levels of noradrenalin (Frazer & Mendels 1977; Heydorn, Frazer, & Mendels 1980; Schildkraut, Winokur, & Applegate 1970).

However these inconsistencies were paid little attention. Reuptake was regarded as a major discovery and Julius Axelrod was later awarded the Nobel Prize for his work on the catecholamine system. The fact that reuptake properties were accorded so much importance, before their significance was fully elaborated, demonstrates that the monoamine hypothesis was influential before it was even properly articulated. The reuptake mechanism was considered important because it allowed imipramine, with its sedative and tranquillising profile of effects, to be incorporated into a more general theory of the biological origin and treatment of depression.

By the mid-60s there was a strong consensus that depression, at least in its severe endogenous form, was caused by an abnormal biochemical state consisting of reduced levels of monoamines in the brain. The theory was set out systematically in a well-known paper by Schildkraut (1965), who concentrated on the role of noradrenalin (Schildkraut 1965). Other authors focused on serotonin (Coppen 1967). Schildkraut asserted that 'some if not all depressions are associated with an absolute or relative deficiency of catecholamines, particularly norepinephrine ... elation may conversely be associated with an excess of such amines' (Schildkraut 1965, p. 509). The primary justification for the theory was the belief that stimulants and antidepressant drugs acted to increase monoamine levels. Schildkraut referred to how the supposed efficacy of imipramine had initially cast doubt on the theory, but the 'riddle' had been solved by Axelrod's research on its ability to block tissue reuptake of noradrenalin.

Despite decades of research, there is no evidence to support the monoamine theory of depression (see Chapter 9). Studies of noradrenalin are inconsistent, with as many finding raised levels in people with depression as those finding reduced levels (Dubovsky, Davies, & Dubovsky 2002). Evidence on serotonin is similarly inconsistent, and eminent mainstream psychopharmacologists admit that there is no evidence of serotonin dysfunction in depression (Lacasse & Leo 2005). Nevertheless, the monoamine hypothesis has survived and remains influential. Contradictory evidence has been overlooked or reframed as supportive. For example, Schildkraut reported research that clearly showed that imipramine decreased noradrenalin levels in the brain, but hypothesised that despite reduced concentrations, the *activity* of noradrenalin might nevertheless be increased (Schildkraut, Winokur, & Applegate 1970).

Subsequently attention switched to neurotransmitter receptors in the 1970s and the monoamine hypothesis was reformulated in terms of monoamine receptors. It was found in animal experiments that several antidepressants reduced the density of beta-adrenoceptors (a type of noradrenalin receptor) in the brain after about two weeks of treatment.

Since this coincided with the commonly accepted two-week lag between starting antidepressants and clinical improvement, it was proposed that the reduction in beta-receptors was the mechanism of their antidepressant action. In line with this proposal, depression was now suggested to be due to '"supersensitive" receptors which need down regulation' (Stahl 1984). The fact that the theory now contradicted its old versions by proposing that depression was due to *increased* activity of the noradrenalin system was glossed over, as was research that showed that other sorts of drugs, including clozapine and thioridazine, also reduced the density of beta-receptors (Gross & Schumann 1982).

Role of the pharmaceutical industry

Subsequent accounts reveal the extent of cooperation between psychiatric researchers and pharmaceutical company personnel in the development of antidepressants (Healy 1996; Lehmann & Kline 1983). Company scientists were involved in providing new compounds for psychiatrists to try and psychiatrists sometimes suggested leads for companies to follow. Nathan Kline subsequently claimed that the industry was sceptical about the market for antidepressants, and was only persuaded to collaborate in research by his own remonstrations (Healy 1997; Lehmann & Kline 1983). However contemporary accounts suggest that by 1961 the industry was 'launching an aggressive search for more antidepressant compounds' (Ayd, Jr. 1961a, p. 32). It may be true that companies were initially reluctant to put their energies into marketing iproniazid, which had been associated with liver toxicity fairly early on, but it also appears that they soon threw themselves into the foray to find drugs for depression. In the *British Medical Journal* in the first two months of 1962, eight different companies placed one or two page adverts for antidepressants, involving seven different drugs or drug combinations. As early as 1961 antidepressant adverts appeared on the back cover of the *British Medical Journal*.

The early marketing campaigns for antidepressants had to establish the idea of depression as a common, medically treatable condition. In order to achieve this, Merck, who finally won the patent for amitriptyline, bought and distributed 50,000 copies of Frank Ayd's book, 'Recognising the Depressed Patient' (Ayd, Jr. 1961b; Healy 1997). In this book, which can be seen as the first full exposition of the modern concept of depression, Ayd suggested that depression was commoner than was generally realised and that it often went undiagnosed. He claimed that one out of every ten people required some sort of psychiatric treatment in their lifetime and that 'of all the psychiatric ills to which man is heir, depression occurs with the most frequency' (Ayd, p. 1). He suggested that depression was most commonly encountered in General Practice, where it could be treated satisfactorily by the General Practitioner. He also suggested that many people who acquired other psychiatric diagnoses were in fact depressed. Like more recent marketing campaigns, Merck sought to create a concept of depression as a *medical* condition, amenable to drug treatment. The concept was also inherently fluid, allowing many more people than before to be pulled into the net of psychiatric treatment.

In the early 1990s, with the launch of the new range of antidepressants such as Prozac (fluoxetine), Lustral or Zoloft (sertraline) and Seroxat or Paxil (paroxetine), the pharmaceutical industry was involved in a number of similar campaigns about depression. The UK Defeat Depression Campaign, run by the Royal Colleges of Psychiatrists and General Practitioners but part-funded by Eli Lilly (makers of Prozac), is a good example and typical of other national depression campaigns. The main message echoed Ayd's book, that depression is an under-recognised problem. The campaign sought to persuade General Practitioners that they should diagnose more people as depressed and prescribe more antidepressants. Campaign literature suggested that 5% of the population suffer from depression at any one time and that around 20% of General Practice attenders have symptoms of depression, with half of these needing treatment (Paykel & Priest 1992). The campaign also aimed to reduce the general public's resistance to taking drugs for depression, stressing that antidepressants were not addictive and distancing them from the recently discredited benzodiazepines. The campaign was particularly concerned to dispel fears of addiction so that people would follow its recommendation that everyone treated with antidepressants, even those with a relatively minor first episode, should continue taking their antidepressants for a further 4–6 months after recovery (Priest et al. 1996). Since most people treated in General Practice were thought to take medication for about three weeks only, this suggestion aimed to achieve a substantial increase in the quantity of antidepressant treatment used. Subsequent publicity about discontinuation effects of antidepressants, especially some SSRIs, has led to an acknowledgement of the difficulties of withdrawing from medication, but there has been no revision of recommendations about the benefits or length of treatment. As a result of the Defeat Depression Campaign and more general marketing, use of antidepressants soared during the 1990s. Between 1992 and 2002 the number of prescriptions issued for antidepressants in the United

Kingdom increased by 235% from 9.9 to 23.3 million (National Institute for Clinical Excellence 2004) (see Figure 8.1 on p. 119).

Many early advertisements referred to the specificity of antidepressants, referring to them as 'specific' and a 'corrective' (see Chapter 4). But the industry was also concerned to capture the market for agents for anxiety that was perceived as a major problem in the 1960s. Therefore, the sedative or anxiolytic properties of antidepressants were often emphasised. Since the 1990s the pharmaceutical industry has promoted an unambiguous message about the biochemical nature of depression and how antidepressants rectify a chemical imbalance. The industry has popularised the idea of antidepressants as a disease-specific treatment and greatly expanded their consumer base. Antidepressants have successfully captured much of the market of drugs for 'everyday nerves', previously occupied by the benzodiazepines (Healy 2004). They are also colonising many other areas including childhood difficulties, eating disturbances and aspects of personality and behaviour such as compulsive shopping and difficulty controlling one's temper, now diagnosable as 'intermittent explosive disorder'.

Professional and political influences

This account of the history of drugs known as 'antidepressants' demonstrates that although there was a perfectly good account of the action of the antituberculous drugs from a drug-centred perspective, a disease-centred notion of their action was formulated that obscured their previously well-known stimulant effects. Similarly, even though the effects of imipramine were transparently contrary to effects induced by other drugs which were thought to counteract the underlying pathology of depressive states, it was nevertheless readily accepted as an 'antidepressant' drug. The concept of a specific drug for depression was embraced despite the absence of any evidence that they acted in a disease-specific way and even before there was any convincing data of their superiority over placebo. The story of the emergence of the antidepressants is therefore further testimony to the strong desire for disease-specific treatments in psychiatry. A drug treatment for a common problem that could be treated outside hospital was just what psychiatry needed in the 1960s. The 'antidepressants' fulfilled this role perfectly. They not only provided a treatment, but with the consensus about their disease-specific action, backed up by the monoamine hypothesis of the chemical nature of depression, they provided a truly medical-seeming treatment. This gave psychiatrists a strong claim to jurisdiction over discontent in the community, in a way that would have seemed more tenuous without a physical treatment to support it.

State support for antidepressants has generally been more passive than it was for the new tranquillisers. Over recent years Western countries have seen a massive increase in numbers of people receiving incapacity benefit as a result of psychiatric illness, mostly depression (Moncrieff & Pomerleau 2000). This has only recently been challenged by governments. In some cases the State has actively supported psychiatric expansion, such as funding the Australian campaign 'beyondblue', which has essentially the same aims and message as the Defeat Depression Campaign. This process of medicalisation can benefit governments by transforming all sorts of problems and disaffections wrought by social and economic changes into psychiatric deviance (Moncrieff 2007).

9
Is There Such a Thing as an 'Antidepressant'? A Review of the Evidence

This chapter reviews the evidence that could establish whether drugs believed to be 'antidepressants' really are disease-specific treatments for depression. The following chapter will consider whether they have any effects that might be useful in depression from a drug-centred perspective.

Although it is widely believed that the efficacy of antidepressants compared with placebo is well established, myself and other critics have been suggesting that this is not the case for some time now (Antonuccio et al. 1999; Greenberg & Fisher 1989; Moncrieff & Kirsch 2005). Our doubts are based on questioning the validity of the research and on demonstrating that the results of this research are not as overwhelmingly positive as they are usually presented.

The first problem with this research is the concept of depression itself. Although recent accounts of psychosis suggest it is not so distinct from normal experience (Bentall 2006), it is still broadly the case that people with psychosis have experiences such as delusions and hallucinations that clearly differentiate them from most other people. But people who are diagnosed as depressed do not usually have any features that categorically distinguish them from other people. The sorts of problems that are diagnosed as depression can vary considerably depending on the use of different diagnostic criteria, the interpretation of those criteria, and public and professional attitudes. Therefore, the first problem with the research is that it is difficult to know what sorts of problems are encompassed under the rubric of 'depression'. For example, many early trials of antidepressants were conducted with psychiatric inpatients but now antidepressant studies recruit people, often through advertisements, who are not even involved in psychiatric services. People who join up after seeing advertisements may do so because they want to be in a trial, sometimes for the pecuniary reward, and may, therefore, have little in common with people with established psychiatric problems.

A related problem is the measurement of outcomes. Rating scales for depression consist of collections of 'symptoms' of depression, but there is no way of validating what these symptoms refer to, because no consistent underlying biological abnormality has been found. It is also difficult to relate rating scale scores to functioning and therefore the actual clinical significance of scores and differences in scores is uncertain. In addition, depression-rating scales do not eliminate the influence of drug-induced effects. For example, all scales in common use contain items that would respond to any drug with sedative properties, such as anxiety, agitation and insomnia. For example, the commonly used 17-item version of the Hamilton Rating Scale for Depression (HRSD) (Hamilton 1960) has a maximum score of 52 and contains three items on sleep difficulties and four relating to different types of anxiety or agitation. The items on sleep alone can score up to 6 points. It is often said that the Hamilton scale was designed with the profile of the tricyclics in mind with their strongly sedative properties (Healy 1997). The designers of a similar scale explicitly state that the scale was contrived in order to maximise the change observed during antidepressant treatment (Montgomery & Asberg 1979).

Amplified placebo effects due to unblinding are likely to be particularly significant in antidepressant trials. People who agree to participate in trials are likely to be committed to the idea that drug treatment will help them. Similarly research personnel usually have a pro-drug bias. I described earlier in Chapter 2 how research shows that people in clinical trials of psychiatric medication can often tell whether they are on the active drug or the placebo because active drugs induce discernible effects such as drowsiness, dry mouth and nausea. If people can discriminate between active drugs and placebo, their expectations of the effects of the two interventions may not be the same. They may have stronger expectations that the active drugs will be helpful and they may have less strong expectations or even negative expectations of the possible effects of having a placebo. Depression and neurotic conditions are likely to be most susceptible to this effect, firstly because patients who enrol in trials are likely to accept the value of medical treatment in a way that some patients with psychosis are less inclined to do. Secondly, anything that increases hope is likely to improve someone's mood since being hopeless is generally considered to be a feature of depression.

Antidepressants versus placebo for short-term treatment

Current textbooks state that antidepressants are 20% to 40% more effective than placebo, achieving an average 60% response rate compared to placebo response rates of between 20% and 40% Dubovsky, Davies, & Dubovsky 2001; Gelder, Mayou, & Cowen 2001). The Royal College of Psychiatrists' information leaflet states that antidepressants produce substantial improvement in 50–65% of people compared with 25–30% of people given placebo tablets (Royal College of Psychiatrists 2007).

There are thousands of randomised trials that compare so-called antidepressant drugs with an inert placebo. A majority of the published trials show that antidepressants are a bit better than placebo, but despite the many possible biases which make positive results more likely, many studies found that antidepressants were no better than placebo and some found that they were worse. Despite the glowing reports of imipramine's effects by Kuhn and others, studies of imipramine are far from convincing. Authors of a review of randomised trials published in 1975 found that 64% of the studies did not find a statistically significant difference between imipramine and placebo, despite categorising data in a way that may have magnified differences (Rogers & Clay 1975). The review also omitted the large negative study conducted by the National Institute of Mental Health (NIMH) described below (Raskin et al. 1970). A large and comprehensive review conducted in 1969 by NIMH concluded that in 'well designed studies the differences between the effectiveness of antidepressant drugs and placebo are not impressive' (Smith, Traganza, & Harrison 1969). More recently a meta-analysis found that 69% of placebo-controlled tricyclic antidepressant (TCA) studies did not show a statistically significant difference (Storosum et al. 2001).

Other meta-analyses produce varying estimates of differences between antidepressants and placebo. Earlier ones tended to suggest differences in effectiveness of the order of 20–30% between antidepressants and placebo (Davis, Wang, & Janicak 1993; Quality Assurance Project 1983). More recent analyses yield lower differences, with several finding differences of only around 10–11% (Bech et al. 2000; Khan, Warner, & Brown 2000; Storosum et al. 2001).

However these categorical figures are misleading, as demonstrated in a widely quoted and influential paper by psychologist Irving Kirsch and colleagues entitled 'The emperor's new drugs' (Kirsch et al. 2002). This analysis was based on a sample of trials submitted to the FDA for approval of a variety of new antidepressant drugs and unlike previous meta-analyses it included unpublished studies. Although in categorical terms the analysis revealed a difference between antidepressants and placebo of 18%, this figure was produced by a difference of only 1.7 points on the Hamilton Rating Scale for Depression. By all assessments of clinical validity, this difference is too small to be meaningful and was referred to as 'vanishingly small' by one of the commentators on the paper (Brown 2002). In addition, a difference as small as this could easily be produced by drug-induced effects such as sedation, amplified placebo effects or other methodological artefacts. The paper's authors concluded that 'the pharmacological effects of antidepressants are clinically negligible' (Kirsch, Moore, Scoboria, & Nicholls 2002, p. 1).

The British Government's National Institute for Clinical Excellence (NICE) review of research on the newer antidepressants produced similar findings but managed to come to different conclusions (National Institute for Clinical Excellence 2004). The review's recommendations were that antidepressants were effective and should be prescribed to everyone with 'moderate' or 'severe' depression. The main analysis of rating-scale scores found a statistically significant difference between antidepressants and placebo, but it was concluded that 'the size of this difference is unlikely to be of clinical significance'. However the same data was then used in an analysis of rates of response and remission by categorising people according to whether they fell either side of a certain level of improvement in rating-scale scores. This analysis produced a relative risk of 0.73 for response to placebo versus antidepressants,[1] which the authors concluded was a clinically significant difference. When myself and others pointed out in the feedback on the draft guidelines that the positive conclusions were based on the very same rating-scale data that, in the primary analysis, had not indicated clinically significant effects, we were ignored. This was particularly pointed because we received a response to other issues we raised. The guideline's authors seemed unable to draw the obvious conclusions from their own data. So they found a way to present it in such a way that allowed them to draw the conclusions they were comfortable with.

It is worth mentioning that two of the largest, most influential and independently funded early trials found little difference between the antidepressants tested and placebo. In the Medical Research Council trial comparing imipramine, phenelzine, ECT and placebo conducted in the United Kingdom (Medical Research Council 1965), it is well known that phenelzine performed poorly. However differences between

Table 9.1 Medical Research Council study results

Symptom	ECT		Imipramine		Phenelzine		Placebo	
	Entry	4 wks	Entry	4 wks	Entry	4 wks	Entry	4 wks
Depressed mood	2.6	0.6	2.4	1.3	2.5	1.7	2.5	1.4
Retardation	1.6	0.3	1.4	0.5	1.6	1.0	1.2	0.6
Suicidal ideas	1.0	0.1	1.0	0.2	1.2	0.6	1.2	0.5
Self-reproach	1.3	0.2	1.4	0.6	0.9	0.8	1.2	0.6
Anxiety	1.9	0.8	1.9	0.9	1.8	1.4	1.8	0.9
Insomnia	1.3	0.3	1.0	0.7	1.0	0.5	1.0	0.6
Anorexia	1.1	0.2	0.9	0.4	1.2	0.5	1.0	0.5
Fatigue	1.1	0.4	1.0	0.5	1.0	0.5	1.2	0.6

imipramine and placebo were also not marked, with no statistically significant difference found for the principle a priori categorical outcome, which was the proportion of patients who showed 'substantial improvement' over four weeks of acute treatment. Instead the main publication highlights the finding that more patients on imipramine than placebo showed 'some improvement' which showed a larger difference. Table 9.1 shows the change in individual symptom scores over four weeks as presented in the paper. It can be seen that although ECT seems to be markedly better than the other treatments, the differences between imipramine, phenelzine and placebo were negligible. The overall rating of the symptom-based scale was not presented.

There was also evidence that the double blind was breached and that investigators could identify the medication patients were taking (Hare 1965).

A large NIMH study comparing imipramine, chlorpromazine and placebo, which was conducted in the United States with a total of 714 subjects, was also essentially negative. The study involved at least 97 different outcomes measured at each of the seven weeks of the trial, yielding a total of almost 700 measures. The paper, which describes the main results, contains no data from any of the scales used, and only presents qualitative impressions of treatment response, which are difficult to interpret. This analysis also excluded 159 black patients who showed a poorer response to imipramine. The paper still only concluded that 'although imipramine did have beneficial effects these effects were generally small' (Raskin et al. 1970). In subsequent publications, results for a few selected items on the scales are given at points in time when they reached statistical significance. However results in two different papers do not correspond. An analysis of differences in response between black and white patients presented 10 items as showing significant differences at week three, compared with only five items in a paper on differences between people with endogenous and neurotic depression (Raskin & Crook 1975, 1976). Since 5% of the 700 measures would be expected to be positive just by chance, or five per week, the results provide little evidence that imipramine had any superior effects.

Are antidepressants effective for severe depression?

Since Kuhn's paper on imipramine, it has been believed that antidepressants are most effective in severe depression. Many people, who are sceptical of their widespread use for milder cases, maintain that antidepressants are nevertheless effective and necessary in severe depression. It has also been suggested that the reason some studies find little difference between antidepressants and placebo is because they are conducted with people with mild depression, who dilute the antidepressant effect (National Institute for Clinical Excellence 2004). The National Institute for Clinical Excellence guidelines on the treatment of depression have gone as far as to suggest recently that antidepressants should not be prescribed to people with mild depression, and should only be used in cases of moderate and severe depression. However there is actually little evidence for the presumption that antidepressants are effective in severe depression.

An early review of the relation between the type of depression and antidepressant response found that evidence for predictors of antidepressant response was sparse and included few controlled studies (Bielski & Friedel 1976). Although they suggested that there was evidence for symptoms associated with an endogenous profile, such as anorexia, retardation and late sleep disturbance being associated with better response, they also noted the inconsistency of studies. They concluded that 'the relationship between severity of illness and tricyclic response is unclear' (p. 1489). A later and larger review by Joyce & Paykel (1989) did not find enough evidence to suggest that sleep and appetite disturbance predicted antidepressant response, and found that studies disagreed about whether endogenous depression responded better or worse to antidepressants than other types of depression. They concluded by suggesting that tricyclic antidepressants might be most useful in the middle range of severity and 'endogenicity'.

More recently a few studies and meta-analyses have examined this issue. A meta-analysis by Angst et al. (Angst, Scheidegger, & Stabl 1993) claimed to show evidence that the efficacy of antidepressants relative to placebo was greater for people who were more severely depressed initially. However the effects were weak and mostly not statistically significant. Another meta-analysis found more impressive gradients of effects, but full data were only provided for 'investigational' antidepressants and not for 'established' antidepressants, whose relationship with severity appeared to be weaker (Khan et al. 2002). A recent analysis found that people on antidepressants showed a greater response with increasing initial severity of depression in contrast to the placebo group whose response rates tailed off at higher severity levels (Kirsch et al. 2007). However even for the most severely depressed subgroup, the benefits of antidepressants over placebo were only around 4 points on the Hamilton rating scale, a difference that is of doubtful clinical relevance and can easily be explained by drug-induced effects. The pattern of response in the antidepressant group may also reflect 'regression to the mean'. This is the phenomenon by which observations naturally tend to gravitate towards the mean value, and hence those people with most severe depression to begin with will tend to show the most improvement. On the other hand, one recent meta-analysis found no effect of initial severity on treatment response (Walsh et al. 2002). The NICE meta-analysis also failed to find a consistent gradient between severity and antidepressant efficacy. However the review still concluded that a relationship had been shown. In fact the middle severity group tended to show the greatest drug-placebo differences in this analysis, but the number of studies in each group was small (National Institute for Clinical Excellence 2004).

Some individual trials of antidepressants that found no overall effects, found a relatively stronger effect in some of the most severely depressed subjects in post hoc analysis (Elkin et al. 1989; Paykel et al. 1988). However post hoc analysis is where the authors look for significant results without predetermining what particular tests are of interest. This sort of analysis is commonly referred to as a 'fishing expedition' and it is well known that it can highlight results that are positive just by chance. Another similar trial conducted in primary care found no association between 'melancholic' depression, that is the most severe depression, and antidepressant efficacy (Malt et al. 1999). These trials were conducted exclusively with people with relatively mild depression and so could not assess the relation over the whole severity range. The meta-analyses too were based mostly on outpatient studies. On the other hand, my own meta-analysis of older trials found that effects in inpatients were small and not statistically significant compared with outpatients, where effects were somewhat larger (Moncrieff 2003a). In addition, it has long been believed that antidepressants are relatively ineffective in severe depression accompanied by psychotic delusions. A study of inpatients found that it was actually greater severity of depression that predicted a worse response to antidepressants and not the presence of delusions (Kocsis et al. 1990). However the fact that the two are associated has led to the impression that it is psychiatric features that mark a lesser response to antidepressants. Recently a large trial of antidepressants versus placebo showed that people experiencing the depressive phase of manic depression, or bipolar disorder, who were also on 'mood stabilisers', showed no better response to antidepressants than they did to placebo (Sachs et al. 2007). Since the mood swings in manic depression are often more severe than other episodes of depression, this trial provides further evidence that, contrary to current opinion, antidepressants are not superior to placebo even in the most severe forms of depression.

Some of the clinical trial evidence suggests that there may be a group of people in the mid range of severity who benefit most from having an active antidepressant compared with a placebo. This would not be expected from a simple biological effect. It is more likely that people within the middle of the severity spectrum have the highest commitment to the idea of the effectiveness of drug treatment and would therefore be most susceptible to non-specific pharmacological and psychological effects. Many people with milder depression probably do not even consider themselves depressed and many do not want to take drug treatment. People with more severe depression, including the sort of people who end up in hospital, may have little faith in any intervention.

Antidepressants versus other drugs

Comparisons between so-called antidepressant drugs and other sorts of drugs do not indicate that antidepressants have a specific effect on depression. Many other drugs show superior effects to placebo or equal effects to antidepressants in randomised trials, as shown in Table 9.2.

The fact that other substances had to compete with ideas about the specificity of antidepressants that were strongly entrenched by the mid-1960s makes these results even more remarkable. The case of benzodiazepines is instructive. In the 1960s, when these were still relatively new drugs, most studies found they were equal or superior to antidepressants

Table 9.2 Randomised trials of other drugs for depression

Type of drug	Study	Results	
Neuroleptics	Davies and Shepherd (1955) Robertson and Trimble (1982)	Reserpine versus placebo Review of 34 randomised controlled trials of neuroleptics in depression	Reserpine superior to placebo Neuroleptic superior to placebo in 10 out of 11 comparisons; superior to antidepressants in 3 comparisons, equivalent in 14, inferior in 2, differential effects in subgroups in 1
Barbiturates	Blashki, Mowbray, and Davies (1971)	Amylobarbitone versus amitriptyline versus placebo	No statistically significant difference between amitriptyline and amylobarbitone for 2 out of 3 depression ratings
Benzodiazepines	Schatzberg and Cole (1978)	Review of 20 studies of benzodiazepines compared with antidepressants	10 out of 20 studies found benzodiazepines were equal to antidepressants or superior to placebo
	Imlah (1985), Feighner et al. (1983), Rickels et al. (1987) Weissman et al. (1992)	Alprazolam versus placebo and imipramine or amitriptyline	Alprazolam superior to placebo and equal or superior to imipramine and amitriptyline
Stimulants	Rickels et al. (1970)	Pemoline and methylphenidate (Ritalin) versus placebo	Both stimulants superior to placebo

(continued)

Table 9.2   (continued)

Type of drug	Study	Results	
	Hare et al. (1964)	Imipramine versus Drinamyl (dexamphetamine plus amylobarbitone)	Equal effects
Buspirone	Robinson et al. (1990)	Five studies of buspirone versus placebo in major depression with anxiety	Buspirone superior overall and for core symptoms of depression as well as anxiety
	Fabre (1990)	Buspirone versus placebo for major depression	Trend towards superiority of buspirone
Opiates	Emrich et al. (1982)	Buprenorphine versus placebo	Buprenorphine superior
Atropine	Moncrieff et al. (1998)	Review and meta-analysis of nine trials comparing antidepressants with an active placebo containing atropine	One study found a significant effect of antidepressant; others found small and non significant differences
St John's wort	Philipp et al. (1999), Szegedi et al. (2005), Kasper et al. (2006)	St John's wort (hypericum) versus placebo, imipramine and paroxetine	St John's wort superior to placebo and equivalent to antidepressants

for people with depression. By the 1970s, most studies found the antidepressant was superior. Despite finding that half of the studies they reviewed showed equal or superior effects with benzodiazepines, by 1978 reviewers Schatzberg and Cole concluded confidently that benzodiazepines 'are less effective than standard antidepressants in the treatment of several types of depressive illnesses' (Schatzberg & Cole 1978, p. 1359). But when a new benzodiazepine, alprazolam, was produced and marketed in the 1980s, studies reported that it was effective in treating depression, and not just depression with anxiety.

Almost all studies comparing antidepressants with neuroleptic drugs found that neuroleptics were equivalent or better (Robertson & Trimble

1982). Two of these studies reported that the antidepressant was superior for patients with "retarded" depression, whereas the neuroleptic was superior for anxious or neurotic patients (Hollister et al. 1967; Raskin et al. 1970). This is readily understandable, given what we know of the drug-induced effects of neuroleptics. Their deactivation effects are likely to compound psychomotor retardation and reduce agitation and anxiety. Reserpine, the drug that was believed to induce a depressive state, was found to be clearly superior to placebo for the treatment of depression in an early trial conducted at the Maudsley hospital in London (Davies & Shepherd 1955).

Despite early convictions that stimulants were ineffective for depression, a large and well-conducted trial by Rickels et al. (1970), involving 120 patients, demonstrated clear superiority of two stimulants over placebo in a four-week trial.

In the early days of antidepressant research, some investigators worried about the possibility of unblinding. In order to reduce this problem they used a placebo containing an active substance to mimic some of the side effects of the antidepressant drugs, instead of the physiologically inert substances that placebos are usually made of such as chalk and lactose. Atropine was the substance used because it produces the same anticholinergic effects that the tricyclic antidepressants produce, such as a dry mouth, constipation and blurred vision, but is not thought to have any specific antidepressant action. However atropine is mildly stimulant, and easily distinguishable from the effects of tricyclic antidepressants, which are strongly sedative, so it is likely that even these studies were not truly double blind. One of the studies used a small amount of a barbiturate as well to produce a mild sedative effect. All but one of these studies found that the differences between the antidepressant and the active placebo were small and not statistically significant. All the inpatient studies found no difference between the active placebo and the antidepressant, and all but one of the outpatient studies found only small differences (Moncrieff, Wessely, & Hardy 1998). The quality of these studies has rightly been criticised and it has been pointed out that most found differences in favour of the antidepressants (Quitkin et al. 2000). However there is evidence that the use of an active placebo was insufficient to disguise the nature of the treatment. For example, one trial reported that side effects were substantially greater with the antidepressants used compared with the active placebo (Hollister et al. 1964). Two trials that asked raters to guess what medication people were taking showed they could guess better than chance (Uhlenhuth & Park 1963; Weintraub & Aronson 1963). In one of these trials there was an association between guessing that patients were taking antidepressants and higher improvement ratings, suggesting that ratings may have been influenced by expectations of treatment (Weintraub & Aronson 1963).

In contrast a large trial of a naturally occurring biological compound called Substance P found no detectable difference from placebo. However the fact that substance P was associated with almost no side effects means that it was probably not distinguishable from an inert placebo. Paroxetine was used as the active comparator in these trials and the published paper suggests that its antidepressant effects were 'confirmed'. In fact the difference between paroxetine and placebo was a miniscule 2–3 points on the Hamilton Rating Scale for Depression (Keller et al. 2006).

As well as the variety of drugs listed in Table 9.2, drugs that are classed as antidepressants have a wide variety of pharmacological actions themselves. A recent meta-analysis showed that there was no distinction between drugs with different types of actions; that they all seemed to have a similar magnitude of effect (Freemantle, Anderson, & Young 2000). This suggests that the superiority that antidepressants and other drugs sometimes show over placebo is not related to a specific pharmacological action. Therefore, it seems likely that it is due to a combination of non-specific pharmacological and psychological factors. The pharmacological factors are the drug-induced effects such as sedation, which may produce temporary relief of some symptoms or features of depression. Alternatively, sedation or the indifference associated with neuroleptics might simply mask or blunt people's emotions (see Chapter 10). The psychological factors are the positive expectations that are associated with knowing that one is taking an active compound; in other words, the amplified placebo effect.

When confronted with this evidence, mainstream psychiatric commentators have either chosen to ignore it, or they have suggested that drugs that are not conventionally recognised as antidepressants may possess 'antidepressant properties' (Robertson & Trimble 1982, p. 173). The trouble with this argument is that if everything that produces some effect in depression is immediately assumed to be an 'antidepressant', with the implication that it has a disease-specific action, then there is no way of distinguishing a specific from a non-specific effect.

Evidence on long-term treatment

The current recommendation is that antidepressants should be continued for 4–6 months after the resolution of an acute episode of depression. This recommendation probably originates with Kuhn's advice but subsequently several long-term studies appeared to show that people are more likely to relapse after stopping antidepressants compared to if they continue to take them. However these studies all use a discontinuation design and involve patients who have done well on antidepressants in the first place. Thus people who have recovered from depression and remained well for some time are randomised either to continue taking their antidepressant, or to have it withdrawn and replaced by an inert placebo. It is now recognised that withdrawal from antidepressants of all classes produces a discontinuation syndrome that among other symptoms includes adverse effects on mood, anxiety and sleep (Dilsaver, Greden, & Snider 1987; Hindmarch, Kimber, & Cockle 2000; Judge et al. 2002). These effects have not been distinguished from recurrence of depression in people who are withdrawn to placebo. Thus some of the relapses in the placebo group may simply be symptoms of drug withdrawal. In addition, discontinuation symptoms are also likely to have a substantial psychological impact. The presence of these symptoms is likely to unblind participants, who will be able to guess whether or not they have been allocated to placebo substitution. Given that people included in such trials are people who have done well with antidepressants in the first place, they are likely to have negative expectations of the outcome of stopping treatment. People who suspect they have been put onto placebo may therefore have a worse outcome because they believe they will do badly.

Viguera and colleagues reviewed 27 discontinuation studies and found that relapse rates were as expected substantially higher in those who had their antidepressants discontinued compared with those who did not (Viguera, Baldessarini, & Friedberg 1998). The increased risk of relapse was much higher in people who had had recurrent episodes of depression. Diagnosing relapse in depression is even more subjective than in psychotic disorders. In the studies reviewed it consisted of a subjectively defined worsening of depression severe enough to warrant resumed antidepressant drug treatment. As with the neuroleptic trials, the meta-analysis showed that the increased risk of relapse was highest immediately after discontinuation and that the difference in relapse rates between people who had their medication stopped versus those who continued fell progressively over time. This suggests that the act of discontinuation itself influenced relapse. However the average time before relapse occurred was much longer than after neuroleptic discontinuation, at around 14 months, and gradual withdrawal did not reduce the risk of relapse compared with abrupt cessation of treatment. Another observation in this analysis was that the time for which people had taken antidepressants and remained stable prior to discontinuation did not influence relapse rates. People who had been stable for only three weeks relapsed at around the same rate after discontinuation as people who had been stable for four years. In fact if anything there was a slight trend for people who had been stable for longer to have higher relapse rates after discontinuation. As people who are stable for longer would normally be at lower risk of a subsequent relapse, this is unexpected and again suggests that the process of withdrawal of the antidepressant itself acts as a precipitant to relapse.

The Harvard group who published this study proposed that pharmacological stress is responsible for relapse after antidepressant discontinuation, the same as they suggest for neuroleptics (Baldessarini, Viguera, & Tondo 1999). There is little evidence that could support or refute this suggestion. One animal study found that rats withdrawn from long-term imipramine had a depressive reaction 40 days later (D'Aquila, Panin, & Serra 2004). On the other hand, the fact that relapses took a considerable time to occur and the fact that no protective effect was observed for gradual discontinuation would argue against this explanation. Psychological mechanisms are likely to be equally or more important in a condition like depression. People who believe that their recovery is attributable to antidepressant drugs are likely to feel anxious and vulnerable if those drugs are withdrawn. The next time they encounter problems they will worry about having a recurrence of their depressive state, in what can soon become a self-fulfilling prophecy. The more often people turn to drugs to help them the greater their insecurity will be. Psychological explanations would fit with the longer time to relapse and might explain how people who have been stable for longer periods are more at risk, since they are likely to be more psychologically dependent on the drugs.

Long-term outcome of depression

Despite the introduction of the antidepressants, the outcome of depression as revealed in research remains pretty poor. This is despite the fact that many less-severe cases are undoubtedly diagnosed now than several decades ago before the introduction of drug treatment. Although most people diagnosed with depression recover initially, a high proportion relapse and the initial episode may be prolonged. Even among milder cases in the community, 50–60% of people have not recovered by one year (Goldberg et al. 1998). In a large follow-up study of people who had recovered, conducted in the United States, 85% relapsed during a 15-year period (Mueller et al. 1999). Among people receiving hospital treatment for depression only 43% of adults and 24% of elderly patients had recovered and remained well after five years (Tuma 2000).

In addition, studies following up people treated in normal conditions, as opposed to controlled trials, show that people who do not take antidepressants have a better outcome than those who do. Two such studies, one conducted in a psychiatric outpatient clinic and one in primary care, demonstrated this effect, even after adjusting the results for the fact that people who were prescribed medication were generally more severely depressed (Brugha et al. 1992; Ronalds et al. 1997). Other studies showed that depressive episodes last longer in people who take antidepressants compared with those who did not (Patten 2004; Posternak et al. 2006). A study of sickness absence found that people who were prescribed antidepressants were less likely to return to work and had more days of sickness absence. The result was strongly statistically significant ($p<.001$) (Dewa et al. 2003), although some of the association is likely to be attributable to the severity of the initial problem. However this result was barely mentioned in the published paper. Instead the paper gives the impression that antidepressants were associated with a better probability of returning to work by focusing on the fact that, among those who were prescribed antidepressants, those prescribed 'recommended doses' did better than those on lower doses.

Epidemiological trends in depression also suggest that the more antidepressants are prescribed, the more prevalent depression is. Sharply rising levels of antidepressant prescribing since the 1990s have been accompanied by increased prevalence of depressive episodes (Patten 2004) and by rising levels of sickness absence for depression (Moncrieff & Pomerleau 2000).

Some authors have suggested a causal relationship between rising antidepressant prescribing and falling suicide rates observed in some countries. A recent analysis by Australian-based researchers with extensive links to companies making antidepressants made this claim in the *British Medical Journal* (Hall et al. 2003). The authors claimed to show that falls in suicide rates were greatest in the age groups in which antidepressant prescribing had risen most. But instead of looking at rates or proportions of prescriptions in different age groups they analysed absolute numbers of prescriptions. I redid the analysis looking at increases in rates of prescriptions. This produced the opposite finding that there was a strong and statistically significant correlation between increased rates of prescription of antidepressants and rising suicide rates (Spearman's correlation coefficients were $\underline{R}=0.86$, $p=.007$ for men;

R=0.76, *p*=.03 for women). This was due to the youngest age group, among whom there has been the most marked rise in consumption of antidepressants, showing a *rise* in suicide rates. In contrast, the elderly, in whom rates of increase of antidepressant use have been less dramatic, have shown a fall in suicide rate (Moncrieff 2003b). In any case suicide is a behaviour that follows very long-term patterns and falls in suicide rates in the elderly started long before the recent hike in antidepressant pre-scribing, from about the 1930s (Gunnell & Ashby 2004; Murphy & Wetzel 1980). In contrast, the suicide rate has been rising in some countries, such as Ireland (World Health Organisation 2006), and in younger age groups (Gunnell & Ashby 2004), despite increased use of antidepressants. Meta-analyses that have examined suicide rates in randomised trials have found no difference in suicide rates between drug and placebo-treated subjects (Khan et al. 2001; Khan, Warner, & Brown 2000; Storosum et al. 2001).

The monoamine theory of depression

Early formulations of the monoamine theory of depression cited two strands of evidence. One was the effects of antidepressant drugs and the other was the effects of reserpine. Skildkraut believed that 'studies have shown a fairly consistent relationship between drug effects on catechloamines, especially norepinephrine, and affective or behavioural states' (Schildkraut 1965, p. 509). He went on to describe how drugs that 'cause depletion and inactivation of norepinephrine centrally produce sedation or depression, while drugs which increase or potentiate brain norepinephrine are associated with behavioural stimulation or excitement and generally exert an antidepressant effect in man' (p. 509).

The idea that antidepressants have a specific action on a biological process is still cited as the main justification for the idea that depression is caused by a biochemical abnormality. A recent review article states that 'The indisputable therapeutic efficacy of these drugs suggests that serotonergic and/or noradrenergic underactivity is the key to the pathophysiology of clinical depression' (Malhi, Parker, & Greenwood 2005, p. 97). However the evidence reviewed above suggests that antidepressant drugs do not exert a specific effect in depression. In addition, although tricyclic antidepressants were found to inhibit reup-take of noradrenalin and serotonin, the significance of this action among their other numerous actions has not been established, and nor has its specificity. In fact, several studies show that instead of increasing nora-drenalin levels, tricyclic antidepressants appear to reduce noradrenalin concentrations (Heydorn, Frazer, & Mendels 1980; Mendels & Frazer

1974; Schildkraut, Winokur, & Applegate 1970; Schultz 1976; Vetulani & Sulser 1975). In addition, amphetamine, cocaine and other stimulants, which are known to increase noradrenalin levels in the brain, are not regarded as effective antidepressants.

The neuroleptic drug reserpine was commonly thought to cause a depressive illness in a high proportion of people who took it and for this reason its sedative effects in animals were used as an animal model of human depression. Since reserpine had been found to reduce levels of serotonin and noradrenalin in the brain (Axelrod 1996), it was suggested that the mechanism of reserpine-induced depression was monoamine depletion (Coppen 1967; Schildkraut 1965). At this time there was relatively little interest in dopamine and so it was not considered a candidate (Axelrod 1996). In the 1950s, it had been found that iproniazid blocked the sedative actions of reserpine (Chessin, Kramer, & Scott 1957), which would be consistent with its stimulant profile. Subsequently Italian researchers claimed that imipramine was also able to reduce the effects of reserpine, which seemed to confirm that the different types of antidepressants had some final common pathway of action on a coherent underlying disease process. This research is generally presented as demonstrating that tricyclic antidepressants block the depressive state induced by reserpine. However the original research only demonstrated that imipramine reduced the hypothermic effect of reserpine and not other effects such as sedation (Garattini et al. 1962). One of these studies showed that chlorpromazine also appeared to block reserpine-induced hypothermia (Costa, Garattini, & Valzelli 1960). This research is curious if one considers that chlorpromazine induces hypothermia and imipramine is closely related to it. It is difficult to know how reliable it was and in any case it did not demonstrate any effect of imipramine on the sedating or depressogenic effects of reserpine. In contrast, another group of researchers found that imipramine appeared to potentiate the sedative effects of reserpine, which would be consistent with it being a neuroleptic-type substance (Lapin et al. 1968).

It is also clear in retrospect that the reserpine-induced state was a state of dopamine blockade, characterised by sedation and inactivity, rather than a valid model of depression (Mendels & Frazer 1974). Whether it commonly caused a true depressive state in humans has also been disputed. One review suggested that it did so in 6% of cases, but mostly in people who had a previous history of depression (Goodwin & Bunney, Jr. 1971). The only controlled study of reserpine on mood found no true cases of depression, but several patients were noted to show signs of 'excessive tranquillisation' or 'pseudodepression' (Bernstein & Kaufman 1960).

Numerous studies of noradrenalin and serotonin activity have been conducted since the 1960s to try and demonstrate the elusive biochemical basis of depression. As with dopamine studies, there has been little attempt to control for other possible influences on neurotransmitter levels. Most studies involved people who were taking or had recently taken antidepressants or other psychotropic drugs that may have affected brain biochemistry. Comparison groups consisted of 'healthy controls' and the effects of stress, anxiety and other factors related to having an acute psychiatric condition were not considered. This research has looked at levels and availability of tryptophan, a chemical precursor of serotonin, effects of depletion of tryptophan and of noradrenalin precursors; serotonin and noradrenergic uptake in platelets; prolactin response to fenfluramine, a drug that is thought to stimulate presynaptic serotonin release; growth hormone response to clonidine, an adrenergic alpha-receptor-blocking drug; serotonin and noradrenergic receptor density in brains of suicide victims; serotonin-receptor binding in living subjects using imaging techniques and arterial assays of noradrenalin and serotonin metabolites. Research on noradrenalin is highly inconsistent with studies showing increased, decreased and normal levels in depressed patients compared with controls (Dubovsky, Davies, & Dubovsky 2001).

Research on serotonin is similarly confusing. For example, some imaging studies found reduced serotonin 1A-receptor binding in drug-free depressed patients, consistent with the hypothesis that there is a deficiency of serotonin activity in depression (Drevets et al. 1999; Sargent et al. 2000). Other studies, however have found no difference between drug-free patients and controls (Meyer et al. 2004) and some found increased binding potential in depressed patients (Parsey et al. 2006; Reivich et al. 2004). Although they are widely thought to show evidence of abnormality, post-mortem findings in the brains of people who committed suicide have also been inconsistent. Many studies have failed to find any differences in serotonin receptors between brains of suicide victims and those of people who have died in other circumstances (Lowther et al. 1997; Matsubara, Arora, & Meltzer 1991; Stockmeier et al. 1997). Tryptophan depletion studies are sometimes claimed to provide 'powerful evidence of a causal link between reduced serotonergic function and depression' (Cleare 2005). Depletion of tryptophan, the chemical precursor of serotonin is thought to lead to a reduction of serotonin, although this cannot be shown empirically because of the impossibility of directly measuring serotonin. Some of these studies showed that dietary tryptophan depletion (by drinking a drink of amino acids devoid of tryptophan, a technique that has been shown to reliably lower blood-tryptophan levels) leads to a transient increase in depressive symptoms in patients who had recovered from depression. However most studies showed that this effect was only present in patients who had been treated with SSRIs and not those treated with other drugs (Delgado et al. 1999). It may, therefore, be related to prior drug treatment, rather than depression itself. Studies with volunteers have not found that dietary tryptophan depletion causes depression (Murphy et al. 2002) and administering large doses of tryptophan as a sole treatment has no effect on depression (Mendels et al. 1975).

Other research into tryptophan depletion was conducted in the 1970s using the chemical parachlorophenylalanine, which has a stronger effect, producing a 60–80% reduction of serotonin metabolites in humans. References to this research have disappeared from the literature but it provides a better exposition of the effects of serotonin deficiency and a ready explanation for the effects seen in patients with the dietary methods. In animals, this technique has been found to induce a state characterised by insomnia, hypersexual behaviour, increased aggression, irritability, increased motor activity and hyper-reactivity to the environment which can be reversed by administration of tryptophan. However it does not produce anything resembling depression. In humans a variety of effects have been found including tiredness, restlessness, unease, anxiety, and at higher doses confusion, agitation and paranoid thinking. Again depression is not a characteristic of this state (Mendels & Frazer 1974). In the dietary studies milder effects of this sort may have been interpreted as a recurrence of depression, bearing in mind that the studies were only set up to look for depression and not other sorts of behavioural change.

However as Jeffrey Lacasse and Jonathan Leo have suggested in a recent article, there is a 'disconnect between the advertisements and the scientific literature' (Lacasse & Leo 2005). The publicity produced by the pharmaceutical industry and the psychiatric profession have convinced much of the general public that a link between serotonin abnormality and depression has been demonstrated. People I speak to are often shocked to hear that the evidence is tenuous and unconvincing. But psychiatric specialists admit that this is the case. The primary American textbook of psychiatry sums up the inconsistency of the evidence: 'studies of serotonin function in depression suggest both hypofunction and hyperfucntion' (Dubovsky, Davies, & Dubovsky 2001, p. 481). A psychopharmacology textbook states that 'so far, there is no convincing evidence that monoamine deficiency accounts for depression; that is there is no real monoamine deficit' (Stahl 2000, p. 601). When interviewed in 2003, award-winning psychopharmacology researcher David Burns said: 'I never saw any convincing evidence that any psychiatric disorder, including depression, results from a deficiency of brain serotonin' (cited in Lacasse and Leo, 2005).

Evidence for disease-centred action of antidepressants

Summarising the evidence reviewed so far reveals that there are no grounds for considering antidepressants to be a disease-centred treatment:

(1) *Is there a demonstrable pathological basis to depression from which the action of 'antidepressant' drugs can be understood?*

Evidence about serotonin and noradrenalin levels in people with depression is inconsistent and confusing and most studies fail to control for the effects of potential confounders, such as previous drug treatment. Overall, there is little evidence to suggest that there is a characteristic abnormality in either of these systems that is associated with depression.

(2) *Do rating scales for depression reliably measure the manifestations of a particular disease process?*

Depression rating scales contain items that are not specific to depression, including sleeping difficulties, anxiety, agitation and somatic complaints. These symptoms are likely to respond to the non-specific sedative effects that occur with most tricyclics and many other antidepressants. Hence changes in rating scale scores may merely reflect drug-induced effects.

(3) *Do animal models of depression reliably select antidepressant drugs?*

It is rarely mentioned that all animal models of depression produce variable results according to where they are conducted. In other words, they are unreliable. In addition to this, they fail to specifically select antidepressants and responses are obtained with drugs that are not generally considered to have antidepressant activity in humans (Bourin, Fiocco, & Clenet 2001). In the forced swim test, one of most common antidepressant screening tests, rats are placed in a tank of water from which they cannot escape. The time until they give up trying to escape is measured, on the assumption that the state of giving up is akin to depression. It is thought that antidepressants should prolong the time to giving up. In this test positive results have frequently been obtained with amphetamines and also occasionally with opiates, antihistamines, some antipsychotics, atropine, pentobarbital, as well as zinc and antibiotics (Bourin, Fiocco, & Clenet 2001; Parra 2003). In line with the underlying assumption that 'antidepressant activity' can be specifically identified or isolated, these results are usually referred to as 'false positives'. Conversely, the SSRIs, widely considered to be specific antidepressants, typically fail to be detected by the forced swim test (Cryan, Markou, & Lucki 2002). Other tests for depression also frequently yield 'false positive' results with non-antidepressant drugs, especially stimulants (Bourin, Fiocco, & Clenet 2001).

(4) *Do antidepressants have superior actions to drugs not generally considered to have specific effects in depression?*

Antidepressants are only minimally different from inert placebos and this difference may be accounted for by amplified placebo effects and other methodological artefacts. In addition, many drugs not normally considered to be antidepressants show comparable effects to antidepressants in studies with depressed people. Drugs that are considered to be antidepressants show a confusing array of pharmacological actions.

(5) *Do studies with healthy volunteers show different or absent effects?*

Antidepressants do not appear to elevate mood in healthy volunteers (see Chapter 10), but neither, as we have seen, is there good evidence that they do so in depressed patients. Although reports of effects of SSRIs suggest that effects on sleep may sometimes differ between patients and volunteers (Mayers & Baldwin 2005), in general side effects of antidepressants in patient trials are consistent with those found in healthy volunteers. For example, tricyclics show sedation and cognitive impairment (Deptula & Pomara 1990; Herrmann & McDonald 1978), while SSRIs show gastrointestinal upset and drowsiness in both patients and volunteers (Dumont et al. 2005).

(6) *Is the outcome of depression improved by the use of antidepressant drugs?*

As reviewed above, outside randomised controlled trials there is little evidence that antidepressants have changed the outcome of depression, and what evidence exists suggests they may possibly have made it worse. Certainly depression is more common today than before antidepressants were introduced and the outcome has not improved. It may be that antidepressants increase the liability to recurrence.

Conclusions

This overview of the research literature on antidepressants shows that despite the strong psychiatric consensus that antidepressants are effective and specific treatments for depression, they are little better than an inert placebo, even in severe depression, and their superior effects can easily be accounted for by drug-induced non-specific effects and amplified placebo effects. Many studies suggest that drugs from other classes can have similar effects in the right circumstances, such as when drug companies put resources behind them. Literature on long-term use suggests that discontinuation of antidepressants makes people more vulnerable to relapse than they might have been if they had never taken them. Research on the outcome of depression shows that antidepressants have done nothing to improve it and may have made it worse. The literature on the monoamine hypothesis of depression does not support the idea that depression is caused by a biochemical abnormality that antidepressants help to reverse. Overall, the model of antidepressants as a disease-specific treatment is not supported by research evidence. In the next chapter I will review the available evidence for what pharmacological effects the various antidepressant drugs produce from a drug-centred perspective and whether they have any potential therapeutic uses for psychiatric problems, particularly depression.

10
What Do Antidepressants Really Do?

The fact that a disease-centred view of the nature and action of antidepressants has dominated psychiatric research since the 1960s means there has been little research into what drug-induced effects these drugs produce. Patient or user literature on their effects is also more often dominated by a disease-centred view than similar literature on neuroleptic drugs, perhaps because no alternative view of their action has ever been established. The first point to appreciate from a drug-centred perspective is that the drugs currently referred to as antidepressants come from many different chemical classes. We would expect them therefore to have quite different profiles of action. I will describe available evidence on two of the main classes of antidepressant drugs.

Tricyclic antidepressants

Tricyclic antidepressants (TCA) are chemically similar to the phenothiazine neuroleptics such as chlorpromazine. Imipramine is structurally almost identical to chlorpromazine but lacks one chlorine and one sulphur atom (see Figure 10.1). Amitriptyline is similar. There are also similarities between the effects they induce. Animal studies have shown that tricyclic antidepressants have some dopamine-blocking properties. However they also antagonise the effects of the neurotransmitter acetylcholine. Since acetylcholine and dopamine have opposing actions in the basal ganglia, the anticholinergic effects of these drugs may counteract their dopamine-blocking qualities to some degree. Indeed, drugs with anticholinergic effects are used to reduce the deleterious effects of reduced dopamine activity in Parkinson's disease and in cases of Parkinson's-like symptoms induced by neuroleptics. Some of the neuroleptics like chlorpromazine also have some anticholinergic action,

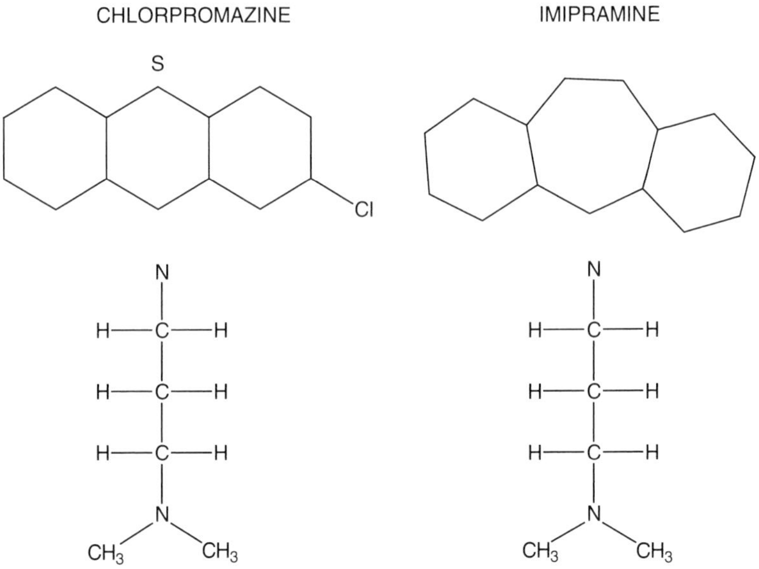

CHLORPROMAZINE

IMIPRAMINE

Figure 10.1   Chemical structure of chlorpromazine and imipramine (taken from Healy 1997, p. 51)

but it is not sufficient to inhibit their dopamine-blocking effects. The tricyclic antidepressants also block histamine receptors, a property they also share with some of the neuroleptics, they block alpha-1 adrenergic receptors and they affect numerous other neurotransmitter systems directly or indirectly (Khan 1999). Although they were shown to block noradrenalin and serotonin reuptake, the actual significance of this action was never confirmed. In particular, it was never shown that it led to a significant increase in availability of noradrenalin or serotonin. In contrast most evidence suggests that the tricyclic antidepressants decrease levels of noradrenalin (see Chapter 9). Thus they combine many pharmacological actions and share many of these with the neuroleptics, but it is uncertain which of these actions predominate in producing their clinical effects.

The anticholinergic effects of tricyclic antidepressants are well recognised and include blurred vision, dry mouth, constipation, increased sweating and confusion at high doses, especially in the elderly. However their strongly sedating effects differentiate them from drugs used primarily for their anticholinergic effects, which are usually mildly stimulant. The sedative effects of tricyclics may result from their blockade of histamine or alpha-1 adrenergic receptors. In common with neuroleptic drugs they are associated with weight gain, an increased liability to seizures and impotence.

Apart from their sedative action it is difficult to know what characteristic psychic effects they induce because of a lack of research designed to investigate this question. A small study conducted in the 1970s comparing effects of four drugs and placebo on volunteers found that the effects of amitriptyline and chlorpromazine on measures of cognitive function and EEG patterns were similar. Both these drugs increased reaction time, reduced co-ordination, and reduced performance on simple cognitive tasks such as mental arithmetic compared with placebo. In contrast diazepam at a dose of 10 mg had little effect on these measures and amphetamine tended to improve them. Both amitriptyline and chlorpromazine decreased feelings of mental well-being and subjects reported feeling fatigued, introverted and less activated. EEG changes showed a shift to slower frequency waves with both chlorpromazine and amitriptyline in contrast to both diazepam and amphetamine, where average frequency increased somewhat compared with placebo (Herrmann & McDonald 1978). Other volunteer studies show that amitriptyline impairs attention, memory and motor speed, increases reaction time and is generally found to be unpleasant (Dumont et al. 2005).

The similarity with chlorpromazine begs the question to what extent do the tricyclic antidepressants cause the deactivation syndrome typical of the neuroleptics? The dominance of the disease-centred view of drug action means that because the tricyclics were designated as antidepressants from early on, there was little investigation of their dopamine-blocking properties. However one study showed that two tricyclic antidepressants, amitriptyline and clomipramine were able to block stimulant-induced stereotyped behaviours in rats in the same fashion as neuroleptics, and that the effects increased after repeated administration (Delini-Stula & Vassout 1979). Imipramine had weaker effects. Several laboratory experiments have shown that long-term treatment with tricyclic drugs, including imipramine, produces supersensitivty of D_2 receptors as shown by an enhanced behavioural response to stimulants, an effect that is more commonly associated with neuroleptics (D'Aquila et al. 2003; Klimek & Maj 1989; Maj et al. 1996). The effect wears off gradually after the drugs are withdrawn (D'Aquila et al. 2003). Neuroleptics are also known to increase the density, as well as the sensitivity of D_2 receptors. Increased density of D_2 receptors in the limbic forebrain but not in the striatum has been shown to occur after long-term tricyclic treatment (Maj et al. 1996). One laboratory experiment showed directly that imipramine blocked the effects of dopamine and other dopamine agonists[1] in the hippocampal tissue of rats (Smialowski 1991).

Clinical neuroleptic-type effects have not been described frequently however. A paper published in 1997 found 30 previously reported cases of extrapyramidal effects and described two more (Vandel et al. 1997). These effects consisted mostly of cases of akathisia or restlessness and myoclonus, which refers to muscle twitching and jerking. Four cases of typical tardive dyskinesia were reported. Only three cases of Parkinson's-type rigidity and reduced movement were recorded. However the authors felt that the incidence of all these effects was probably much higher than the small number of case reports suggested because clinicians failed to look for it. Dose may also explain the apparent lack of Parkinson's-type symptoms with tricyclics. Typical doses of tricyclic antidepressants are 75–150 mg and maximum doses are nowadays around 200 mg. Chlorpromazine is rarely prescribed at doses below 200 mg in psychosis and doses of up to 1000 mg are not unusual. Other antipsychotics are also prescribed at doses well above the equivalent of 200 mg of chlorpromazine. Although dosing has decreased recently, higher doses were more fashionable until recently and doses of haloperidol of the order of 60 mg were not unusual. By current estimations this translates into chlorpromazine equivalents of 2000 mg! Therefore, if tricyclic antidepressants, such as imipramine and amitriptyline, and chlorpromazine are equipotent drugs, we have little idea of their comparative effects at similar doses. The animal studies suggest they may well produce effects associated with dopamine blockade.

Whether or not they produce the deactivation syndrome, tricyclics' main psychic effect at currently used clinical doses is profound sedation. Although there is some variation between different tricyclics, they are all sedative to some degree. However textbooks often misleadingly refer to some as being 'activating', although there is no good evidence for this (Marangell et al. 2001). As with other drugs, tolerance develops leading to a decline in the sedative effects, to some extent, with repeated use.

Subjective descriptions of the experience of taking tricyclic antidepressants confirm that the main effect is sedation, which some people find useful for insomnia, but others find difficult to tolerate. Some people also describe feeling 'drugged'. One participant in an Internet chat room described his experience of taking imipramine as a 'drug-induced fog', (Antidepressant Web 2006). Someone who had been prescribed amitriptyline described how 'my mind was extremely foggy and I could not gather my thoughts or organisational skills to do daily household duties' (Askapatient.com 2007, accessed 17.03.07). A volunteer study, which compared the effects of amitriptyline with those of an opiate drug, buprenorphine, described how both drugs 'rendered subjects drowsy, feeble, mentally slow and muzzy' (Saarialho-Kere et al. 1987). The sedative effect may be experienced as useful for someone who is acutely anxious or agitated, and it does promote sleep. This may be why low dose tricyclic antidepressants were popularly prescribed in General Practice. However tricyclics are toxic to the heart and cardiovascular system in the same way as neuroleptics. They frequently cause a potentially dangerous drop in blood pressure, conduction defects, arrhythmias and most are highly toxic if taken in overdose. Their utility as sedatives has never been properly investigated. In particular they have not been compared systematically with other sedative drugs in terms of efficacy and safety. Benzodiazepines are generally safer because they do not have the same toxic effects on the heart, but addiction may be more of a problem. Comparative research is required to see if the tricyclics have any useful role as sedative drugs in their own right.

So overall it is difficult to know what sort of drugs the tricyclic antidepressants are. They combine many different types of pharmacological action. They show some similarities to neuroleptics, to whom they are closely related structurally and there is some evidence that they too block the effects of dopamine. However there is not enough data currently to determine whether they share the neuroleptics most characteristic property of psychomotor deactivation. Most of them are powerful sedatives but it is not clear that they have any advantages over the use of safer sedatives like benzodiazepines.

Selective Serotonin Reuptake Inhibitors (SSRIs)

Although by definition, all SSRI antidepressants are believed to inhibit serotonin reuptake, they also have a variety of effects on other neurotransmitter systems. Fluoxetine, for example, has been shown to decrease brain dopamine levels in some animal studies (Smith et al. 2000). They also differ from each other in their profiles of action on different systems.

Despite the recent furore they have inspired, volunteer studies show that SSRIs have only minor effects compared with placebo. A large review of such studies by Dumont and colleagues found that there were almost no statistically significant differences from placebo. However the authors suggested that a single low dose of an SSRI might produce a slight stimulant effect, although none of the pertinent results was statistically significant even after combining data from different studies (Dumont et al. 2005). The stimulant effect was observed primarily on what is called the Critical Flicker Fusion test, in which the lowest frequency of a flickering light that is perceived by the subject as a stable light is determined. This is employed as a test of attention, but it is known to be sensitive to the diameter of the pupil. Since SSRIs increase pupillary diameter, this may account for the test results, without necessarily indicating that they improve attention. Studies that have controlled for pupil size have found that Critical Flicker Fusion test results are depressed by SSRIs (Schmitt et al. 2002). Longer-term studies have also found that SSRIs depress Critical Flicker Fusion performance with or without controlling for pupil diameter, indicating an impairment of attention with long-term use (Ramaekers, Muntjewerff, & O'Hanlon 1995; Schmitt et al. 2002).

Other findings that indicate possible stimulant effects are slightly improved memory at low doses (higher doses were associated with the opposite effect), increased rate of tapping (a test of motor speed) and a reduction in sleep. Reaction times in contrast are impaired overall and especially at high doses. EEG patterns show slightly increased beta wave activity indicating a possible stimulant pattern at low doses with increased slow waves, indicating a sedative pattern, at higher doses. However again these results were not statistically significant, meaning they could have occurred by chance. In contrast to classical stimulant drugs, which produce a feeling of well-being, Dumont et al.'s review found that low dose SSRIs were not different from placebo and higher doses were experienced as subjectively unpleasant. This latter finding was the only statistically significant result in the whole review (Dumont et al. 2005).

Few longer-term volunteer studies have been conducted. Those that exist suggest that SSRIs have sedating effects and mildly impair some aspects of cognitive functioning. We have already mentioned that in the long term they reduce attention as measured by the Critical Fusion Flicker test. A comparative study of sertraline and another recently introduced antidepressant, reboxetine, conducted by David Healy and colleagues and lasting for two weeks, showed that sertraline treatment reduced concentration, increased fatigue, reduced vigour and reduced quality of life scores. It had no effects on mood, anxiety or mood intensity (Tranter et al. 2002). Reboxetine in contrast, which is from a different pharmacological class of drug, appeared to have mildly stimulant effects. It improved concentration, reduced fatigue but also had no impact on quality of life. Like sertraline, it did not affect mood or anxiety ratings. A small observational study of working people taking SSRIs found some impairment of aspects of memory compared with non-SSRI users, even after controlling for levels of anxiety and depression (Wadsworth et al. 2005).

Other general effects experienced by volunteers on SSRIs compared with placebo are similar to side effects noted in clinical trials. They include drowsiness, headache, nausea, diarrhoea, dizziness, general malaise, tremor, restlessness and insomnia (Lader et al. 1986; Raptopoulos, McClelland, & Jackson 1989; Saletu et al. 1991). SSRIs are known to be associated with impaired sleep. Healthy volunteer studies consistently report impaired sleep (Mayers & Baldwin 2005). In clinical trials around 25% of patients report insomnia (Winokur et al. 2001) but some patient studies find sleep improves overall on SSRIs (Mayers & Baldwin 2005).

It has sometimes been suggested that SSRIs reduce emotional responsiveness, and this has been suggested to be how they might 'work' in depression. However there is actually little data to support this. One study of patients and three recent studies with volunteers have examined this possibility. In the first volunteer study, participants took a single dose of reboxetine. Reboxetine was associated with slightly higher recognition of happy faces and slightly higher 'happiness intensity'. However differences were not large and the results would be consistent with it having a mildly euphoric or stimulant effect (Harmer et al. 2003). A second study compared effects of citalopram with reboxetine and placebo (Harmer et al. 2004). This time there were small differences in recognition of some negative emotional expressions with people on both antidepressants being less able to recognise anger, disgust and fear but not sadness. Subjects on drugs also recalled more positive words than subjects on placebo. Subjects taking citalopram showed a reduced startle response to negative emotional expressions compared with placebo. However all differences were small and multiple tests were conducted, raising the possibility that the associations occurred by chance. Again Reboxetine was associated with increased feelings of energy, consistent with a stimulant effect. Another study of elderly volunteers carefully traced their emotional reactions to events over a three-week period of taking SSRIs (paroxetine or sertraline) or placebo. There was no drug-related effect on mood or emotional variability over the study. From a complex statistical analysis the authors concluded that the antidepressants were associated with a decrease in negative emotional reactions to negative events (Furlan et al. 2004). However there was no direct difference between the drug and placebo groups on this measure. A small study of 15 patients referred for treatment of sexual side effects of SSRI treatment[2] found that 12 of them complained of 'clinically significant blunting of several emotions' (Opbroek et al. 2002, p. 415). However as well as the small sample in this study, there are problems with its generalisability due to the fact that patients were selected because of complaints of sexual dysfunction. There was also no control for the effects of depression.

Some anecdotal descriptions of reduced emotional responsiveness exist. On one website for people taking antidepressants I found several reference to 'being dulled' and 'personality suppression'. One woman put it like this: 'I can't cry anymore and sometimes I feel the real me has disappeared ... I feel empty' (Antidepressant Web 2006, accessed 18/10/06). In the scientific literature there are several case reports of apathy in adults and children after long-term use of SSRIs. A review of these reports suggested that apathy, indifference and lack of motivation may emerge in patients who take SSRI drugs long term. These effects appeared in people with a mixture of diagnoses and were not associated with sedation or signs of depression. In all cases reported, the effects resolved or improved with discontinuation of the drug or reduction of the dose (Barnhart, Makela, & Latocha 2004). Contributors to the principal American textbook of psychiatry confirmed the existence of this syndrome in their clinical experience and likened it to the symptoms that develop when the frontal lobes of the brain are damaged. This syndrome is known as 'frontal lobe syndrome' and is characterised by apathy, disinhibited behaviour, demotivation and personality change similar to the effects of lobotomy (Marangellet al. 2001, p. 1059). The interesting question that has yet to be addressed is whether these possible effects of SSRIs are specific. Do the SSRIs have a characteristic emotional blunting effect like the neuroleptics could be said to have? Or are we merely observing the non-specific effects of chemical intoxication? The drug ketamine is also noted to reduce emotional recognition, for example (Abel et al. 2003). All psychoactive drugs are likely to coarsen our emotional responses to some extent. The question is whether SSRIs have any additional inhibiting effect on emotional experience.

Although stimulant effects in volunteer studies are not obvious, clinical studies of SSRIs report what are called 'activation' effects. These include insomnia, agitation, anxiety, nervousness and restlessness. Studies by Eli Lilly employees found that between 21% and 28% of patients taking fluoxetine (Prozac), an SSRI, experienced one of these effects, with highest rates among people taking higher doses (Beasley, Jr. et al. 1991b, 1991c). However in one study 21% of patients taking imipramine, a tricyclic antidepressant, also reported activation effects (Beasley, Jr. et al. 1991c, 1992) and other studies have found that up to 25% of placebo-treated patients also report activation events (Beasley, Jr. & Potvin 1993). However Eli Lilly papers revealed that the company identified a problem with agitation early on and in early trials all patients randomised to fluoxetine were prescribed a benzodiazepine to help prevent it (Scott 2006, p. 231). The reality of the effect is confirmed by the dropout rate for agitation in clinical trials which is around 5% for patients receiving SSRIs as against only 0.5% for placebo. David Healy and colleagues suggest these effects are a form of akathisia akin to the motor and psychic restlessness associated with neuroleptics (Healy, Herxheimer, & Menkes 2006).

Several reports have raised the possibility that SSRI antidepressants are associated with extrapyramidal movement disorders. Akathisia is the type most commonly reported, but cases of Parkinsonism, dystonia (acute rigidity), dyskinesia (abnormal involuntary choreic movements) and tardive dyskinesia have also commonly been reported, both in the scientific literature and in company files (Gerber & Lynd 1998). However there are difficulties with interpreting the literature, such as the use of concomitant neuroleptic drugs by some patients. A population-based study found a modest increased incidence of these effects in people taking SSRIs compared with people taking other antidepressants (Gony, Lapeyre-Mestre, & Montastruc 2003; Schillevoort et al. 2002). In addition, it is unclear whether the akathisia described is really the same as neuroleptic induced akathisia. Most volunteer studies do not report clear-cut extrapyramidal effects or activation effects other than insomnia. However some case reports of volunteers' individual experiences confirm findings from patient reports. In the Tranter et al. (2002) study two volunteers described an akathisia-like reaction and a Parkinson's-like jaw stiffness with sertraline. In addition, data from GlaxoSmithKline shows that 'hostile events', which could be related to activation, occurred in 1.1% of volunteers taking SSRIs compared with none taking placebo (Healy, Herxheimer, & Menkes 2006). Healy and colleagues (2006) note that although low, this figure is remarkable because hostile events are rare in volunteer trials.

Many cases that are referred to as antidepressant-induced mania could also be cases of agitation or 'activation'. It is part of psychiatric folklore that antidepressants of all classes can cause mania. A drug-centred perspective makes this difficult to believe of the tricyclic antidepressants, with their strong sedating properties and evidence that some of them have dopamine-blocking properties. Anticholinergic drugs can be associated with psychosis and confusion, but although tricyclic antidepressants possess marked anticholinergic activity, they do not share the stimulant profile of classical anticholinergic drugs. It is easier to believe that SSRIs might induce a manic episode due to their possible activating properties.

However despite the long-standing consensus, there is no good evidence that any antidepressants can induce a true episode of mania. This belief has been based on descriptions of high rates of mania in people with manic depression who take antidepressants. However better quality-controlled studies do not demonstrate higher rates of mania in people treated with antidepressants compared with people who are not on antidepressants (Visser & van der Mast 2005).

Overall it is difficult to characterise the effects of the SSRIs. Firstly, in most cases they appear to have fairly trivial physiological and subjective effects. They may have a mild stimulant effect after a single dose but this is uncertain, especially because of problems with interpretation of the Critical Fusion Flicker test of attention. In the longer term they may be associated with sedating effects and mild cognitive impairment in some realms. However they do appear to possess a sort of activating effect, in that they impair sleep and cause restlessness and agitation in a proportion of patients. This seems to be qualitatively different from the activation associated with classical stimulants. There is some evidence that they cause emotional blunting or an apathy syndrome with long-term use. However no studies have explored the effects of antidepressants in relation to other drugs in this respect and they have also been associated with emotional disinhibition (Garland & Baerg 2001). We know that the neuroleptic drugs induce a characteristic state of psychic indifference and this seems to be an intrinsic part of their action. What is uncertain is whether SSRIs and other antidepressants also produce a characteristic state of this sort, or whether their effects on emotional reactions are simply a non-specific consequence of being drugged.

SSRIs, suicide and violence

For well over a decade now there have been suggestions that the SSRI and other newer antidepressants might induce suicidal ideas or behaviour in some people. In 1990 details of six patients who had developed intense suicidal thoughts after starting fluoxetine (Prozac) were published in an article in the *American Journal of Psychiatry* (Teicher, Glod, & Cole 1990), followed by similar case reports (Rothschild & Locke 1991). A series of papers produced by Eli Lilly employees then claimed to find no connection, some even suggesting that SSRIs were associated with a lower rate of suicidal ideation than other antidepressants (Beasley, Jr. et al. 1991a). However the efforts of campaigners kept the issue alive and in the early years of the 21st century drug-regulatory bodies in the United States and United Kingdom issued warnings of a possible link between antidepressants and suicidal behaviour first for children and then for adults.

However the connection remains controversial. Finding quantitative evidence of links between drugs and suicide is difficult because of the rarity of suicide. It is well established that there is a very high risk of someone committing suicide in the month after they have been prescribed an antidepressant of any sort, but it is usually assumed that this is unrelated to the drug treatment (Jick, Kaye, & Jick 2004). Two meta-analyses of data from randomised trials in adults indicated small increases in suicide attempts or self-harm in people on SSRIs compared with placebo (Fergusson et al. 2005; Gunnell, Saperia, & Ashby 2005). Several studies of children and adolescents found an increase in suicidal behaviour with at least some SSRI antidepressants (Dubicka, Hadley, & Roberts 2006; Olfson, Marcus, & Shaffer 2006; Whittington et al. 2004; Wohlfarth et al. 2006). Some analyses have found slightly increased rates of suicide or suicidal behaviour among people who were prescribed the SSRIs fluoxetine and paroxetine compared with other antidepressant drugs, but the differences did not reach levels of statistical significance (Jick, Kaye, & Jick 2004; Jick, Dean, & Jick 1995). However other studies found no difference between different classes of antidepressants (Fergusson et al. 2005; Martinez et al. 2005). In addition, some meta-analyses did not find increased rates of suicide or suicide attempts associated with use of SSRIs compared with placebo (Khan et al. 2003).

David Healy has questioned the data from placebo-controlled trials on the basis that people in the placebo group have usually been withdrawn from an antidepressant before starting the placebo (Healy & Whitaker 2003). Since there is a suggestion that withdrawal from some antidepressants might also increase the risk of suicide, he argues that the suicide rate in the placebo group might be higher than would be expected in a group of people who had had no drug treatment, at least early on in the study. Comparisons between SSRIs and people who had not had previous drug treatment might indicate higher differences in suicidal behaviour. When Healy and Whitaker (2003) analysed Khan et al.'s (2003) data distinguishing suicidal acts that occurred in the early placebo washout phase of the trial and adding some further data, they produced figures that suggested a statistically and clinically significant increase in suicide and suicidal acts in patients on SSRIs compared with placebo. The odds of suicide while taking an SSRI were increased more than four times and the odds of non-fatal suicidal acts by more than twice.

Several authors, including David Healy, have suggested that the induction of suicidal ideas is related to the ability of SSRIs to induce activation or an akathisia-like state. The idea is that the agitation makes people do desperate things. Acts of violence and hostility have also been linked to use of SSRIs. Again, quantitative evidence is difficult to find because, like suicide, extreme violence is rare. However evidence from case reports of violent incidents, including legal reports and data from drug-monitoring agencies suggest that a link between SSRIs and violence is at least a possibility. The association, if it exists, may again be attributable to activation or agitation; or it may be due to emotional blunting effects, whether these be specific to SSRIs or generic to all psychoactive drugs.

The arguments are likely to continue and may be difficult to resolve quantitatively, although evidence suggesting a link between antidepressants and suicidal behaviour, at least in children, seems to be accumulating. The case reports, especially those where restlessness, agitation or akathisia were clearly involved and suggest a comprehensible mechanism for suicidal or dangerous acts, are also compelling. It may always be difficult to be certain about the connection, or to estimate the prevalence of SSRI-induced suicidal or violent acts. However because the events are so serious by nature, even a small and uncertain effect should make people cautious about the use of these drugs.

Are antidepressants useful in depression?

It should have become clear in this chapter that we are uncertain about the nature of the effects of antidepressant drugs and how those effects are produced. This is because the disease-centred model of drug action has focused attention on the drugs' effects on what are taken to be manifestations of the 'disease' of depression, as measured by rating scales of dubious validity. Similarly the disease-centred model has directed basic pharmacological research away from finding out what overall physiological effects the drugs produce and concentrated on their effects on particular neurotransmitter systems and receptors, predetermined by theories about the biochemical nature of depression. Thus we have no clear idea how tricyclic antidepressants produce their most profound effect, sedation. It may be due to their effects on histamine transmission, possibly combined with blockade of alpha-1 adrenergic receptors, but there has been little interest in clarifying this issue because it does not fit with accepted psychiatric disease models. Their capacity for reuptake of noradrenalin and serotonin have been selected among their many actions because they fitted into the monoamine theory of depression, but their pharmacological significance has not been established, especially in relation to the drugs' many other actions. Similarly, SSRIs have numerous and diverse actions in the brain and how the drugs' subjective effects are produced is not known.

Evidence suggests that for people without mental health problems, antidepressant drugs are unpleasant to take and make them feel worse. The evidence reviewed in the previous chapter suggests that we have no reason to believe that they elevate mood in patients either.

A drug-centred view of the treatment of depression must start by listing the possible effects that drugs are known to induce. We know that many drugs can induce euphoria in the short term, including alcohol, opiates, stimulants, benzodiazepines and others. However this effect is strongly dependent on context. In other words, someone has to be in the right environment and in the right state of mind for the euphoria to occur. In the wrong environment or state of mind, the same effects can be experienced as unpleasant. In addition, the body develops tolerance to the effect so that higher and higher doses are required to produce it. This is the basis of addiction to drugs such as opiates and alcohol. People have to increase the dose to achieve the effect they desire and cannot stop or reduce the drug because the body's adaptations to it give rise to an unpleasant and sometimes dangerous withdrawal syndrome when the drug is removed. Other drug-induced effects that might be relevant to someone with depression, include sedation of various types, emotional indifference and physiological stimulation.

However it is difficult to believe that any of these effects could be particularly useful in depression, especially in the long term. It would also seem ethically dubious to recommend that someone who is depressed should take a drug in order to blunt or numb their emotional responses, even though a drug with these properties might look extremely effective when judged by depression-rating scales. The use of drugs with sedative effects may be justified in the short term in people who have severe agitation or anxiety associated with depression. A case could be made that people who are depressed, especially those that have been depressed for a long time, might benefit from use of a euphoriant drug to remind them of the experience of feeling pleasure. In the 1950s Hans Lehmann prescribed a combination of an opiate and amphetamine to chronically depressed people on the basis that 'chemically induced states of euphoria might reactivate their ability to experience pleasure and enable them to free themselves from their hopeless anhedonia' (Lehmann & Kline 1983, p. 216). However euphoriant effects are short-lived and may be nullified by the adverse circumstances that are likely to accompany ongoing depression. Similarly, people who are depressed and lethargic might find the effects of stimulant drugs helpful, even in a single dose, to remind them of the benefits of activity. Overall, however when approached in this way, it seems unlikely that any drug-induced effects will be very useful or ethically acceptable in people who are depressed.

Drugs that are currently referred to as antidepressants have no obvious place in the treatment of depression according to this approach. Tricyclic antidepressants could be used to produce short-term sedative effects where these are desired and have probably been used in this way for many years by General Practitioners. But because of their toxic effects on the heart, benzodiazepines are probably safer, as long as care is taken about the length of time for which they are prescribed and adequate warnings given about their addictive potential. The SSRIs produce no effects that look likely to be useful in depression. They cause unpleasant agitation in a proportion of patients and, although it is difficult to prove conclusively, an increase in suicidal and violent tendencies may be associated with this effect. Therefore, I can think of no good reason to prescribe them at all.

Apart from the adverse physical effects of antidepressant drugs, they have damaging psychological effects that should cause just as much concern. The idea that your emotional state has been caused by a bio-chemical imbalance in your brain is profoundly disempowering. Because of the disease-centred implications of the notion of an antide-pressant, every time an antidepressant is prescribed it conveys this message. The promotion of antidepressants has convinced millions of people to 'recode their moods and their ills' in terms of their brain chemistry (Rose 2004) (see Chapter 4). Depression websites bear witness to people's anxiety about relapsing back into depression if they ever stop drug treatment. Many correspondents on the Antidepressant Web, for example, talked of the 'slippery slope down to depression again' that they feared if they tried to withdraw from antidepressants (Antidepressant Web 2006).

If people believe that it is brain chemicals that have made them depressed and that they only improved because a drug helped to rectify a chemical defect or imbalance, then they are likely to fear the recur-rence of depression with every difficult period in their lives. In addition, they are not likely to recognise the things that they did to help them-selves out of depression, because they attribute their recovery to a drug. If in contrast they had managed to get through the period without taking a drug that they thought sorted out their biochemistry, they would have had an experience of self-efficacy that could build their confidence and help them to face future problems with greater strength. I know that most doctors and health professionals want to help people to help themselves over depression in this way. What they fail to realise is that every prescription they issue conveys a message of hopelessness and powerlessness. Every time they recommend antidepressants they contradict the message they should be reinforcing about the ability of human beings to overcome adversity.

11
The Idea of Special Drugs for Manic Depression (Bipolar Disorder)*

Drugs and manic depression

Lithium was introduced into modern psychiatric practice in the 1950s and for decades it was the only drug that was thought to have a specific effect on the psychiatric condition known as manic depression. At first it was viewed as a specific treatment for an acute episode of mania and later it was proposed to have prophylactic properties against recurrence of future episodes. It continues to be recommended for the treatment of acute mania, although it is rarely used alone in such circumstances. It is most commonly prescribed for the prophylaxis, or prevention of recurrence, of manic-depressive episodes.

In the 1980s it was suggested that some anticonvulsant drugs may have similar efficacy and specificity. The stated rationale for this was an analogy between manic depression with its discrete and recurrent episodes and the paroxysmal nature of epilepsy. The anti-epileptic drug, carbamazepine, started to be used both for treatment of acute mania and prophylaxis, and subsequently sodium valproate and other anticonvulsants have been marketed for use in manic depression. In the early 21st century Eli Lilly started conducting studies of the prophylactic effect of a drug that was primarily designated as an antipsychotic agent, their blockbuster drug Zyprexa (olanzapine). Since the 1990s drugs indicated for manic depression are often referred to as 'mood stabilisers', a term which appeared subsequent to the licensing and

*I have chosen to use the older term manic depression where I can, instead of the more modern 'bipolar disorder'. Manic depression is a vivid and useful descriptive term, whereas bipolar disorder is not descriptive and suggests an analogy with physical systems such as electricity, which conveys unfounded implications about the nature of the condition.

promotion of sodium valproate for treatment of manic depression (Harris et al. 2003; Healy 2006). However there is no consensus about what this term means. Although it implies that the drugs concerned have some specific property that reduces or evens out mood fluctuations, there is little research to establish whether they have an effect of this sort. The term is essentially a new way of referring to drugs that are believed to be specifically effective in manic depression. However the implication that these drugs have a more general mood-stabilising quality has helped to widen their use. Although many professional authorities still consider that lithium is the most effective, the influence of marketing of other drugs, combined with lithium's recognised drawbacks, mean that other drugs are now more commonly used in people with manic depression.

There has never been a convincing disease-specific explanation of how lithium or other drugs might act in manic depression. Various ideas have been proposed at different times. John Cade, the man usually credited with 'discovering' lithium's therapeutic application, suggested at one time that manic depression might be caused by lithium deficiency, but the idea never caught on since lithium is barely present in the human body and has no biological role. Electrolyte disturbances, effects on nerve cell second-messenger proteins and nerve cell membranes have all been proposed, but there is still no generally accepted disease-centred theory of how lithium or other drugs reverse the presumed biological basis of manic depression. Researchers continue to search for a unifying theory of the mechanism of action of all the diverse drugs that are now being used as 'mood stabilisers', but nothing credible has yet emerged (Harwood & Agam 2003).

From the 1970s long-term drug treatment has been recommended for most people suffering from manic depression. Currently the major American textbook recommends that 'patients with bipolar disorder require lifelong prophylaxis with a mood stabiliser' (Marangell et al. 2001, p. 1115). The benefits of drug treatment are believed to be so obvious that there is rarely any discussion of alternative strategies. People with manic depression have to be strong willed to go against the psychiatric consensus and refuse long-term drug treatment.

From manic depression to a 'bipolar spectrum'

Manic depression, now known as bipolar disorder, used to be regarded as a relatively rare condition, perhaps affecting up to 1% of people at some point during their lifetime. However over recent years the concept has been expanded. Starting in the 1990s, and coinciding with the investigation of drugs that were more profitable than lithium for use in manic depression, papers began to appear which suggested that bipolar disorder was more common than previously thought. The concept of bipolar II disorder had been framed back in the 1970s, but was used little outside the United States. It is not described in the World Health Organisation's International Classification of Disease version 10, published in 1992, for example, but only listed under the heading 'Other Bipolar Affective Disorders'. Bipolar II disorder is a supposedly milder form of the classical condition, in which the patient suffers primarily from depression, but experiences mild episodes of mania, which are not severe enough to require hospital admission. More recently the idea of bipolar spectrum disorder has been proposed, consisting of 'lifelong temperamental dysregulation' accompanying depressive episodes (Akiskal 1996). The prevalence of classical manic depression is now estimated at 5% of the population, with an additional 11% suffering from bipolar II disorder. A total of 24% of the population are said to suffer from some disturbance on the 'bipolar spectrum' (Angst et al. 2003).

Although the epidemiological research has not been produced by drug companies, the industry's promotional material echoes and reinforces these messages. For example, literature on the website of Abbott laboratories, the producers of Depakote (the commercial brand of sodium valproate) suggests that bipolar disorder 'is more common than you think' (Abbott Laboratories 2006). It emphasises that bipolar disorder is a 'brain disorder' that may 'happen as a result of structural and chemical changes in the brain' and emphasises the need for long-term treatment 'just like diabetes'. The website contains a questionnaire for prospective patients to fill in to assess whether they qualify as having bipolar disorder, and urges people to show the questionnaire to their doctors (questionnaire accessed 6/11/06). Eli Lilly sponsor a website containing a similar questionnaire. In 2002 they ran a television advertisement in the United States featuring a young woman involved in activities such as dancing at a night club and energetically painting her apartment (described in Healy [2006]). These activities were portrayed as signs of mania or hypomania and the advert was aimed at encouraging people to recognise themselves as having bipolar disorder. This advert appeared shortly after olanzapine received a licence for use in manic depression. Several other atypical antipsychotics have a licence for the treatment of mania or bipolar depression. In an increasingly competitive market place, the manufacturers are keen to find further indications for these extremely profitable drugs and the flexible concept of 'bipolar disorders' offers such an opportunity.

What had once been a relatively rare disorder, for which there was considered to be only one very specific treatment is now regarded as a widespread problem with an array of new drug treatments. In addition, the concept of the mood stabiliser allows drugs for manic depression to be used in many other situations in which there appears to be some instability of mood. Since almost by definition acute psychiatric disorders involve extreme emotional responses, almost any psychiatric patient can qualify for treatment with a mood stabiliser. My clinical experience suggests the use of these drugs among psychiatric patients has expanded considerably.

The emergence of lithium as a psychiatric treatment

The history of lithium illustrates the professional appeal of the disease-centred paradigm of drug action. No disease theory has ever been able to justify lithium's proposed therapeutic action, and its toxic effects are well recognised and on a continuum with the effects of therapeutic doses. Yet the consensus that lithium is a disease-specific treatment is near impregnable. As described in the next chapter, lithium is a highly toxic substance and the signs and symptoms of full-blown toxicity appear at doses very close to those used to achieve therapeutic effects. Because of this lithium therapy can only appear in drug-centred terms as a highly dangerous procedure. In the early days of lithium use some psychiatrists recognised this and deplored the 'treatment of manic patients by lithium poisoning' (Wikler 1957). Yet lithium came to be seen as a disease-specific treatment and despite subsequent dissent, the consensus on this point is as strong as ever.

Lithium's popularity owes little to the pharmaceutical industry, since profits that can be derived from a simple element are limited. Its appeal and significance lie in the presumed specificity of lithium for manic depression and the evidence this seems to offer that a biological basis for this condition might be identifiable. In a retrospective view of lithium's significance, published in 2001, Mochens Schou commented that lithium established 'recurrent manic-depressive illness as a treatable condition and psychiatry as a medical discipline' (Schou 2001, p. 28). Another recent review paper was entitled 'The psychopharmacologic specificity of the lithium ion: origins and trajectory' (Soares & Gershon 2000). After 50 years of fruitless research in this area the authors could still propose that lithium's marked specificity for manic depression 'may prove to be very useful for elucidating the pathophysiology of the disorder' (p. 20). Neil Johnson, a sympathetic historian of lithium explained lithium's importance in the following eulogising terms:

> If affective disorder could be eliminated by the simple expedient of administering a chemical substance, did this not suggest that the basis of these disorders might take a chemical form? And not only that; might affect, mood, emotion, and the whole gamut of human conscious experience be translated into chemical terms? At a stroke, the elusive "aetherial" Freudian psyche was replaced as the primary object of attention by the polyphasic physico-chemical system called the brain. Psychiatry came of age and took its place among the biological sciences.
>
> (Johnson 1984, p. xiv)

In the same way that the neuroleptics came to be regarded as an effective and specific treatment for schizophrenia, lithium came to represent a cure for the other major psychiatric disorder of the Kraepelinian dichotomy,[1] manic depression. Lithium's supposed specificity has helped to legitimate this dichotomy and with it the whole enterprise of medical diagnosis in psychiatry. Without it the treatments for mania and schizophrenia would appear indistinguishable (as they more or less are), the justification for diagnosis would be undermined and the whole disease-centred conception of modern psychiatric drug treatment would start to look fragile. The specificity of lithium in mania and tranquillisers in schizophrenia were cited as justification for the process of medical diagnosis in psychiatry in response to antipsychiatry critiques in the 1970s (Spitzer 1976).

In order to understand how the modern consensus on lithium could arise, it is necessary to know its history. Although Neal Johnson's account endorses the modern disease-centred view of lithium treatment, it is nevertheless revealing (Johnson 1984). The element named lithium was discovered in 1818 at around the time that medical practitioners were engaged in a struggle for professional recognition. As the emergent profession became increasingly united and confident, it was able to propagate new explanatory theories with greater credibility than before. When uric acid crystals deposited in the joints were discovered to be the cause of gout, uric acid became a fashionable substance, and everything from rheumatism to cardiac problems to mental conditions were attributed to it. When it was suggested that lithium could dissolve uric acid stones, it was used as a treatment for gout and the numerous other conditions ascribed to uric acid. Some medical practitioners used it to treat depression but it does not appear that it was frequently used in psychiatry at this time.

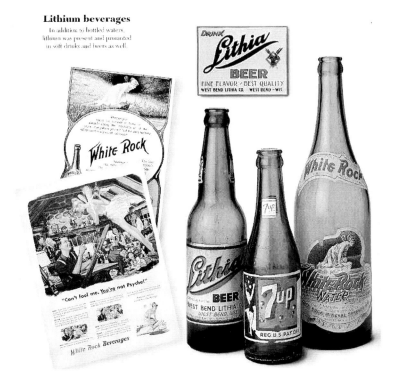

Illustration 11.1 Lithium drinks

Lithium became a popular medicinal substance under the influence of the uric acid hypothesis. Proprietary medicines, 'tonics' and fashionable mineral spas were advertised as containing lithium and other recommended antidotes to uric acid. Lithium was even put into beer and the drink 7 UP started life as a lithium drink (Healy 2002) (see Illustration 11.1).

However laboratory experiments showed that it did not in fact dissolve uric acid crystals, and its use started to decline. Uric acid also dropped out of fashion. However old ideas and practices can take a long time to die out. Lithium continued to be prescribed for gout, arthritis, rheumatism and other complaints. It was listed as a recommended treatment for these conditions until the 1930s in major pharmacopoeias. Even when these publications admitted there was no 'rational foundations for the use of these (lithium) salts', they still listed indications for lithium use and instructions on how to administer it

(Johnson 1984). It remained available in hospital pharmacies into the 1950s and preparations containing lithium could be obtained over the counter as late as the 1970s in the United Kingdom (Johnson 1984).

The importance of this history is that it meant there was a precedent for the use of lithium as a medicine. It also meant that lithium was readily available for experimentation in the pharmacies of psychiatric hospitals. Therefore when John Cade, an Australian psychiatrist, suggested that lithium might be a useful treatment in people with mania in the 1940s, it did not seem curious. Cade also experimented with use of the elements strontium and cerium in the treatment of psychiatric disorders, but they never caught on in the same way because there was no prior history of medicinal use.

In 1946 John Cade started experimenting with urine from patients with mania to search for toxins that he believed must be the basis of the condition. By his own account, Cade was an enthusiast for research into the biological underpinnings of psychiatric disorders. He told Johnson that during his time in a Japanese prisoner of war camp, 'I could see that so many of the psychiatric patients suffering from the so-called functional psychoses appeared to be sick people in the medical sense. This fired my ambition to discover their aetiology' (Johnson 1984, p. 34). Cade thought that a toxic substance bound to urates might be the cause of mania and mixed patients urine with lithium to dissolve the urates before injecting the mixture into guinea pigs. When he found that the guinea pigs were sedated by this mixture, he thought that lithium might have a therapeutic effect in manic patients. It has subsequently been suggested that he was actually observing signs of severe toxicity in the guinea pigs since they received large doses of lithium (Johnson 1984, p. 36).

In 1949 Cade published a paper describing his experience of treating 10 patients with mania with lithium. He announced dramatic effects and importantly claimed that the effects were specific to mania. This claim was made on the basis of a very brief description of the response of some patients with schizophrenia who were said to have shown 'no fundamental improvement' although some of them became 'quiet and amenable' (Cade 1949, p. 351). In addition, the delusions and hallucinations experienced by one of the patients diagnosed as manic failed to improve with lithium. All the patients with mania were said to have improved in terms of becoming 'quieter'. Cade also noted the return of symptoms after lithium withdrawal. On the basis of these observations Cade concluded that 'the effect on patients with pure psychotic excitement – that is true manic attacks – is so specific that it leads to speculations as to the possible etiologic significance of a deficiency of lithium ions in the genesis of the disorder' (Cade 1949). However after looking at Cade's clinical notes on this experiment, Johnson suggests that the results were more ambiguous. Toxic effects and 'side effects' were more frequent and severe than the impression conveyed in the published paper. The notes record that one patient died, two others had to discontinue lithium because of severe toxicity and one patient refused to take it, none of which is reported in the published article. Side effects were recorded 41 times in the clinical records but only 13 times in the published version. Johnson also found that in the clinical notes the distinction between toxic effects and so-called therapeutic effects was often not clear-cut. However in the published paper Johnson notes that 'therapeutic advantages and toxic side effects were fairly sharply demarcated' (p. 41). Toxic effects were covered only briefly and incidentally towards the end of the paper. Johnson concludes that this 'enhanced the chances that the findings would be taken seriously' and that if Cade had accurately reported all the side effects he had noted, 'it is doubtful whether his work would have been accorded more than a passing consideration' (p. 41).

Cade's observations were noted by other Australian and European psychiatrists. Much early European work on lithium characterised it as a treatment for 'psychomotor excitation' or 'agitated states' (Teulie, Follin, & Begoin 1955; Vartanian 1959), implying that it was employed according to a drug-centred rationale on the basis of its sedative characteristics. It was Danish psychiatrist Mogens Schou, who became lithium's most ardent advocate, who elaborated the disease-centred theory of lithium treatment in relation to the condition of manic depression. Schou also had an interest in biological psychiatry and had a brother who suffered from depression. He started to use lithium with his patients in the 1950s and in 1954 published the results of a partially controlled trial of lithium in patients with mania. Since the 1950s he has published numerous papers on lithium and tirelessly argued for its benefits. As David Healy has suggested without his efforts it is doubtful that lithium therapy would ever have caught on (Healy 2002).

In the 1950s it appears that it was only a small coterie of psychiatrists who were using and researching lithium. Schou and lithium's other early disciples frequently noted a lack of interest in lithium (Gershon & Yuwiler 1960; Schou et al. 1954) and the view that lithium treatment consisted of inducing toxicity was not disreputable (Wikler 1957). In contrast to the neuroleptics and antidepressants, lithium was not mentioned in major psychiatric textbooks until the late 1960s. Figure 11.1 shows that publications on its use in psychiatry before this point were few.

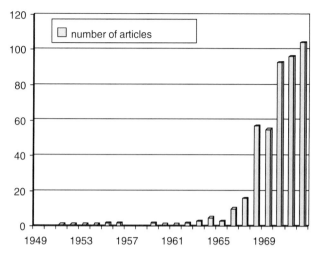

Figure 11.1   Articles retrieved by searching for 'lithium and affective disorder' on *Medline*

In 1963 Schou set out a clear statement of the disease-centred view of lithium treatment (Schou 1963). He characterised lithium, and imipramine as well, as 'compounds with an action specific to a disease rather than to a symptom' (p. 803). He maintained that lithium did not just sedate people like the new tranquillisers, but lead to the complete normalisation of mood. He argued that patients 'do not feel or give the impression of being drugged or doped' (p. 805) and that lithium had no effects on the 'normal mind' (p. 807), denying in particular that it caused apathy or impaired intellectual function. Despite his confident assertions of its disease-specific nature, he admitted that the mode of action of lithium was 'completely unknown' (p. 808). Others echoed these statements, referring to lithium as 'remarkably specific' (Hartigan 1963, p. 810). One of the first North American psychiatrists to publish on lithium suggested that it was the first specific drug in psychiatry (Williamson 1966). Many authors believed that due to its specificity lithium would 'shed more light on the biological mechanisms possibly involved in manic depressive illnesses' (Pearson & Jenner 1971, p. 533).

Through the 1960s the idea of lithium treatment was spreading. In 1967 Schou and his colleague Poul Baastrup published a paper alleging the benefits of lithium for the prophylaxis of manic depression, based on a series of case histories (Baastrup & Schou 1967). In this paper they produced a graph showing how episodes of mania or depression appeared to be less frequent after lithium was started than before. In 1968 Michael Shepherd and Barry Blackwell of the Maudsley Hospital in London criticised this paper in the *Lancet* medical journal and threw doubt on the still emergent consensus about lithium's benefits and specificity (Blackwell & Shepherd 1968). However by the late 1960s lithium is mentioned in British psychiatric textbooks for the first time and in one, *Clinical Psychiatry*, it inspired a whole section on the aetiological significance of electrolyte disturbance in affective disorders (Mayer-Gross, Slater, & Roth 1960).

The criticisms of Baastrup and Schou's work included the suggestion that for many of the patients studied there was actually little difference in the course of the condition before and after lithium was started. Blackwell and Shepherd suggested that Baastrup and Schou had mistakenly regarded some single episodes prior to starting lithium as multiple episodes, thus exaggerating the apparent reduction of episodes after lithium was initiated (Blackwell & Shepherd 1968). It was also suggested that episodes of affective disorder might naturally 'cluster', that is people might experience a number of closely spaced episodes that then became less frequent (Saran 1969). If this were the case the results of Baastrup and Schou's study would provide no evidence for the benefits of lithium, since any reduction of episode frequency after lithium was commenced could simply represent the natural course of the disorder.

Around this time some Swiss researchers became interested in lithium and, together with Schou, they publicised the notion that the natural untreated history of manic depression is for the episodes to get closer and closer together. For a long time this was regarded as an established fact about the course of manic depression and it is still stated that without treatment 'the illness will progress to a more malignant course' (Marangell, Silver, Goff, & Yudofsky 2001, p. 1115). The idea is frequently used to emphasise the necessity and benefits of drug treatment. Its appearance around 1970 suggests that it was inspired as a defence against the criticisms of Baastrup and Schou's paper on prophylaxis. Although the idea is repeatedly asserted to be true, it is actually difficult to trace any evidence for it. The original papers presented results of regression analyses that demonstrated that people who had more previous episodes had shorter cycle duration (Angst et al. 1970). But all this shows is that people who have lots of episodes relapse more quickly! It does not confirm that cycle length progressively shortens as was claimed. One subsequent paper showed that interval length between episodes decreased slightly up to the fourth episode. No data was given for subsequent episodes (Dunner et al. 1979). In contrast, a retrospective study of untreated patients found evidence of clustering, with a reduced risk of further episodes in people who had experienced previous ones (Winokur 1975). A later paper by one of the Swiss researchers, Jules Angst, showed that manic depression may remit or 'burn out' in around a quarter of patients (Angst 1986). Clinically it is apparent that the course of manic depression varies considerably between individuals. In some there is a tendency for there to be a flurry of episodes at the onset of the condition and in many people it settles down somewhat in later life. However the idea that manic depression generally shows a 'malignant course' is still widely believed, commonly quoted and used to justify lifelong drug treatment (Marangell et al. 2001, p. 1115).

During the 1970s several clinical trials appeared to confirm lithium's efficacy for the treatment of mania and the prophylaxis of manic-depressive episodes. Remaining doubts about it disappeared for a time. In the 1990s research suggested that lithium discontinuation could precipitate mania. Following from this observation, I published two papers questioning the methodology of the early clinical trials, especially the use of the discontinuation design, and suggesting that the case for the use of lithium was still not proven (Moncrieff 1995, 1997). Since that time three major trials have compared lithium with placebo in manic depression for the first time since the 1970s. Despite the fact that their results are not uniformly positive and methodological concerns remain, the consensus on lithium has strengthened and its efficacy is now regarded as unquestionable (Young & Newham 2006).

The idea of a 'mood stabiliser'

Harris and colleagues have pointed out that the epilepsy drugs, carbamazepine and sodium valpromide (closely related to sodium valproate) were being used in psychiatry in the 1970s in France and Japan because of their sedative properties (Harris et al. 2003). The obvious limitations of lithium, both in terms of lack of effectiveness and adverse effects, meant that there was interest in alternative drug treatments for manic depression. In 1980 a paper in the *American Journal of Psychiatry* suggested that carbamazepine might be an effective acute and prophylactic treatment for mania (Ballenger & Post 1980). One of the paper's authors, Robert Post and colleagues subsequently developed a theory of 'kindling' in manic depression. Kindling is a proposed phenomena in epilepsy in which each fit increases the sensitivity of the brain to further fits. Post argued that the common assumption that episodes of manic depression get closer and closer together was evidence that a kindling type process operated in manic depression as well. Post's theory was principally based on drawing an analogy between manic depression and epilepsy on the basis that they were both recurrent phenomena that were thought to originate in the brain. Post acknowledged that there was no evidence to support a biological link between epilepsy and manic depression and proposed that the kindling theory was a 'model' to explain 'syndrome progression' (Post et al. 1998, p. 153). However the idea that there is a real link vaguely persists in the psychiatric consciousness linked with the use of anti-epileptic drugs. For example, a recent paper on the mechanism of action of anticonvulsants states: 'Bipolar disorder, like epilepsy, is episodic in nature. It should not be surprising then that anticonvulsants such as carbamazepine and valproate have proven efficacy as mood stabilisers' (White 2003).

Although it was only a model, the idea of kindling superficially appeared to provide a disease-specific justification for the use of anticonvulsants in manic depression. It also opened up the possibility of defining a sort of drug that would reduce emotional reactivity, in the same way that anticonvulsants are believed to reduce the brain's nervous excitability. In this sense kindling gave birth to the notion of a mood stabiliser. However as David Healy has pointed out, it was not until Abbott laboratories started to research and market sodium valproate for manic depression that the idea of a mood stabiliser really took root (Healy 2006).

There is no consensus on what a 'mood stabiliser' refers to. It was recently pointed out in a *British Journal of Psychiatry* editorial that the only evidence base for the term is the research on effects of drugs in acute mania and the prophylaxis of manic depression. However the term implies something both more and less specific than this. The American textbook defines a mood stabiliser as a drug that can 'stabilise mood oscillations, regardless of etiology' (Marangell et al. 2001, p. 1104). The concept of a mood stabiliser, therefore, implies the idea of a drug that can act on the biological basis of emotional instability in a range of situations and diagnoses, rather than a drug that is specific for a single diagnostic condition. The randomised trials have been conducted in people diagnosed with manic depression because that is a recognised clinical condition that is relatively easy to define. In this context 'mood stabilisers' are regarded as having specific effects in contrast to other drugs such as benzodiazepines and neuroleptics (other than ones now designated as mood stabilisers!). But the concept lends itself well to marketing to people with other diagnoses and to the general population. The idea of a drug that can control emotional instability, smooth out life's ups and downs, has huge potential appeal. Drug company campaigns such as those described at the beginning of this chapter suggest that the pharmaceutical industry is well aware of the possibilities. This marketing will surely persuade some people to view ordinary emotional variation as signs of a pathological condition that needs to be rectified by drug treatment.

The new generation of neuroleptic drugs licensed for the treatment of mania and manic depression is also being promoted according to a disease-centred model. On the bipolar section of its Zyprexa (olanzapine) website, Eli Lilly describes how medication 'treats the illness directly' (Eli Lilly 2006). When used for acute mania the neuroleptics are now often referred to as 'antimanics' (National Institute for Clinical Excellence 2006). Since the publication of studies purporting to show olanzapine's efficacy for the prophylaxis of manic depression, it is referred to as a 'mood stablliser'. This is despite the fact that the tranquillising and sedative properties of neuroleptics provide a perfectly good explanation for their effects in mania.

In the next section, I will review the major research on lithium and other drugs currently used as 'mood stabilisers'. Despite the greater sophistication of recent research, its interpretation is as much evidence of wishful thinking as the presentation of Cade's early experiments with lithium.

12
Evidence on the Action of Lithium and 'Mood Stabilisers'

The nature of lithium

Lithium is an alkali metal in the same chemical group as sodium and potassium. Like many other metals it is profoundly toxic to the human body at relatively small doses. It is particularly toxic to the nervous system, the gastrointestinal system and the kidneys. Full-blown lithium toxicity is characterised by diarrhoea, vomiting, incontinence and numerous neurological abnormalities including tremor, ataxia (loss of balance), dysarthria (slurred speech), muscle rigidity, myoclonus (jerking movements), drowsiness and disorientation. In the final stages it produces seizures, coma, kidney failure, cardiovascular collapse and death. All drugs can impair bodily functioning at high doses, but lithium causes these severe effects at doses that are not much higher than those used for treatment. In my view this justifies referring to lithium as a particularly toxic substance in relation to other medical drugs.

The fact that therapeutic doses are only just lower than toxic doses and actually overlap with them also suggests that the so-called therapeutic effects of lithium are mild manifestations of lithium's characteristic toxic effects. In animal studies it is acknowledged that it is difficult to distinguish between toxic and 'pharmacological' effects (Ananth, Ghadirian, & Engelsmann 1987). Volunteer studies show that, at ordinary clinical doses, lithium impairs intellectual and motor performance, prolongs reaction times and reduces learning ability and memory. Such effects suggest a mild state of neurological impairment (Judd et al. 1977b; Kropf & Muller-Oerlinghausen 1979; Squire et al. 1980; Stip et al. 2000). Subjectively lithium induces an unpleasant or dysphoric state associated with anxiety and lethargy and 'a loss of interest in interacting with others or the environment' (Judd et al. 1977a). One set of researchers noted that 'lithium leads to decreased vigilance and reduced spontaneous activity' (Muller-Oerlinghausen et al. 1979). Volunteer studies have found no evidence that lithium reduces or stabilises mood variability (Barton, Jr. et al. 1993; Calil, Zwicker, & Klepacz 1990).

Most studies that have compared patients functioning on and off lithium find negative effects of lithium on memory and information processing, reduced mental speed as well as indications of impaired creativity as measured by word association tests (Honig et al. 1999; Kocsis et al. 1993). However patients are often not aware of their mental slowness (Honig et al. 1999).

There seems no reason, therefore, to eschew the description of lithium therapy as 'the treatment of manic patients by lithium poisoning', in the words of an early critic (Wikler 1957). Anticonvulsants do not share the toxicity profile of lithium, but by virtue of their use to prevent epileptic fits, they all exert depressant effects on the activity of the central nervous system. With this profile of drug-induced effects in mind, let us examine the research on whether lithium or other drugs currently used in manic depression act in a disease-centred way and consider whether they have any real benefits.

The evidence for lithium as a specific treatment for acute mania

Given the sedation associated with its neurological toxicity, lithium could be predicted to reduce levels of excitement and activity in people with acute mania. However its utility is likely to be limited by its toxic potential. There are few well-designed trials of lithium versus placebo for the treatment of acute mania, and none that conduct sufficiently long follow-up to look at the ultimate outcome. In fact there were no proper randomised controlled trials conducted until the 1990s, despite the fact that lithium had been accepted as an effective treatment for mania since the 1950s. The most rigorous of a motley collection of early studies found that lithium was superior to placebo for the first two weeks of a four-week trial but not for the last two weeks. Five of the 28 patients, 18%, developed toxic reactions (Stokes et al. 1971). It was not until 1994 that a fully randomised trial comparing lithium with placebo for the treatment of acute mania was published. This trial was set up to evaluate sodium valproate and was supported by its manufacturer, Abbott laboratories. Its results give at best only weak evidence for the superiority of lithium over placebo. Although lithium-treated patients had lower Mania Rating Scale scores than placebo-treated patients, this only reached statistical significance at one of four measurement points during the trial. Fifty six per cent of the lithium group discontinued treatment early for reasons other than recovery compared with 61% of the placebo group. There was no record of the use of supplementary medications such as benzodiazepines during the trial (Bowden et al. 1994).

There is little evidence that lithium is superior to other drugs with sedative actions for the treatment of acute mania. Benzodiazepines, neuroleptics and anticonvulsants have all been tried in mania and none have been found to be inferior to lithium. Two small studies of clonazepam in mania found it was superior to lithium (Chouinard 1988; Chouinard, Young, & Annable 1983). All new- and old-generation neuroleptics have been found to be more effective than placebo (Perlis et al. 2006). Comparisons of lithium with the sedative anticonvulsants carbamazepine and sodium valproate show similar effects (Bowden et al. 1994; Freeman et al. 1992; Lerer et al. 1987; Small et al. 1991).

Trials that have compared neuroleptic drugs with lithium for the treatment of acute mania generally find that neuroleptics are superior for very overactive patients, presumably because lithium's toxicity limits the amount of sedation that can be achieved (Braden et al. 1982; Garfinkel, Stancer, & Persad 1980; Prien, Caffey, Jr., & Klett 1972). In a large American study comparing lithium with chlorpromazine, involving over 200 participants, the authors emphasised how difficult it was to manage the severely manic patients allocated to lithium. Many had to be secluded to try and keep them in the trial (Prien, Caffey, Jr., & Klett 1972). An exception is a Japanese trial in which lithium was found to be superior to chlorpromazine, but patients had only moderate symptoms after a long washout period. In addition, the mean dose of chlorpromazine was a modest 250 mg compared with a relatively high mean dose of lithium of 1.1 g (Takahashi et al. 1975).

Two studies have directly addressed the question of lithium's specificity for mania or affective psychosis, as it is sometimes called. In one of these studies a group of 78 patients admitted with an acute psychotic episode diagnosed as mania, schizophrenia or schizoaffective disorder were randomised to receive lithium or chlorpromazine. The authors hypothesised that patients diagnosed as manic would respond better to lithium and those diagnosed with schizophrenia would respond better to chlorpromazine. In contrast they found that there was no difference in the effects of the different drugs on people with different diagnostic labels and that the only discernible effect was the inferiority of lithium in severely disturbed patients (Braden et al. 1982). A similar study published in 1988 claimed to show that lithium had specificity for manic symptoms, although not manic or affective disorders as such (Johnstone et al. 1988). In this study 105 patients with acute psychosis were randomised to lithium or the neuroleptic pimozide. Again whether the patient was diagnosed with schizophrenia, schizoaffective disorder or pure mania did not predict the response to the different drugs. The authors' claims were based not on a direct analysis of drug effects on symptoms, which presumably did not show any differences, but on a complex analysis of symptom change in subgroups of patients classified according to their predominant mood. The fact that this complex analysis was necessary in the first place suggests that there was little difference between the two drugs' effects. In addition, numbers of patients in the different groups do not match up, suggesting that patients might have been selectively omitted from the analysis. In any case, the results, which are presented graphically, are not convincing. If anything they show that pimozide was a little more effective for 'positive symptoms' and that lithium had few superior effects. The large American trial of the treatment of mania also found no evidence that lithium was superior to chlorpromazine for affective-type symptoms in manic patients. Indeed, in the most overactive patients, chlorpromazine was superior to lithium for some typically manic symptoms including grandiosity and excitement (Prien, Caffey, Jr., & Klett 1972).

Lithium is rarely used as the only treatment for acute mania, a practical acknowledgment of its limitations. If it is used at all it is combined with a neuroleptic and other sedatives are frequently prescribed as well. Trials comparing effects of lithium and carbamazepine in acute mania reveal that substantial doses of benzodiazepines or barbiturates were used in addition to the study drugs (Freeman et al. 1992; Small et al. 1991). However the belief in lithium's specificity for manic depression means it is still deemed an effective treatment and it is still recommended for mild to moderate cases of mania (National Institute for Clinical Excellence 2006).

The evidence for lithium as a prophylactic of manic depression

Trials that compare the relapse rate among people treated with lithium and people treated with placebo are thought to have established the efficacy of lithium for the prevention of recurrence in manic depression. However all these studies were actually discontinuation studies or involved discontinuing lithium in at least some subjects. Many earlier studies especially involved people who had taken lithium for many years and were then randomised either to continue lithium, or to have lithium abruptly replaced by placebo. The existence of withdrawal-related relapse is now well established in relation to lithium and manic depression (Franks, Macritchie, & Young 2005). Numerous studies have shown that the risk of relapse, especially manic relapse, is particularly high in the period after stopping lithium (Baldessarini, Tondo, & Viguera 1999; Cavanagh, Smyth, & Goodwin 2004; Perlis et al. 2002; Suppes et al. 1991). As time goes on the risk falls. Two French researchers suggested that 50% of people have a manic relapse within two weeks of stopping lithium abruptly (Verdoux & Bourgeois 1993). Gradual cessation appears to lower the risk (Baldessarini et al. 1997; Faedda et al. 1993), although one small study did not find this protective effect (Yazici et al. 2004). The strongest evidence that discontinuation precipitates relapse comes from several studies which demonstrate that the risk of relapse was higher after discontinuation than it was prior to the commencement of lithium therapy (Baldessarini, Tondo, & Viguera 1999; Cundall, Brooks, & Murray 1972; Suppes et al. 1991). Therefore, discontinuation studies do not establish prophylactic efficacy, they only document the adverse effects of lithium withdrawal.

The mechanism for withdrawal-induced relapse is unclear. It has mainly been documented in people with a pre-existing diagnosis of manic depression. Given lithium's toxic effects it seems plausible that withdrawal may cause a rebound state of excitability of the nervous system that may predispose people to develop an episode of psychosis or mania. In theory an effect of this sort might occur in people without a history of manic depression. One open study of lithium augmentation for depression found that 2 out of 15 subjects (13.3%) developed a manic episode within four months after lithium was discontinued. Faedda and colleagues pointed out that this rate of mania is higher than the rate at which manic episodes would be expected to develop in depressed people with no prior history of mania and suggested that it could be a consequence of lithium withdrawal (Faedda, Tondo, & Baldessarini 2001). However in general lithium is only prescribed to people with severe psychiatric disorders, in which case any episode of disturbance following withdrawal is likely to be attributed to the underlying problem. Although there is no clear documentation of this reaction occurring with lithium used for gout and other disorders prior to the 1950s, it was likely that it was used at much lower doses, since toxicity was also less common than currently (Johnson 1984). However it is also likely that people with a history of manic depression, and possibly other psychotic disorders, may be particularly vulnerable to discontinuation-induced effects.

Although it is now widely acknowledged that lithium discontinuation can induce relapse, the full implications of this phenomenon have been avoided. In 2001 the principle American textbook of psychiatry ignored it altogether. It even cited one of the papers that demonstrated the occurrence of withdrawal-related relapse (Suppes et al. 1991) as evidence in support of its recommendation of lifelong drug treatment for manic depression (Marangell et al. 2001, p. 1115).

The problems of lithium discontinuation are recognised in recent meta-analyses of the prophylactic efficacy of lithium and studies that employ a classical discontinuation design are excluded. Table 12.1 lists studies included in the latest meta-analysis (Geddes et al. 2004). However as mentioned above, even these studies all involve lithium discontinuation to some degree. Therefore, the higher rates of mania in

Table 12.1   Characteristics of placebo-controlled prospective trials of lithium prophylaxis

Study and year	Design	Interventions	Proportion of patients who were on lithium at entry to the trial
Prien et al. (1973)	205 participants, recently manic, 2-year follow-up	Lithium vs placebo	100% (all patients stabilised on lithium prior to randomisation)
Kane et al. (1982)	22 participants, up to 2-year follow-up	Lithium vs lithium plus imipramine vs imipramine vs placebo	100% (all patients stabilised on lithium for 6 months prior to randomisation)
Bowden et al. (2000)	372 participants, recently manic 1-year follow-up	Lithium vs sodium divalproex vs placebo	33%
Bowden et al. (2003)	175 participants, recently manic, 1-year follow-up	Lithium vs lamotrigine vs placebo	21%
Calabrese et al. (2003)	463 participants, recently depressed, 1-year follow-up	Lithium vs lamotrigine vs placebo	20%

the placebo group may be the result of lithium discontinuation, rather than the natural history of the condition in some cases. For example, in the early study by Robert Prien and colleagues, which was a continuation of the study of treatments for acute mania, all patients were stabilised on lithium after recovery from their acute episode. In the small study by Kane et al. they were stabilised on lithium for six months before randomisation. In addition, the Prien study was not fully blinded. The treating physicians were aware of the allocated treatment and were instructed to increase the dose of lithium if there were signs of relapse. Thus the lithium group can be viewed as receiving early treatment for manic episodes that the placebo group did not receive.

In the latest trials high rates of dropout are another potential source of bias. In the trial of lamotrigine (a new anticonvulsant) 43% of participants left the study early for reasons other than relapse (Bowden et al. 2003). In the sodium valproate trial 40% terminated early without relapsing (Bowden et al. 2000). None of these patients are followed up further and so there is no information about their relapse history. Patients who relapse are also dropped, and so there is no subsequent history for them either. In statistical jargon, these studies have not performed a full 'intention to treat' analysis. They have not collected the same information on everyone who was allocated to the different groups. It may be, for example, that drug-treated patients dropout for reasons related to adverse effects, but then relapse after they have dropped out, leading to an underestimation of the relapse rates in the drug-treated group. Not doing an intention to treat analysis potentially subverts the protection from systematic bias conferred by the process of randomisation. A further problem is the sort of patients that are selected for modern day trials. They appear to have less-severe conditions than the classical profile of manic depression, since many of them have not been hospitalised for manic episodes. Full-blown mania is usually a severe condition that would normally require inpatient admission. Several authors have suggested that this may bias studies against lithium and other drugs, since there is a general perception that lithium is most effective in people with severe classical manic depression. However this perception is not supported by the data. In fact, evidence suggests the opposite; that lithium appears most beneficial in people with milder conditions (Engstrom et al. 1997; Hartong et al. 2003; Tondo, Baldessarini, & Floris 2001) without complicating factors (Greil et al. 1998).

The first recent placebo-controlled study of lithium prophylaxis did not find any difference between lithium, sodium valproate and placebo in rates of recurrence of manic or depressive episodes (Bowden et al. 2000). Another recent trial found that lithium was superior to placebo and lamotrigine in preventing manic episodes with 18% of patients taking lithium having a manic episode versus 40% on placebo. However the results indicate that almost all this increased risk occurred in the first eight months after randomisation, with the majority of relapses occurring in the first few weeks. The graphs presented in the paper indicate that there were no manic relapses in the placebo group after about the ninth month of the trial to its conclusion at 16 months. This suggests that a discontinuation effect was operating, as otherwise relapses would be expected to be evenly spaced over the follow-up period. In contrast, relapses in the lithium group are evenly spread throughout the length of the trial. The published report of this study does not consider the possibility of a discontinuation effect despite this suggestive pattern of relapse (Bowden et al. 2003). The other most recently published trial compared lithium, placebo and lamotrigine in patients who had experienced a recent depressive episode. Overall differences between all treatments were small. Lamotrigine was superior to placebo in terms of the proportion requiring treatment for depression, but there was no difference between lithium and placebo in this respect. The proportions of patients relapsing with any mood episode was similar for lithium at 46% and placebo at 54%. Lithium was superior to placebo in terms of rates of intervention for mania, but mania occurred in only 16% of the placebo group and 8% of the lithium group. Dropout rates for reasons other than relapse were above 30% for all treatment groups. As in the other trials, a proportion of patients were taking lithium during the run-in to the trial, making them vulnerable to discontinuation effects (Calabrese et al. 2003). Therefore, there have been no studies that have eliminated the bias introduced by lithium discontinuation effects entirely.

Is anything better than placebo for prophylaxis?

Since the 1980s there has been a belief that drugs that were first used for epilepsy, such as carbamazepine, sodium valproate and lamotrigine may also be specific treatments for manic depression. This idea was mooted because the paroxysmal nature of epilepsy was suggested to be analogous to the recurrent cycling nature of manic depression. Several studies have compared lithium and carbamazepine. Overall these show similar effects – although some studies have attempted to show differences in different subgroups of patients (Hartong et al. 2003). Sodium valproate was no better than placebo or lithium for prevention of manic-depressive episodes in the only randomised controlled trial of this drug to date, funded by its manufacturers (Bowden et al. 2000). The new anticonvulsant lamotrigine has been claimed to have superior effects on depressive relapses compared with placebo and lithium in two studies sponsored by its makers GlaxoSmithKline (Bowden et al. 2003; Calabrese et al. 2003).

Several trials of olanzapine for prophylaxis of manic depression have now been conducted, funded by Eli Lilly, and claim to show positive evidence of efficacy. A comparison with lithium demonstrated little difference between the two treatment groups overall, although olanzapine appeared to be better at preventing recurrence of mania (Tohen et al. 2005). The only placebo-controlled trial that has been published showed superiority of olanzapine, but there was evidence of a discontinuation effect. Fifty per cent of the placebo group relapsed within 22 days of randomisation and almost all the excess risk of relapse was confined to the first three months of the study (Tohen et al. 2006). All patients were treated with olanzapine initially and since no gradual discontinuation schedule was mentioned, it appears that it was stopped abruptly at the point of randomisation for patients allocated to placebo.

However the greatest doubts about the effectiveness of any drug treatment for manic depression emerge from the data on the natural history of manic depression. Comparing studies done in different eras is difficult because of changing diagnostic practice. We know that most mental disorders are diagnosed more frequently nowadays than they were in the early 20th century. Therefore, studies of the pre-lithium era shown in Table 12.2 were either conducted retrospectively using modern diagnostic criteria, or data has been selected to reflect modern experience. Thus data from the Lundquist study showing low rates of relapse among people with a single manic episode was excluded, since this may not be classical manic depression as characterised today (Lundquist 1945). However these studies show remarkably consistent relapse rates of around 50% in two-and-a-half to three years (Harris et al. 2005; Lundquist 1945; Winokur 1975). In the modern era patients not treated with lithium do as well as those who are (Coryell et al. 1997; Markar & Mander 1989). Relapse rates in patients treated with lithium vary, but in most cases they are higher than rates of relapse prior to the introduction of lithium.

Recent follow-up studies focus on patients who comply with lithium for long periods, thereby selecting patients whose outcome is relatively benign. People who comply with any treatment, including placebo, are known to have better outcomes than non-compliers in a range of medical conditions, including even reduced mortality (Simpson et al. 2006).

Table 12.2   Studies of relapse frequency in manic depression

Study	Number in study	Design	Subject	Period of observation	Outcome
Pre lithium era:					
Lundquist (1945)	36	Retrospective	Subjects with at least 2 episodes of mania admitted in the 1920s	3 years	50% relapsed
Winokur (1975)	100	Retrospective	Patients with mania admitted between 1934–1944	Mean 3.2 years	48% relapsed
Harris et al. (2005)	37	Retrospective	Patients admitted with manic depression in the 1890s	10 years	On average patients relapsed every 2.5 years (4 admissions in 10 years)
Naturalistic follow up studies from post lithium era:					
Dunner et al. (1979)	140	Retrospective	Patients from a lithium clinic prior to starting lithium	Mean 11.4 years	Mean of 0.54 episodes per patient per year
Markar & Mander (1989)	83	Retrospective	Recurrent affective disorder (41 on lithium, 42 not on lithium)	2 years	60% relapse both groups
Coryell et al. (1997)	181	Prospective	Patients recovered from a mood episode	2 years	59% of patients treated with lithium continuously relapse, *vs* 61% of those who completed study without lithium

Lithium-treated patients

Dunner et al. (1976)	96	Prospective	Patients on long-term lithium attending a lithium clinic	2 years	46% relapsed
Angst (1986)	215	Prospective	Admissions for bipolar I and II disorder 1959–63 (presumably mostly drug-treated)	Mean 20 years	Median 10 episodes
Coryell et al. (1989)	117	Prospective	Admissions for depression in people with bipolar I and II disorder (most subjects on lithium for some time)	2 years 5 years	70–89% relapsed 90–95% relapsed
O'Connell et al. (1991)	248	Prospective	Attenders at lithium clinic (all on lithium >1 year)	1 year	44% relapsed
Maj et al. (1998)	402	Prospective	Patients starting lithium	5 years	62% of 247 patients who took lithium continuously relapsed. 35 discontinued for lack of efficacy
Tondo et al. (2001)	360	Prospective	Patients compliant with lithium for 1 year. Those with long relapses (>12 weeks) excluded	Mean 6 years of lithium treatment	Mean of 0.81 episodes per year

(Continued)

Table 12.2 (Continued)

Study	Number in study	Design	Subject	Period of observation	Outcome
Harris et al. (2005)	70	Retrospective	Patients admitted with manic depression during the 1990s	10 years	On average patients relapsed every 1.6 years (mean of 6.3 admissions in 10 years)
Trials:					
Prien et al. (1973)	205	RCT*: lithium vs placebo	Patients admitted with mania	2 years	43% relapse on lithium, 80% on placebo
Bowden et al. (2000)	372	RCT*: lithium vs sodium valproate vs placebo	Patients with recent manic episode	Up to 1 year	31% relapse on lithium, 24% on sodium valproate, 38% on placebo
Bowden et al. (2003)	175	RCT*: lithium vs lamotrigine vs placebo	Patients with recent manic episode	Up to 18 months	39% relapse on lithium, 47% on lamotrigine, 70% on placebo
Tohen et al. (2005)	214	RCT*: lithium vs olanzapine	Patients with recent episode of mania	Up to 1 year	39% relapse on lithium, 30% on olanzapine
Tohen et al. (2006)	225	RCT*: olanzapine vs placebo	Patients with recent manic or mixed episode	Up to 48 weeks	47% relapse on olanzapine, 80% on placebo

*RCT = randomised controlled trial

Why this should be so is not known. It may be due to other factors that are associated with both compliance and better outcome. Being from a higher social class, being married and having greater social support are all likely to be relevant. In Maj et al.'s study people who complied with lithium treatment for five years still relapsed at a rate of 62% and the figure would be higher if it included the 35 people who discontinued lithium for perceived lack of efficacy. People who were taking no mood-stabilising drug at the final follow-up had equivalent outcomes to those on lithium (Maj et al. 1998). Coryell et al. (1997) found that people who complied with lithium treatment for almost two years still relapsed at a rate of 59%, which was almost identical to the rate of recurrence among people not taking lithium. Tondo et al. (2001) selected long-term compliers and also strangely excluded subjects who had a relapse that required treatment for more than 12 weeks. The average recurrence rate (that is the recurrence rate for 50% of the sample) was still almost one episode per year! For mania alone, the average episode rate was 0.36 per year, suggesting that 50% of the sample had one episode in less than three years (Tondo, Baldessarini, & Floris 2001).

In prophylactic trials, relapse rates in drug-treated groups are between 24% and 47% in trials that last for one year and 43% in the only study conducted over two years (Prien, Caffey, Jr., & Klett 1973). No studies have lasted for longer. These rates are not lower than rates of relapse found prior to the introduction of lithium. Relapse rates in placebo groups are higher than the natural risk of recurrence suggested by the data. This is further evidence that the apparent superiority of drug treatment is attributable to a discontinuation effect, which makes people on placebo fare worse than if they had never had any drug treatment, rather than a real prophylactic effect.

Lithium and suicide

It is frequently claimed that lithium reduces the risk of suicide in people with manic depression. Meta-analyses of numerous diverse studies claim to show that people with manic depression or depression who take lithium have lower suicide rates than people who do not (Baldessarini et al. 2006). However the studies included in these analyses yield conflicting results. For example, a large British study found that people taking lithium had suicide rates that were 36 times higher than general population rates (Norton & Whalley 1984). In addition, those studies that find an association between lithium and reduced rates of suicide exclude people who discontinue lithium and others that are lost to follow-up. They are, therefore, studies of suicide in long-term lithium compliers. Since compliers are known to have better outcomes than non-compliers, they are likely to have a lower risk of suicide to begin with by virtue of being the sort of people who comply with treatment. In addition, there is evidence that lithium discontinuation increases the risk of suicide, and suicides among people who have recently stopped lithium have wrongly been counted as suicides among non-lithium-treated people. Two studies found that suicide rates were increased substantially in the first year after lithium discontinuation, but tailed off thereafter and that suicide rates were higher after lithium discontinuation than before lithium was started (Baldessarini, Tondo, & Hennen 1999; Tondo et al. 1998). Abrupt cessation of lithium increased risk more than gradual discontinuation (Baldessarini, Tondo, & Hennen 1999). This may be a direct effect of lithium withdrawal, related to the increase in morbidity that it can cause. Or it may be that people who are depressed, hopeless and about to commit suicide stop their drug treatment just before they do so. In either case, suicides in this group should be counted as suicides associated with lithium treatment or at least discounted. Strangely, the researchers who produced evidence of lithium discontinuation and its relation to suicide rates, the same group who demonstrated the adverse effects of discontinuing other psychiatric drugs, seem to have forgotten their previous research. Their latest review concludes that lithium has specific antisuicidal properties and makes no mention of potential confounding by discontinuation effects (Baldessarini et al. 2006).

The least biased evidence on whether lithium and other mood stabilisers have antisuicidal properties comes from randomised controlled trials and this is negative. A large amount of data from studies of drug treatment of acute mania and relapse prevention found no difference in rates of suicide or suicide attempts between patients randomised to take mood stabilisers, including lithium, and those randomised to placebo (Storosum et al. 2005).

Do mood stabilisers fulfil criteria for disease-centred action?

1. **Pathophysiology of the disorder:** There is no commonly accepted theory about the biological origins of manic depression or bipolar disorder that would explain the actions of any currently used 'mood stabiliser' in disease-centred terms.
2. **Rating scales:** Rating scales for mania and depression contain items that would respond to non-specific effects induced by drugs.

Mania rating scales in particular are likely to show improvement after treatment with any drug with sedative effects.

3. **Animal models:** There are no widely accepted animal models of manic depression.

4. **Volunteer studies:** Volunteers taking lithium show signs of mild lithium toxicity. Patient studies also note these effects, such as mental slowing and dysphoria, which are designated as 'side effects'. The data is consistent with the interpretation that it is lithium's neurotoxic effects that result in reductions in manic symptoms.

5. **Comparison with non-specific drugs:** Studies that compared lithium with older neuroleptics for the treatment of acute mania or psychosis generally found that the neuroleptic was better tolerated and, therefore, more effective in the most severely disturbed patients. There is no evidence that lithium's effects are specific to affective psychosis and little evidence that it has selective effects on affective symptoms. Unsurprisingly, given that mania is characterised by heightened arousal and activity, all sedative drugs that have been trialled in mania have been found to be more effective than placebo, including several anticonvulsants, neuroleptics and benzodiazepines. There are no studies comparing the long-term use of drugs thought to have specific prophylactic effects with drugs that might have non-specific effects.

6. **Long-term outcome:** Many naturalistic studies suggest that the outcome of manic depression is not better now than it was before the introduction of lithium and other mood stabilisers. If anything, the data suggest that the outcome is slightly worse nowadays, although this may partly reflect changing diagnostic practice, particularly lower thresholds for diagnosing a disorder.

Are lithium and other drugs for manic depression useful?

From a drug-centred perspective, it is logical to expect that drugs with sedative properties will be useful in the treatment of mania. The fact that a wide range of different types of sedative drugs have been shown to have more or less equivalent effects is not surprising. However if sedative effects are what is primarily required, then benzodiazepines may be preferable to the use of neuroleptics, lithium and anticonvulsants. Benzodiazepines are already widely used in people with mania, but always in combination with 'mood stabilisers' or neuroleptics and they have received little attention in their own right. Although two small company-funded randomised trials conducted in the 1980s suggested that clonezepam was more effective than lithium, further research was never conducted or at least published (Chouinard 1988; Chouinard, Young, & Annable 1983). This might mean that clonezepam was not as promising as first thought, or that the company switched its marketing strategy. Anecdotally some people with manic depression describe the beneficial effects of temporary use of benzodiazepines when the early warning signs of impending mania occur. However tolerance might reduce their effectiveness if mania persists for months, as it often does, and they would need to be tapered slowly on recovery to avoid discontinuation symptoms.

It is conceivable that sedative drugs might also be able to reduce recurrences of mania, although bodily adaptations or tolerance might counteract their effects. It is more difficult to see how they could prevent episodes of depression, except by dulling the senses and blunting the emotions. However long-term studies and drug trials do not provide strong evidence that any drugs reduce the incidence of recurrence because of the confounding effects of discontinuation and other methodological issues. Evidence suggests that the use of lithium and other 'mood stabilisers' have not improved the long-term course of manic depression and may actually have made it worse, possibly because of the increased risk of relapse on discontinuation of lithium. The evidence on discontinuation implies that, for lithium at least, anything other than several years of treatment is likely to increase the risk of relapse above the rate at which it would occur without any treatment (Goodwin 1994). But most people find lithium and the alternatives unpleasant to take and evidence shows that the majority of people stop taking lithium within a short period. A large study of a health maintenance database found that the median duration of lithium use was only 72 days and that only around 10% of patients took it for more than a year (Johnson & McFarland 1996).

Manic depression is a potentially devastating condition. Sufferers are often desperate to find anything that will reduce its virulence and professionals are desperate to have something to offer. According to the drug-centred approach the main question is whether the adverse effects associated with taking any sort of psychotropic drug on a long-term basis are worth the uncertain and probably small benefit. Even without developing severe toxicity, lithium has adverse effects on kidney function, causes weight gain and impairs intellectual abilities. Sodium valproate is associated with endocrine abnormalities, weight gain and occasionally serious blood problems and liver toxicity; carbamazepine with serious blood disorders and liver disease. Olanzapine, now one of the first-line drugs recommended for long-term treatment of manic depression, is associated, as we saw in Chapter 7, with metabolic disruption and brain atrophy with long-term use.

Psychotherapeutic approaches to managing manic depression have recently become fashionable. These approaches help people to identify possible precipitants and early warning signs of mania and depression so that they can adjust their lifestyle to reduce the likelihood of a relapse and seek help early if one is impending. Although early studies reported positive findings, a large trial found that cognitive behaviour therapy did not prevent relapse in people with manic depression (Scott et al. 2006). However it can be argued that helping people to feel more empowered and less at the mercy of uncontrollable moods is important whether or not it decreases relapse. In addition, this approach has only been advocated as an adjunct to drug treatment and has never been evaluated in its own right. Psychiatric professionals seem unable to conceive of the possibility of not taking long-term medication for manic depression. Despite this, many sufferers do manage to do without it.

The portrayal of drugs for manic depression as specific treatments is misleading. It obscures the real questions about the pros and cons of treatment, the process of weighing up a lifetime of emotional blunting and cognitive impairment with a possible small reduction in the risk of recurrence. By clouding these questions it may act as a hindrance to people's own efforts to exert some mastery over this frightening condition.

13
Democratic Drug Treatment: Implications of the Drug-Centred Model

In this chapter, I look at the implications of accepting the drug-centred model of psychotropic drug action for the theory and practice of psychiatry. Firstly I examine what the drug-centred model means for our understanding of the nature of psychiatric conditions. Then I look at what psychiatry could be like if it based its approach to drug treatment on a drug-centred model, and how drug research and development would differ from their current emphasis.

Models of 'mental illness'

Psychiatry and its central idea that madness and distress are biological diseases that can be explained and treated by physical means, has long been a target of controversy. Criticism of psychiatry has been voiced by a range of academic disciplines, including philosophy and sociology, as well as dissident psychiatrists and psychiatric service users or 'survivors'. Much of the criticism has focused on the logical inconsistencies in the concept of mental illness and the social forces that have led to its adoption. Psychiatrist Thomas Szasz famously described the concept of mental illness as a myth or a metaphor. Szasz argues that whereas a diagnosis of physical disease generally indicates a specific physical pathology, a diagnosis of mental illness is simply a description of aberrant behaviour (Szasz 1970). Foucault also refers to the 'heterogeneity' between psychiatry and clinical medicine (Foucault 2006, p. 12). The transcription of deviant behaviour into medical conditions serves important functions. It authorises certain actions such as the incarceration and restraint of the disturbed individual and the dedication of funds for the care and maintenance of the economically dependent. It also conceals the moral and political judgements that are embedded in these actions

(Ingelby 1982). The concept of mental illness as a medical phenomenon, therefore, facilitates a disguised form of social control. As Szasz describes: 'The mandate for contemporary psychiatry ... is precisely to obscure, indeed to deny the ethical dilemmas of life and to transform these into medicalised and technicalised problems susceptible to "professional" solutions' (Szasz 1970, p. 11). Or in Foucault's words: 'Psychiatry is a moral practice, overlaid by the myths of positivism', where positivism refers to an empirical scientific framework (Foucault 1965, p. 276).

Other psychiatric critics have challenged the notion that psychiatric conditions are meaningless manifestations of disordered brain function, and suggested that psychiatric 'symptoms' can be seen as meaningful, albeit bizarre and dysfunctional responses to the social world. Scottish psychiatrist R.D. Laing attempted to render the experience of psychosis in terms of a meaningful response to the family environment and as an existential retreat from the demands of the modern materialist world (Laing 1965, 1967). Recent accounts have also emphasised the importance of recognising meaning in order to understand psychiatric disturbance and to aid recovery (Bracken & Thomas 2005).

The drug-centred model of psychiatric drug action does not inherently contradict the biological view of psychiatric disorders. Although I have demonstrated that there is no evidence that psychiatric conditions are caused by a biochemical imbalance, and that drugs in current use do not act on the neurological basis of these conditions, these facts in themselves do not preclude the future discovery of the biological origins of mental disorders and the future development of disease-specific drugs. However the disease-centred model of drug action is one of the main foundations of the biological account of psychiatric problems. Biological models of psychosis and depression, for example, have been constructed by assuming that drugs act by reversing the underlying pathology, or part of it, and drugs' effects are still regarded as the strongest evidence to support these models. For example, a recent article on depression suggested that 'the indisputable therapeutic efficacy of these drugs (antidepressants) suggests that serotonergic and/or noradrenergic underactivity is key to the pathophysiology of the condition' (Malhi, Parker, & Greenwood 2005, p. 97). Discussions of the dopamine hypothesis of schizophrenia still cite the action of neuroleptic drugs. Without the disease-centred model of drug action the view that psychiatric conditions, like other medical diseases, arise out of specific and identifiable physical defects has little support. Independent evidence that there are specific biochemical deviations in the brains of people with various psychiatric diagnoses is weak and inconsistent. In addition, even if there were evidence of this sort, it would not demonstrate that the biochemical aberration was the cause of the psychological state. It might just as well be the consequence, or merely the correlate of the subjective experience, and it is surely simplistic to assume that there is a one-to-one relation between our complex emotions and biochemical states. For example, we know that adrenalin, the 'fight or flight' hormone as it is known, is produced in situations characterised by many different emotions. It is produced when someone is feeling aggressive during a fight or a battle, when someone is frightened, acutely anxious or euphoric. It hardly makes sense to say that adrenalin is the cause of these varying emotional reactions. It is better to view it as the body's response to a situation involving increased arousal and as such it is a correlate of many different emotions.

Genetic research is also quoted as irrefutable evidence of there being a biological substrate to mental conditions. However several critics have argued that the genetic contribution to psychiatric conditions such as schizophrenia and alcoholism is overstated (Joseph 2003; Rose, Lewontin, & Kamin 1984). In his recent book, Jay Joseph argues that the twin and adoption studies that are claimed to demonstrate a genetic component to schizophrenia are flawed and points out that molecular genetic studies have failed to detect any genes that are strongly associated with the disorder (Joseph 2003).

Therefore, undermining the basis of the disease-centred model of drug action presents a challenge to the medical model of mental illness and the argument that psychiatry is a branch of medicine like any other. As such it presents a direct threat to the predominant view the psychiatric profession holds about itself and its activities. However psychiatry has always been an eclectic activity, encompassing countervailing theories and styles. Although I have argued that the medico-biological view has been its underlying core, many other approaches have been popular and influential. In the mid-20th century American psychiatry was strongly influenced by the ideas of Adolf Meyer. Although his views accommodated a more traditional medical approach, he emphasised the importance of 'understanding the life story of the individual patient' rather than reducing people's problems to a diagnostic category (Double 2006, p. 185). Psychoanalysis and psychotherapeutic approaches also stress understanding each person in terms of the unique influences on their development, especially their relationships with other people. The movement loosely referred to as 'social psychiatry' emphasised the influence of the social environment on an individual's emotions and behaviour. Innovations such as therapeutic communities were inspired by the idea that forming supportive social relationships was key to improving someone's functioning, rather than adjusting their brain chemistry.

There are, therefore, many precedents, both within and outside of psychiatry, for understanding madness and distress as manifestations of the interaction between the variety of human propensities and the challenges of modern living. A drug-centred model is well suited to this sort of approach. It provides a framework for the judicious use of drugs without having to attribute someone's problems to a brain disease. The use of drugs to induce temporary states that might bring relief from intense psychological torment is compatible with viewing psychiatric disturbance as an extreme but meaningful response to the world. Whether practitioners require a full medical degree for this approach, even if it does involve the use of drugs from time to time, is debatable.

Democratic drug treatment according to a drug-centred model

So what would psychiatric drug treatment look like if it were based on a drug-centred model of drug action? It could be argued that prior to the 1950s a drug-centred approach resulted in a similar pattern of drug use to today. Large amounts of drugs were used for purposes of restraint and sedation but little attention was given to these effects. However changes in the social climate have changed the nature of interactions between professionals and their clients, including psychiatrists and their patients. Up until the last few decades, psychiatric patients were regarded as so afflicted and helpless that almost any intervention could be justified in the name of treatment. Hazardous research and physical 'treatments' were conducted on them with scant regard for their safety. There was little thought about what the patient wanted or what they thought of the treatments they received. But today people are better informed about medical and psychiatric interventions and expect to be involved in discussions about treatment options. The Internet provides both a source of official information and a forum for the exchange of personal experience of drug use in the burgeoning number of drug 'chat rooms'. Professional autonomy has also been eroded by management controls, guidelines and greater demands for public accountability. Currently patient or consumer choice is driving the restructuring of medical services and professionals are appraised according to the views of their clients. In this climate a drug-centred model could become a force for a more democratic practice of psychiatry.

The drug-centred model of drug action implies a different sort of relationship between psychiatric service users and prescribers. Instead of acting like a medical doctor, telling the patient what disease they have and what is the appropriate treatment, the psychiatrist or prescriber needs to act more as a pharmaceutical advisor. They should inform people about the range of effects a drug can induce, both those that might be useful and those that are likely to be harmful in order to help people to evaluate the benefits of taking a particular drug for themselves. However the user's experience of a drug's effects will be the key determinant of the drug's utility and thus they become a more equal partner in the consultation. Rather than being the passive recipient of a regimen prescribed by someone else, they make an active decision about whether drugs will be helpful in their own situation. Thus the drug-centred model promotes a process of 'shared decision making', in which professionals collaborate with service users to help them use drugs in a way that will facilitate and not impede the recovery of 'valued social roles' (Deegan & Drake 2006). Many people already use medication in this way of course, adapting prescribed regimens to suit their own individual needs by taking drugs sporadically or not at all, rather than continuously, and adjusting the dose according to their subjective experience.

This new relationship between psychiatrists and their clients has echoes of the relationship between patron and apothecary prior to the development of modern medical therapies (Rosenberg 1977). The power of the psychiatrist would be less than it is today and people's expectations of the outcome of treatment would be lower. Psychiatry would be a more modest enterprise, no longer claiming to be able to alter the underlying course of psychological disturbance, but thereby avoiding some of the damage associated with the untrammelled use of imaginary chemical cures.

A reciprocal and democratic approach to drug treatment based on a drug-centred model requires the clarification of two things: Firstly, it is necessary to know what patients and others want from a psychiatric intervention. Secondly, we must be clear about what effects different drugs are, and are not, able to produce. Discerning what people really want from psychiatrists is difficult because people's expectations have now been influenced by the widespread promotion of the idea of the biological origin of distress and the concomitant disease-centred model of drug treatment. Thus people will consult a doctor because they already believe they have a biochemical imbalance and need drugs to rectify it. In this situation it is important to elucidate what precise problems have led someone to consider themselves in this light and to seek medical intervention. The principles of rehabilitation for alcohol and drug users can provide some lessons here. Recovering addicts are encouraged to identify what effects they are looking for from drugs, why they want them and what alternatives are possible. For example, drug users sometimes seek euphoria and indifference to dampen down painful memories of childhood abuse and can be helped to develop less destructive ways of bearing their past experiences.

The effects that different sorts of drugs can induce need to be matched to the problems that people are experiencing. People who are highly aroused and overactive, including people with an acute psychotic or manic episode, may benefit from taking something with sedative properties. However the problem of pharmacological tolerance means that sedative effects may weaken and higher and higher doses may be required. Excessive preoccupation with mental events such as delusions, hallucinations and obsessional or anxious thoughts might be reduced in the short term by drugs with deactivating properties or those that induce emotional indifference. Again tolerance may lead to a diminution of this effect with prolonged use. The decision about whether to use a drug of this sort would ultimately depend on balancing possible benefits in terms of reducing symptom intensity with the numerous adverse effects. Even in the short term neuroleptics commonly cause acute dystonia,[1] Parkinson's disease-type symptoms, weight gain and impotence and less frequently severe and life-threatening conditions such as neuroleptic malignant syndrome[2] and blood disorders. More candid use should perhaps be made of the benzodiazepine drugs, which are relatively safe and not experienced as unpleasant. They are already commonly used for emergency sedation when someone is acutely disturbed and potentially dangerous, and also widely prescribed in conjunction with other drugs on a long-term basis. As described in Chapter 6, they have also been shown to reduce psychotic symptoms as effectively as neuroleptics in a few trials. However they are known to induce pharmacological tolerance and physical dependence, and like most other drugs, their long-term use is accompanied by adverse consequences (Ashton 1986). Some studies suggest that long-term use may be associated with brain shrinkage similar in nature to that observed with neuroleptics (Lader, Ron, & Petursson 1984; Schmauss & Krieg 1987), but other studies have not replicated this finding (Busto et al. 2000; Perera, Powell, & Jenner 1987).

According to the disease-centred model of drug action, long-term use of drugs after recovery from an acute episode is justified because, by counteracting the neurological process that produces the symptoms, drugs may prevent the disorder from re-emerging. Since the drug-centred model suggests that drugs merely suppress symptoms by inducing states of intoxication and do not impinge on the mechanism that gives rise to the symptoms, it follows that long-term treatment is unlikely to be able to prevent the recurrence of the condition in some guise. Even if it is accepted that there are some advantages to maintenance treatment, the cost benefit ratio does not look favourable in most cases. The best studies available in psychosis or schizophrenia suggest that the reduction in the risk of relapse brought about by drug treatment is 16–17% and this may still be an overestimate because of discontinuation effects (Carpenter, Jr. et al. 1990; Crow et al. 1986). All drugs suggested to have prophylactic efficacy in conditions such as schizophrenia and manic depression have generalised sedative effects, impair or slow up mental faculties and are experienced as unpleasant; effects that are likely to impede a return to normal life. They hasten death, cause neurological impairment and some cause serious metabolic disruption. High rates of non-compliance suggest that many patients decide that they would rather take the risk of relapse than accept a life time of drug-induced disabilities.

It is important to acknowledge, however that there are people who become extremely disturbed for long periods of time. A chemical straight jacket such as that produced by the neuroleptic drugs with their Parkinson's-inducing effect may be preferable to other methods of restraint, although it may be impossible to achieve this effect in the long term, given the body's ability to counteract the effects of drugs. However if drugs are to be used in this way we must be honest about what is being done. We must admit that the drugs will not cure some underlying disease, even if one does exist. We must be sure that there are no better options and that the individual's behaviour is violent or disruptive enough to warrant the use of chemical control. Thankfully, even prolonged periods of madness usually burn out with time, so everyone should have the chance to have their medication reduced or withdrawn when they calm down. Currently however people remain on drugs because improvement is always attributed to the effects of treatment and because of the difficulties of stopping medication.

Many of the situations that people are in when they seek psychiatric intervention are unlikely to be helped by the range of effects that current drugs are known to induce. Some problems may be exacerbated by drugs. It is difficult to see how drugs with sedative and deactivating properties can do anything other than compound the negative symptoms of schizophrenia, for example, despite claims from the manufacturers of some newer neuroleptics such as amisulpride that their drugs are especially effective for negative symptoms. The role of drug treatment in people seeking help for 'depression' and other difficulties is also minimal. The reduced emotional sensitivity associated with the use of any psychoactive substance may bring temporary relief to someone who is very distressed, but it is unlikely to help them to uncover and deal with the source of their problems. What people who are depressed or unhappy really need is help and support from other human beings (Scott 2006). Being drugged is a barrier to developing the relationships and the activities that help people to recover.

Drug-centred drug research

The disease-centred model of drug action has restricted our understanding of the effects of drugs used in psychiatry by directing attention to the effects of drugs on a hypothetical disease process and neglecting other areas. For example, although there is ample research about effects of the new generation of antipsychotic drugs on the numerous different dopamine and serotonin receptors, it is almost impossible to find out their effects on such basic physiological parameters such as pulse rate and blood pressure and there is little interest in their potentially significant effects on the histamine, cholinergic and noradrenalin system. Therefore we are uncertain about the basic nature of many of the drugs prescribed for psychiatric complaints. Studies with volunteers that could establish these effects are conducted by the pharmaceutical companies and are limited to establishing obvious acute toxic reactions. In addition, most are not even published (Cohen & Jacobs 2007). There is also little research into the important consequences of long-term drug use including withdrawal syndromes, tolerance, and cognitive and behavioural effects. There has been almost no interest in the impact of the use of prescribed psychotropic drugs on people's social relations and functioning in arenas such as work, family life and personal relationships.

The first requirement of research based on a drug-centred model would be to establish the range of global effects associated with different drugs and the impact of these effects. Ideally this would require volunteer studies with multiple observers, including people who know the volunteers well who can comment on drug-induced changes. Volunteers would need to take the drug for protracted periods as in clinical practice and then be followed through a period of withdrawal. This would help to establish the effects of withdrawal and enable the volunteers to evaluate the experience of being on the drug when they are in a drug-free state again (Cohen & Jacobs 2007). This is particularly important, since the state of altered consciousness produced by ingesting drugs, however subtle, may interfere with someone's ability to make judgements about their capabilities and desires. Peter Breggin has called this effect 'spellbinding' and described how people 'underestimate the degree of drug-induced mental impairment' (Breggin 2006). As he points out we are well aware that this effect occurs with alcohol, but there has been little recognition of its significance in relation to drugs used as psychiatric treatments. However there is evidence that people treated with lithium cannot recognise their cognitive impairment, and that people taking neuroleptics are often unaware of certain effects such as reduced or abnormal movement (Gerlach & Larsen 1999).

Knowledge based on a drug-centred model would differentiate psychoactive effects of drugs more finely than we do today. It would distinguish between the different quality of sedation induced by classical neuroleptics, the newer or 'atypical' neuroleptics, benzodiazepines, tricyclic antidepressants, opiates, etc. Benzodiazepines and opiates, for example, have sedative actions that are accompanied by euphoria and relaxation, whereas older neuroleptics, tricyclic antidepressants and SSRIs produce sedation that is experienced as unpleasant and may be accompanied by agitation. The characteristics of the sedation produced by some of the newer antipsychotic drugs is not yet clear. Attention would be paid to whether the activation effects induced by SSRIs are subjectively similar to the effects of stimulant drugs, whether they are more akin to the akathisia caused by neuroleptics or whether they are a distinct type of effect. The various effects of drug-induced states on emotional responses would also be delineated. The emotional disinhibition caused by alcohol and benzodiazepines could be distinguished from the indifference and demotivation associated with neuroleptics and from the non-specific reduction in emotional sensitivity that is likely to occur under the influence of any sort of mind altering substance.

A drug-centred model of drug action would lead to a new classification of psychotropic drugs according to their characteristic global effects and their chemical class, rather than their effects on a hypothetical disease. Historically an elementary drug-centred classification of drug action distinguished drugs on the basis of whether they had primarily sedative or stimulant effects. Table 13.1 presents a crude attempt at a more sophisticated drug-centred classification based on our limited existing knowledge.

Table 13.1   Drug-centred classification schema

Chemical class	Characteristic global effects
Butyrophenones, e.g., haloperidol	Parkinson's like effects of reduced movement (akinesia) and mental activity, emotional indifference, demotivation accompanied by dysphoria and restlessness (akathisia)
Phenothiazines and related drugs, e.g., chlorpromazine (Largactil/ Thorazine). Some tricyclic antidepressants, e.g., amitriptyline	Same effects as butyrophenones accompanied by other effects including stronger sedation
Dibenzodiazepine derivatives and thienobenzodiazepines, e.g., clozapine, olanzapine	Milder Parkinsonian effects plus strong sedation and metabolic changes
Benzodiazepines, e.g., diazepam (Valium), nitrezepam (Librium) and lorazepam	Sedation, euphoria, disinhibition, muscle relaxation
Barbiturates	Sedation, euphoria, disinhibition
Opiates	Sedation, analgesia, euphoria, emotional indifference
Central nervous system stimulants, e.g., amphetamine, methylphenidate (Ritalin) and cocaine	Physiological stimulation, i.e., increased arousal, reduced sleep, increased heart rate accompanied by euphoria
SSRIs, e.g., fluoxetine (Prozac), paroxetine (Seroxat, Paxil)	Mild drowsiness, occasional agitation, possible emotional indifference, gastrointestinal effects

Cohen and Jacobs have suggested that the classical clinical trial is useless for evaluating the effects of psychiatric drugs. In trials the complex experience of drug taking is rendered in terms of outcome measures with a limited focus accompanied by a cursory enquiry into adverse effects. In this way the researcher or clinician structures the patients' opportunities to report their experience and trials that detect 'improvement' cannot distinguish between whether the improvement consists of a genuine return to normal functioning or whether it reflects the effects of being drugged (Cohen & Jacobs 2007). In contrast, qualitative and unmediated accounts of patients' experience, such as those found in Internet chat rooms, provide an important source of information in the absence of detailed volunteer studies. Indeed, this is currently the only source of information about many aspects of the use of psychiatric drugs. However pharmaceutical company propaganda and the diffusion of the idea of the chemical imbalance have coloured how people experience their medication, sometimes preventing people from perceiving the full nature of the psychoactive effects of the drugs they take.

The drug-centred model and the politics of psychiatry

If the data presented in preceding chapters is accepted, the adoption of the drug-centred model of drug action should lead to a substantial reduction in the use of psychiatric drugs. In particular I have argued that the long-term use of psychiatric drugs is not justified by current evidence and that the benefits are rarely likely to outweigh the disadvantages. However the pharmaceutical industry has proved adept at taking commercial advantage of different accounts of drug action and would no doubt attempt to capitalise on the possibilities of a drug-centred approach. In the 1960s, drugs were advertised for their drug-induced properties for a wide range of situations. Stimulant or 'antilethargic' effects were recommended for the menopause, the postnatal period and for 'old age'. Tranquillisers were also widely marketed for use in older people. Benzodiazepines were successfully pressed onto a large proportion of the female population of many Western nations from the 1960s until the 1980s. However concerns about the exploitation of a drug-centred model by the pharmaceutical industry should be balanced by the bonanza that it has made out of the disease-centred model, especially since the 1990s. The industry needs to be better regulated whatever model of drug action predominates. There need to be much tighter reigns on the claims it can make to patients and doctors, the sort of promotion that is acceptable and the industry's influence on academic research and publication.

Current mental health legislation is based on the view that psychiatric conditions are analogous to medical diseases and require and respond to specific treatments. Compulsory hospitalisation of psychiatric patients is usually justified by the notion that they suffer from a condition that can be viewed as an illness that requires medical treatment to cure or reverse it. Compulsory treatment such as forced drugging and ECT is justified on grounds that these are medical treatments for particular diseases. The disease-centred model of drug action is therefore embedded in psychiatric law. Since this model implies that drug treatment is fundamentally benign, because it is reversing an abnormal biological state, use of psychiatric drugs is subject to little scrutiny and then only usually when patients actively object to it. Psychiatric practice is permeated with the involuntary use of drugs. Some patients actively resist drug treatment and may be held down and forcibly injected. Many more patients are pestered, pressurised and cajoled into taking drugs, often with threats that they will not be able to leave hospital until they do. In the United States, patients can be made subject to a system known as 'financial leverage', in which they are not given social security payments unless they adhere to a treatment programme, which often includes taking prescribed medication. In some states 15–19% of psychiatric patients are subjected to these conditions (Appelbaum & Redlich 2006; Monahan et al. 2005).

Adopting a drug-centred model of drug action would require a different sort of legislation and a different attitude to involuntary drug treatment. Every drug used against a person's will would need to be justified to an official independent body in terms of the effects it was intended to achieve and the need for those effects. Increases in dose would need to be defended and there would need to be regular reviews of whether continued use of chemical restraint was necessary. It would always have to be demonstrated that the suggested benefits of the drugs on behaviour and mental state outweighed the damage they might induce.

As psychiatric critics such as Thomas Szasz have pointed out, psychiatry has been used by the state as a smokescreen behind which to hide some of its thorniest problems: How, in a democratic liberal society premised on the equality of rights of all individuals, is it possible to manage people whose behaviour is difficult, disturbing and disruptive without fulfilling the usual requirements for the sanctions of the criminal law? How does modern society deal with adult dependents and police non-participation in the work place (Szasz 1994)? By transferring these issues to the authority of the medical profession, they have been transformed into technical rather than political problems. These issues, which should be at the heart of public debate, have become medical disorders requiring specialist medical intervention. However in contrast to Szasz's anti-statist views, I believe the State needs to acknowledge the political nature of the problems posed by madness and discontent and take a lead in formulating a fair and democratic response. Asylum, sanctuary and even control and containment have a role, but they need to be seen for what they are so that they can be openly debated and properly scrutinised.

Although abandoning the disease-centred view challenges some of the most fundamental principles of modern psychiatry, it also opens the way to a more honest practice and one which requires its own specialist knowledge. Adopting a drug-centred model of drug action would require psychiatrists to become more informed about the effects of different psychoactive drugs, and to become attuned to evaluating the subjective experiences of their patients in a more equal and reciprocal relationship. Where their function was to participate in mechanisms of social control this would be openly acknowledged and rigidly controlled, rather than veiled, as currently, under the cloak of medicine.

14
The Myth of the Chemical Cure

The ideology of psychopharmacology

The data surveyed in this book suggest that psychiatric drug treatment is currently administered on the basis of a huge collective myth; the myth that psychiatric drugs act by correcting the biological basis of psychiatric symptoms or diseases. We have seen that for the three main classes of drugs used in psychiatry there is no evidence to substantiate this view. Instead, the evidence suggests that these drugs induce characteristic abnormal states that can account for their so-called therapeutic effects. This book has been about how and why this myth of psychiatric drugs as 'chemical cures' was constructed and sustained.

The disease-centred model of understanding psychiatric drug action can be viewed as an ideology, or false consciousness, in the Marxist sense. Like other forms of ideology, it presents itself as an objective, impartial body of knowledge determined only by the facts of the world, whereas it actually conveys a partial view of human experience and activities that are motivated by particular interests. The institution of psychiatry, aided and abetted by the pharmaceutical industry and ultimately backed by the state, has constructed a system of false knowledge about the nature of psychiatric drugs. This ideology acts to obscure the actual effects these drugs produce. By focusing on the action of drugs on the putative neural basis of psychiatric disorders, the disease-centred model has obscured the abnormal physical and psychic states necessarily produced by ingesting psychoactive chemicals of any sort.

The way that vested interest have embedded themselves into the fabric of our knowledge about psychiatric drugs demonstrates the symbiosis between power and knowledge highlighted by Foucault (2006). Power helped to construct the idea of the drug as a chemical cure and the body of knowledge that it has generated. Its influence operates at every level and in every strand of the production of this knowledge. It determines what theories are adopted, what questions are asked and how they are researched, and what questions are ruled out of bounds. It influences the day-to-day conduct of research from the selection of subjects, designation of diagnosis, assessment of outcomes and collection of data and it shapes the way that data are analysed, presented and publicised. In turn this knowledge has itself become an instrument of psychiatric power. It has facilitated the particular form of social control that is embodied in psychiatric practice, by construing psychiatric restraint as the medical cure of a mental disease. It has helped to disperse psychiatric power throughout the population by concealing the moral nature of psychiatric judgements. People have become willing recipients of the idea that their problems emanate from a chemical imbalance in their brains. The idea has diffused into the public consciousness, fundamentally changing the way we view ourselves and the nature of our experience (Rose 2004). Elsewhere I have argued that this view of ourselves as chemically flawed renders us vulnerable to increasing economic exploitation and diverts our attention from the social causes of our discontent (Moncrieff 2007).

However this is not a relativist account of psychiatric knowledge. Relativist and post-modern analyses are ultimately unsatisfactory because, by suggesting that all forms of knowledge are ultimately ungrounded, there is no basis for deciding between different theories of the nature of madness and how to manage it. In contrast, I believe that although human interests and influence can never be expunged from the process of investigation, the form of the world determines the possibilities of knowledge. The nature of reality can be more or less accurately represented, and sometimes it is misrepresented because it does not fulfil the requirements of the parties that produce official 'knowledge'. If these parties are powerful and there are no equally powerful groups to challenge them, then the false knowledge becomes established as real knowledge.

Consequences of the disease-centred model

As preceding chapters have documented, over the 1950s and 60s views of drugs used in psychiatry changed dramatically. When they were first introduced, the neuroleptics were regarded as producing their therapeutic effects by creating a neurological disease akin to Parkinson's disease. However within a decade, they were being presented as 'magic bullets' that produced improvement through acting directly on the biological basis of a psychiatric disease. This transformation did not occur because of the overwhelming weight of supportive evidence. It occurred because the desire for it to be true shaped the data that were produced and how this data were represented. In this way a picture was painted in which the drugs became miracle cures responsible for emptying the asylums and transforming the outlook of psychiatric conditions. The benefits of drugs came to dominate psychiatric thought and it was rapidly concluded that they needed to be continued indefinitely. The fact that psychiatric conditions may improve spontaneously was forgotten and other ways of helping people became secondary concerns. As this view took hold the original knowledge about the effects these drugs induce was forgotten and their neurological toxicity was redesignated as an incidental side effect that bore no relation to the mechanism of their therapeutic action.

Drugs used in depression underwent a similar metamorphosis. Early ideas about the benefits of inducing stimulant effects changed as drugs came to be regarded as specifically targeting the biochemical basis of a depressive illness. The anti-tuberculous drugs, iproniazid and isoniazid, which were clearly stimulants, were rebranded as 'antidepressants' and imipramine was promoted as an antidepressant with barely any acknowledgement of its psychoactive effects. Again, this change was achieved by a selective presentation of data that ignored general drug-induced effects or repackaged them as side effects. Although it took rather longer to catch on, lithium became known as a specific agent for the treatment of manic depression, even though its clinical effects are obviously on a continuum with its toxic effects.

The disease-centred model of drug action, the myth that psychiatric drugs are curative or restorative treatments, has led to their indiscriminate prescription to millions of people often for decades on end. It is likely that many people exposed to the harmful physical and psychological effects of these drugs derive no benefit from them. For example, the long-term use of neuroleptic drugs is based on flawed studies, which cannot distinguish true prophylactic effects from the problems induced by drug withdrawal. Even the initial benefits of neuroleptic treatment may be lost due to bodily adaptations and many people find the experience of the Parkinson's disease-like state they induce, which is responsible for the therapeutic effects in most cases, worse than their original symptoms.

In addition, there is evidence that the neuroleptic drugs produce neurological and psychiatric disturbance in their own right. The abnormal movements associated with tardive dyskinesia, a condition they are known to induce with long-term use, are probably just one manifestation of a general state of brain damage that also involves cognitive dysfunction and behavioural disturbance. This possibility is supported by findings that neuroleptic drugs are associated with shrinkage of brain matter after a relatively short period of treatment. It is too early to say whether the newer generation of antipsychotics really cause a lesser degree of brain impairment than the older drugs. Rates of tardive dyskinesia are lower but still not negligible.

The problems associated with coming off psychiatric medication may also be responsible for exacerbating the chronicity of psychiatric problems. Hence the 'revolving door' patient, who keeps relapsing after stopping their drugs may in fact be suffering from the problems induced by medication withdrawal. If these effects were recognised for what they were they might be manageable. For example, someone may need to taper their medication more slowly, or may require a short period of additional treatment or simply some reassurance until the withdrawal-related problems subside. However problems that occur after discontinuing drugs are inevitably diagnosed as a recurrence of the initial condition and viewed as confirmation of the need for lifelong treatment.

The idea that drugs can reverse the basis of psychiatric conditions prevents society from developing other ways to deal with serious psychiatric disturbance. It allows governments to cut back on supported care for the mentally ill, for example. A census taken in the United Kingdom in 2006 found that 30% of inpatients had been in hospital for more than a year (Commission for Healthcare Audit and Inspection 2007). Modern drugs are not liberating the mentally ill. And yet there is now almost no provision of long-term care by the United Kingdom's National Health Service, except for offenders. Instead people with ongoing problems languish on 'acute' wards designed for people with short-lived disturbance, or they are farmed out to the private sector, where the quality of care is variable. The misconception that mental illness can be cured by drugs discourages the provision of decent services that recognise and respect difference and disability and promotes instead the notion that people can be drugged into some sort of conformity or passivity.

As far as antidepressant drugs are concerned, randomised trials have found that they are barely distinguishable from a placebo and it has never been established that they have a specific action on the neurobiology of mood. The small degree of superiority over placebo in some trials may easily be attributable to amplified placebo effects or drug-induced effects such as sedation that can be achieved by many other sorts of drugs. In contrast to neuroleptics, where the disease-centred model has obscured the powerful and toxic nature of their effects, in the case of SSRIs the model has enabled drugs with relatively few psychoactive effects to be presented as potent treatments. However we remain uncertain about the exact nature of the effects they induce and particularly whether they may occasionally provoke a state that predisposes people to aggressive or suicidal behaviour.

Despite this situation, the marketing of antidepressants has persuaded a large proportion of the population of Western countries to take prescribed drugs to deal with the problems of living. Diverse situations from relationship break-ups to job difficulties to sexual abuse and severe trauma have been transformed into chemical problems. Individual human beings with their unique life histories and personal characteristics are reduced to biochemical entities and in this way the reality of human experience and suffering is denied. The message that drugs can cure your problems has profound consequences. It encourages people to view themselves as powerless victims of their biology and stores up untold misery for the future when people come to realise that their problems have not gone away but have failed to develop more constructive ways of dealing with them. It sets a precedent for the use of chemical solutions that may encourage people to find solace in recreational drugs when the prescription drugs prove inadequate. At another level it allows governments and institutions to ignore the social and political reasons why so many people feel discontented with their lives (Moncrieff 2007).

One of the worst consequences of the disease-centred model is the rising use of prescription drugs in children, who form an increasing section of the market for antidepressants and neuroleptic drugs as well as stimulants like Ritalin. By suggesting that drugs reverse an underlying problem, the disease-centred model conceals the limitations of drugs and the damage they can do, which is likely to be magnified many times in children with their developing brains and personalities. The prescription of drugs also appears to confirm that the problem lies in the individual child and thus obscures the way that modern Western society has problematised childhood (Timimi 2002).

In reality psychiatric patients are often prescribed a whole cocktail of drugs, often at high doses. Many take a combination of neuroleptics, so-called mood stabilisers and benzodiazepines, all of which have sedative effects that dampen down and restrict nervous system activity in different ways. A British government report published in 2007 suggested that up to one in three psychiatric patients was being overtreated with drugs

(Healthcare Commission 2007). Other surveys have found that 25% of patients on neuroleptics are prescribed higher than recommended doses (Harrington et al. 2002). In addition, patients have to be prescribed drugs to counteract the physical and psychological consequences of their psychiatric medication. Hence many are now taking statins, antidiabetic medications and anti-obesity drugs to alleviate the metabolic disturbance caused by some of the newer neuroleptics, olanzapine and clozapine in particular. Anticholinergic drugs are frequently prescribed to combat severe and debilitating Parkinson's disease-like symptoms, the manifestation of the dopamine blockade caused by the neuroleptics. And antidepressants are prescribed in an attempt to combat the inevitable depression that accompanies the effects of so many sedative drugs. It is not surprising, therefore, that psychiatric inpatients wards are full of people who are obviously 'drugged' and spend much of their time asleep, or that many patients seek out illegal drugs especially cannabis and stimulants to try and counteract the effects of taking so many sedatives.

In retrospect the physical treatments of the mid-20th century, such as insulin coma therapy and frontal lobotomy, stand revealed as dangerous and degrading procedures perpetrated on vulnerable people in the name of medical progress. In the same way the multiple and long-term drugging of modern day psychiatric patients will surely some day be acknowledged as a dangerous fraud. At least the physical procedures were restricted by their cumbersome nature to those who were severely disturbed enough to require hospital admission. Drug treatment, in contrast, can be pressed onto a much larger proportion of the population, spreading the tentacles of psychiatric power ever further out into society.

The creators of the myth

The evidence presented in this book demonstrates the eagerness of the psychiatric profession to embrace the myth of disease-specific treatments. This is understandable, given the profession's long-standing battle to align itself squarely as a branch of the medical profession. Thus psychiatric disorders have generally been conceptualised as biological conditions and physical interventions have been at the heart of psychiatric therapeutics, despite the influence of psychoanalysis and social psychiatry at times in parts of the world. In the 19th century the emergence of psychiatry was intimately linked to its control of the asylum system, but the fact that these institutions made the chronicity of mental disorders highly visible, led to them becoming a source of professional embarrassment. From the beginning of the 20th century psychiatry sought to relocate its practice in general hospitals and outpatient departments. Drug treatments, especially if they could be presented as acting on a disease process, were well suited to this new environment. They also helped to give psychiatry a strong claim to jurisdiction over discontent in the community against other contenders such as social workers and psychologists.

The psychiatric profession was supported in its aims by a State that was seeking technical solutions for various social problems. Psychiatry offered the possibility of transforming the complex political problem of how to manage psychiatric disturbance into a medical and technical issue. Although the early 20th-century British State embraced the notion of social intervention and was highly authoritarian in some regards, it still had to attend to the deeply ingrained liberal ideals of the 19th century, which regarded government with suspicion and prized individual liberty. Therefore, the ability to remove difficult issues of social control from the political arena was appealing. Later in the century these imperatives merged with financial incentives to close down the Victorian asylums. The new drugs, with their reportedly miraculous effects, were an important part of the rationale for changes in the mental health system that were introduced during the 1950s and 1960s. They helped justify both the turn towards community care and the development of more medicalised legislation.

Joan Busfield has pointed out how the pharmaceutical industry helps to create a 'culture in which the use of drugs is encouraged even when this is unhelpful, counterproductive and even harmful' (Busfield 2006, p. 300). It is able to create such a culture by the power it exerts over the 'fact making' process through its conduct of research and orchestration of publicity about drugs. The industry and the knowledge it helps to produce have played an important role in establishing drugs as the dominant form of psychiatric treatment since the middle of the 20th century. The scale of some of the advertising campaigns in the 1950s and 1960s indicates that the industry already regarded psychiatry as a potentially fertile market. However the relation of the pharmaceutical industry to views on psychotropic drug action is complex. At different times it has suited the industry to promote psychiatric drugs both as producing drug-induced states such as stimulation and sedation, and as having disease-specific actions. However since the 1990s the industry has thrown its weight behind a disease-centred model of the nature of psychiatric drug treatment. Psychiatric conditions are attributed to hypothetical 'chemical imbalances' and medications are promoted for their ability to correct an abnormal biochemical state. This change may have been a reaction to the scandal of the mass prescribing of benzodiazepines that was revealed in the 1980s, since these drugs are not generally regarded as having a disease-specific action. With the commercial muscle of the pharmaceutical industry promoting it, the idea that our emotions and problems originate in abnormal biological processes that can be rectified by drugs has achieved greater credibility than ever before. People have started to interpret their experiences in terms of their brain chemicals. As social scientist Nikolas Rose suggests, we have become a society of 'neurochemical selves' and millions of people worldwide are now convinced that they need to take psychiatric drugs to be normal (Rose 2004).

Identifying the interests that have shaped and distorted what passes as knowledge about psychiatric drugs creates opportunities for 'resistance', in Foucault's terms. These opportunities can help to shape a different form of knowledge and activity freed from the constraints of those particular interests. The drug-centred model provides a basis for such a knowledge. It puts the modest and usually temporary benefits of drugs in perspective and exposes the damage that drug use inflicts. It allows people to determine for themselves whether drugs bring more benefits than harms, without the scientific illusion that they reverse the nature of the problem. It helps to lift the veil of medical jargon, exposing our miracle cures as psychoactive chemicals, which distort normal brain function by producing a state of intoxication. And by revealing the involuntary use of drugs as a form of chemical control it points the way to a more honest and humane response to psychiatric disturbance.

Notes

2 An Alternative Drug-Centred Model of Drug Action

1. Sedative drugs such as diazepam (Valium) and lorazepam, commonly used for acute tranquillisation and also used recreationally by some drug misusers.
2. An 'intention to treat' analysis is an analysis of outcome of the original groups produced by randomisation with everyone analysed according to the treatment they were intended to receive.
3. The half-life is a measure of the time it takes to eliminate 50% of the drug from the body and it is a measure of the speed of action and elimination of a drug.

3 Physical Treatments and the Disease-Centred Model

1. I am indebted especially to Robert Whitaker (2002) and Leonard Roy Franks (1978) for material on the history of insulin coma therapy and ECT.
2. At the beginning of the 20th century, Emil Kraepelin, a German psychiatrist divided severe psychiatric disturbance into two conditions: dementia praecox, which became known as schizophrenia, and manic depression.

5 The Birth of the Idea of an 'Antipsychotic'

1. Movement disorders such as Parkinson's disease-like symptoms caused by dysfunction of the extrapyramidal region of the brain that includes the basal ganglia.
2. A drug-induced effect consisting of motor and psychological restlessness.
3. Thorazine was the brand name for chlorpromazine in the United States.
4. Negative symptoms of schizophrenia is a term used to refer to symptoms such as apathy, social withdrawal and reduced emotional responsiveness associated with this diagnosis.

6 Are Neuroleptics Effective and Specific? A Review of the Evidence

1. Successful treatment was defined as a Clinical Global Impression scale score of 3, mild, or above, or a score of 4, moderately ill, plus improvement of two plus points from baseline.

2. A funnel plot is when studies are plotted according to their size and effect. Studies should be spread out symmetrically around the average effect. If smaller negative studies are not published the plot is asymmetrical.
3. The fluid in the nervous system.

7 What Do Neuroleptics Really Do? A Drug-Centred Account

1. Droperidol is an older neuroleptic, which was commonly used but is now withdrawn due to cardiac toxicity.
2. Tolerance is when the effects of drugs are counteracted by bodily adaptations.
3. Grey matter refers to the nerve cell bodies, white matter to the nerve cell fibres.
4. The thalamus is a mass of grey matter situated in the forebrain that is involved in arousal, movement and acts as a relay between different parts of the brain.
5. Anticholinergic drugs are prescribed to people on neuroleptics to reduce extrapyramidal symptoms and they are thought to impair cognitive function.
6. Dyslipidaemia refers to abnormalities of blood lipids (fats), particularly raised cholesterol and increased triglycerides.

8 The Construction of the 'Antidepressant'

1. Known as norepinephrine in North America.
2. Neurasthenia was a common diagnosis throughout the early and mid-20th century, which described a state of chronic fatigue and weakness. It is still listed in the International Classification of Disease and still used in some parts of the world, such as China.

9 Is There Such a Thing as an 'Antidepressant'? A Review of the Evidence

1. Relative risk is the ratio of the risk (in this case the risk of 'response') in one group compared to another.

10 What Do Antidepressants Really Do?

1. A dopamine agonist is a drug that stimulates dopamine receptors.
2. SSRI drugs are associated with sexual problems such as anorgasmia and delayed ejaculation.

11 The Idea of Special Drugs for Manic Depression (Bipolar Disorder)

1. See Chapter 3, note 2.

13 Democratic Drug Treatment: Implications of the Drug-Centred Model

1. Acute dystonia is sudden and severe muscular spasm which can infrequently be life threatening.
2. Neuroleptic malignant syndrome is a condition of increased muscle tone, hyperthermia, delirium and dysregulation of the autonomic nervous system which has a significant mortality.

References

Abbott Laboratories. www.depakoteer.com/bipolar_patient/index.html. 06.11.2006.

Abel, K. M., Allin, M. P., Kucharska-Pietura, K., David, A., Andrew, C., Williams, S., Brammer, M. J., & Phillips, M. L. 2003, 'Ketamine alters neural processing of facial emotion recognition in healthy men: an fMRI study', *Neuroreport*, vol. 14, no. 3, pp. 387–391.

Abi-Dargham, A. 2004, 'Do we still believe in the dopamine hypothesis? New data bring new evidence', *Int.J.Neuropsychopharmacol.*, vol. 7, suppl. 1, pp. S1–S5.

Abi-Dargham, A., Gil, R., Krystal, J., Baldwin, R. M., Seibyl, J. P., Bowers, M., van Dyck, C. H., Charney, D. S., Innis, R. B., & Laruelle, M. 1998, 'Increased striatal dopamine transmission in schizophrenia: confirmation in a second cohort', *Am.J.Psychiatry*, vol. 155, no. 6, pp. 761–767.

Abi-Dargham, A., Mawlawi, O., Lombardo, I., Gil, R., Martinez, D., Huang, Y., Hwang, D. R., Keilp, J., Kochan, L., Van Heertum, R., Gorman, J. M., & Laruelle, M. 2002, 'Prefrontal dopamine D1 receptors and working memory in schizophrenia', *J.Neurosci.*, vol. 22, no. 9, pp. 3708–3719.

Abi-Dargham, A., Rodenhiser, J., Printz, D., Zea-Ponce, Y., Gil, R., Kegeles, L. S., Weiss, R., Cooper, T. B., Mann, J. J., Van Heertum, R. L., Gorman, J. M., & Laruelle, M. 2000, 'Increased baseline occupancy of D2 receptors by dopamine in schizophrenia', *Proc.Natl.Acad.Sci.U.S.A*, vol. 97, no. 14, pp. 8104–8109.

Abse, D. W., Dahlstrom, W. G., & Tolley, A. G. 1960, 'Evaluation of tranquillizing drugs in the management of acute mental disturbance', *Am.J.Psychiatry*, vol. 116, pp. 973–980.

Ackner, B., Harris, A., & Oldham, A. J. 1957, 'Insulin treatment of schizophrenia: controlled study', *Lancet*, vol. 2, pp. 607–611.

Adler, C. M., Elman, I., Weisenfeld, N., Kestler, L., Pickar, D., & Breier, A. 2000, 'Effects of acute metabolic stress on striatal dopamine release in healthy volunteers', *Neuropsychopharmacology*, vol. 22, no. 5, pp. 545–550.

Aitken, M. & Holt, F. 2000, 'A prescription for drug marketing', *The McKinsey Quarterly*, vol. 22nd March 2000, p. 82.

Akiskal, H. S. 1996, 'The prevalent clinical spectrum of bipolar disorders: beyond DSM-IV', *J.Clin.Psychopharmacol.*, vol. 16, no. 2, suppl. 1, pp. 4S–14S.

American Psychiatric Association 1980, *Task force report: tardive dyskinesia*, American Psychiatric Association, Washington, DC.

American Psychiatric Association. Schizophrenia, 1996.

American Psychiatric Association. Lets talk facts about depression. 2005.

Ananth, J., Ghadirian, A. M., & Engelsmann, F. 1987, 'Lithium and memory: a review', *Can.J.Psychiatry*, vol. 32, no. 4, pp. 312–316.

Andersson, U., Eckernas, S. A., Hartvig, P., Ulin, J., Langstrom, B., & Haggstrom, J. E. 1990, 'Striatal binding of 11C-NMSP studied with positron emission tomography in patients with persistent tardive dyskinesia: no evidence for altered dopamine D2 receptor binding', *J.Neural Transm.Gen.Sect.*, vol. 79, no. 3, pp. 215–226.

Angell, M. 2004, *The truth about the drug companies: how they deceive us and what to do about it.* Random House, New York.

Angst, J. 1986, 'The course of affective disorders', *Psychopathology*, vol. 19, suppl. 2, pp. 47–52.

Angst, J., Gamma, A., Benazzi, F., Ajdacic, V., Eich, D., & Rossler, W. 2003, 'Toward a re-definition of subthreshold bipolarity: epidemiology and proposed criteria for bipolar-II, minor bipolar disorders and hypomania', *J.Affect.Disord.*, vol. 73, no. 1–2, pp. 133–146.

Angst, J., Scheidegger, P., & Stabl, M. 1993, 'Efficacy of moclobemide in different patient groups. Results of new subscales of the Hamilton Depression Rating Scale', *Clin.Neuropharmacol.*, vol. 16, suppl. 2, pp. S55–S62.

Angst, J., Weis, P., Grof, P., Baastrup, P. C., & Schou, M. 1970, 'Lithium prophylaxis in recurrent affective disorders', *Br.J.Psychiatry*, vol. 116, no. 535, pp. 604–614.

Anonymous. Warley Hospital Brentwood. The first hundred years 1853–1953 incorporating into the second century 1953–1963, 1990. Brentwood, Essex, Warley Hospital.

Antidepressant Web 2006, 'The Antidepressant Web', www.socialaudit.org.uk/_disc/cgi-bin/discuss.pl.

Anton-Stephens, D. 1954, 'Preliminary observations on the psychiatric uses of chlorpromazine (largactil)', *J.Ment.Sci.*, vol. 100, no. 419, pp. 543–557.

Antonuccio, D. O., Danton, W. G., DeNelsky, G. Y., Greenberg, R. P., & Gordon, J. S. 1999, 'Raising questions about antidepressants', *Psychother.Psychosom.*, vol. 68, no. 1, pp. 3–14.

Appelbaum, P. S. & Redlich, A. 2006, 'Use of leverage over patients' money to promote adherence to psychiatric treatment', *J.Nerv.Ment.Dis.*, vol. 194, no. 4, pp. 294–302.

Armstrong, D. 1983, *Political Anatomy of the Body*, Cambridge University Press, Cambridge.

Arnt, J. 1982, 'Pharmacological specificity of conditioned avoidance response inhibition in rats: inhibition by neuroleptics and correlation to dopamine receptor blockade', *Acta Pharmacol.Toxicol.(Copenh)*, vol. 51, no. 4, pp. 321–329.

Ashton, H. 1986, 'Adverse effects of prolonged benzodiazepine use', *Adverse Drug Reaction Bulletin*, vol. June 1986, no. 118, pp. 440–43.

Askapatient.com 2007, www.askapatient.com/viewrating.asp?drug=20592&name=ZYPREXA-.

Aviram, U., Syme, S. L., & Cohen, J. B. 1976, 'The effects of policies and programs on reduction of mental hospitalization', *Soc.Sci.Med.*, vol. 10, no. 11–12, pp. 571–577.

Axelrod, J. 1996, 'The discovery of amine reuptake,' in *The Psychopharmacologists*, D. Healy, ed., Chapman & Hall, London, pp. 29–50.

Axelrod, J., Whitby, L. G., & Hertting, G. 1961, 'Effect of psychotropic drugs on the uptake of H3-norepinephrine by tissues', *Science*, vol. 133, pp. 383–384.

Ayd, F. J., Jr. 1961a, 'A critique of antidepressants', *Dis.Nerv.Syst.*, vol. 22, no. 5, Pt 2, pp. 32–36.

Ayd, F. J., Jr. 1961b, *Recognising the Depressed Patient*, Grune & Stratton Inc., New York.

Baastrup, P. C. & Schou, M. 1967, 'Lithium as a prophylactic agents. Its effect against recurrent depressions and manic-depressive psychosis', *Arch.Gen. Psychiatry*, vol. 16, no. 2, pp. 162–172.

Baker, A. A., Game, J. A., & Thorpe, J. G. 1958, 'Physical treatment for schizophrenia', *J.Ment.Sci.*, vol. 104, no. 436, pp. 860–864.

Baldessarini, R. 1985, 'Drugs and the treatment of psychiatric disorders,' in *The Pharmacological Basis of Therapeutics*, A. Gilman et al., eds, Macmillan, New York, pp. 387–445.

Baldessarini, R. J., Kando, J. C., & Centorrino, F. 1995, 'Hospital use of antipsychotic agents in 1989 and 1993: stable dosing with decreased length of stay', *Am.J.Psychiatry*, vol. 152, no. 7, pp. 1038–1044.

Baldessarini, R. J., Tondo, L., Davis, P., Pompili, M., Goodwin, F. K., & Hennen, J. 2006, 'Decreased risk of suicides and attempts during long-term lithium treatment: a meta-analytic review', *Bipolar.Disord.*, vol. 8, no. 5, Pt 2, pp. 625–639.

Baldessarini, R. J., Tondo, L., Floris, G., & Rudas, N. 1997, 'Reduced morbidity after gradual discontinuation of lithium treatment for bipolar I and II disorders: a replication study', *Am.J.Psychiatry*, vol. 154, no. 4, pp. 551–553.

Baldessarini, R. J., Tondo, L., & Hennen, J. 1999, 'Effects of lithium treatment and its discontinuation on suicidal behavior in bipolar manic-depressive disorders', *J.Clin.Psychiatry*, vol. 60, suppl. 2, pp. 77–84.

Baldessarini, R. J., Tondo, L., & Viguera, A. C. 1999, 'Discontinuing lithium maintenance treatment in bipolar disorders: risks and implications', *Bipolar.Disord.*, vol. 1, no. 1, pp. 17–24.

Baldessarini, R. J. & Viguera, A. C. 1995, 'Neuroleptic withdrawal in schizophrenic patients', *Arch.Gen.Psychiatry*, vol. 52, no. 3, pp. 189–192.

Baldessarini, R. J., Viguera, A. C., & Tondo, L. 1999, 'Discontinuing psychotropic agents', *J.Psychopharmacol.*, vol. 13, no. 3, pp. 292–293.

Ball, J. R. & Kiloh, L. G. 1959, 'A controlled trial of imipramine in treatment of depressive states', *Br.Med.J.*, vol. 2, no. 5159, pp. 1052–1055.

Ballenger, J. C. & Post, R. M. 1980, 'Carbamazepine in manic-depressive illness: a new treatment', *Am.J.Psychiatry*, vol. 137, no. 7, pp. 782–790.

Ban, T. 1996, 'They used to call it psychiatry', in *The Psychopharmacologists Volume 1*, D. Healy, ed., Altman (Chapman and Hall), London, pp. 587–620.

Barnhart, W. J., Makela, E. H., & Latocha, M. J. 2004, 'SSRI-induced apathy syndrome: a clinical review', *J.Psychiatr.Pract.*, vol. 10, no. 3, pp. 196–199.

Barton, C. D., Jr., Dufer, D., Monderer, R., Cohen, M. J., Fuller, H. J., Clark, M. R., & DePaulo, J. R., Jr. 1993, 'Mood variability in normal subjects on lithium', *Biol.Psychiatry*, vol. 34, no. 12, pp. 878–884.

Batki, S. L. & Harris, D. S. 2004, 'Quantitative drug levels in stimulant psychosis: relationship to symptom severity, catecholamines and hyperkinesia', *Am.J.Addict.*, vol. 13, no. 5, pp. 461–470.

Beasley, C. M., Jr., Dornseif, B. E., Bosomworth, J. C., Sayler, M. E., Rampey, A. H., Jr., Heiligenstein, J. H., Thompson, V. L., Murphy, D. J., & Masica, D. N. 1991a, 'Fluoxetine and suicide: a meta-analysis of controlled trials of treatment for depression', *Br.Med.J.*, vol. 303, no. 6804, pp. 685–692.

Beasley, C. M., Jr., Dornseif, B. E., Pultz, J. A., Bosomworth, J. C., & Sayler, M. E. 1991b, 'Fluoxetine versus trazodone: efficacy and activating-sedating effects', *J.Clin.Psychiatry*, vol. 52, no. 7, pp. 294–299.

Beasley, C. M., Jr., Sayler, M. E., Bosomworth, J. C., & Wernicke, J. F. 1991c, 'High-dose fluoxetine: efficacy and activating-sedating effects in agitated and retarded depression', *J.Clin.Psychopharmacol.*, vol. 11, pp. 166–174.

Beasley, C. M., Jr. & Potvin, J. H. 1993, 'Fluoxetine: activating and sedating effects', *Int.Clin.Psychopharmacol.*, vol. 8, no. 4, pp. 271–275.

Beasley, C. M., Jr., Sayler, M. E., Weiss, A. M., & Potvin, J. H. 1992, 'Fluoxetine: activating and sedating effects at multiple fixed doses', *J.Clin.Psychopharmacol.*, vol. 12, no. 5, pp. 328–333.

Bech, P., Cialdella, P., Haugh, M. C., Birkett, M. A., Hours, A., Boissel, J. P., & Tollefson, G. D. 2000, 'Meta-analysis of randomised controlled trials of fluox-etine v. placebo and tricyclic antidepressants in the short-term treatment of major depression', *Br.J.Psychiatry*, vol. 176, pp. 421–428.

Belmaker, R. H. & Wald, D. 1977, 'Haloperidol in normals', *Br.J.Psychiatry*, vol. 131, pp. 222–223.

Bennett, A. E. 1945, 'An evaluation of the shock therapies', *Dis. Nerv.Sys.*, vol. 6, p. 21.

Bentall, R. 2006, 'Madness explained: why we must reject the Kraepelinian para-digm and replace it with a 'complaint-orientated' approach to understanding mental illness', *Med.Hypotheses*, vol. 66, no. 2, pp. 220–233.

Berenson, A. Eli Lilly said to play down risks of top pill. *New York Times*, 17.12.2006. New York.

Bernstein, S. & Kaufman, M. R. 1960, 'A psychological analysis of apparent depression following Rauwolfia therapy', *Journal of Mount Sinai Hospital*, vol. 27, pp. 525–530.

Berridge, C. W. 2006, 'Neural substrates of psychostimulant-induced arousal', *Neuropsychopharmacology*, vol. 31, pp. 2333–2340.

Bhanji, N. H. & Margolese, H. C. 2004, 'Tardive dyskinesia associated with olanzapine in a neuroleptic-naive patient with schizophrenia', *Can.J. Psychiatry*, vol. 49, no. 5, p. 343.

Bielski, R. J. & Friedel, R. O. 1976, 'Prediction of tricyclic antidepressant response: a critical review', *Arch.Gen.Psychiatry*, vol. 33, no. 12, pp. 1479–1489.

Bilder, R. M., Goldman, R. S., Volavka, J., Czobor, P., Hoptman, M., Sheitman, B., Lindenmayer, J. P., Citrome, L., McEvoy, J., Kunz, M., Chakos, M., Cooper, T. B., Horowitz, T. L., & Lieberman, J. A. 2002, 'Neurocognitive effects of cloza-pine, olanzapine, risperidone, and haloperidol in patients with chronic schizo-phrenia or schizoaffective disorder', *Am.J.Psychiatry*, vol. 159, no. 6, pp. 1018–1028.

Bilder, R. M., Reiter, G., Bates, J., Lencz, T., Szeszko, P., Goldman, R. S., Robinson, D., Lieberman, J. A., & Kane, J. M. 2006, 'Cognitive development in schizo-phrenia: follow-back from the first episode', *J.Clin.Exp.Neuropsychol.*, vol. 28, no. 2, pp. 270–282.

Blackwell, B. & Shepherd, M. 1968, 'Prophylactic lithium: another therapeutic myth? An examination of the evidence to date', *Lancet*, vol. 1, no. 7549, pp. 968–971.

Blashki, T. G., Mowbray, R., & Davies, B. 1971, 'Controlled trial of amitriptyline in general practice', *Br.Med.J.*, vol. 1, pp. 133–138.

Bockoven, J. S. & Solomon, H. C. 1975, 'Comparison of two five-year follow-up studies: 1948 to 1952 and 1967 to 1972', *Am.J.Psychiatry*, vol. 132, no. 8, pp. 796–801.

Bola, J. R. & Mosher, L. R. 2003, 'Treatment of acute psychosis without neuroleptics: two-year outcomes from the Soteria project', *J.Nerv.Ment.Dis.*, vol. 191, no. 4, pp. 219–229.

Bond, C. H. 1915, 'The position of psychiatry and the role of the general hospitals in its improvement.', *J.Ment.Sci.*, vol. 61, pp. 1–17.

Borison, R. L. & Diamond, B. I. 1978, 'A new animal model for schizophrenia: interactions with adrenergic mechanisms', *Biol.Psychiatry*, vol. 13, no. 2, pp. 217–225.

Bourin, M., Fiocco, A. J., & Clenet, F. 2001, 'How valuable are animal models in defining antidepressant activity?', *Hum.Psychopharmacol.*, vol. 16, no. 1, pp. 9–21.

Bourne, H. 1953, 'The insulin myth', *Lancet*, vol. 265, p. 1259.

Bowden, C. L., Brugger, A. M., Swann, A. C., Calabrese, J. R., Janicak, P. G., Petty, F., Dilsaver, S. C., Davis, J. M., Rush, A. J., Small, J. G., Garza-Trevino, E. S., Risch, C., Goodnick, P. J., & Morris, D. D. 1994, 'Efficacy of divalproex vs lithium and placebo in the treatment of mania. The Depakote Mania Study Group', *JAMA*, vol. 271, no. 12, pp. 918–924.

Bowden, C. L., Calabrese, J. R., McElroy, S. L., Gyulai, L., Wassef, A., Petty, F., Pope, H. G., Jr., Chou, J. C., Keck, P. E., Jr., Rhodes, L. J., Swann, A. C., Hirschfeld, R. M., & Wozniak, P. J. 2000, 'A randomized, placebo-controlled 12-month trial of divalproex and lithium in treatment of outpatients with bipolar I disorder. Divalproex Maintenance Study Group', *Arch.Gen.Psychiatry*, vol. 57, no. 5, pp. 481–489.

Bowden, C. L., Calabrese, J. R., Sachs, G., Yatham, L. N., Asghar, S. A., Hompland, M., Montgomery, P., Earl, N., Smoot, T. M., & DeVeaugh-Geiss, J. 2003, 'A placebo-controlled 18-month trial of lamotrigine and lithium maintenance treatment in recently manic or hypomanic patients with bipolar I disorder', *Arch.Gen.Psychiatry*, vol. 60, no. 4, pp. 392–400.

Bowes, H. A. 1956, 'The ataractic drugs: the present position of chlorpromazine, frenquel, pacatal and reserpine in the psychiatric hospital', *Am.J.Psychiatry*, vol. 113, pp. 530–539.

Bracken, P. & Thomas, P. 2005, *Post Psychiatry: Mental Health in a Post Modern World.* OUP, Oxford.

Braden, W., Fink, E. B., Qualls, C. B., Ho, C. K., & Samuels, W. O. 1982, 'Lithium and chlorpromazine in psychotic inpatients', *Psychiatry Res.*, vol. 7, no. 1, pp. 69–81.

Bralet, M. C., Yon, V., Loas, G., & Noisette, C. 2000, 'Cause of mortality in schizophrenic patients: prospective study of years of a cohort of 150 chronic schizophrenic patients', *Encephale*, vol. 26, no. 6, pp. 32–41.

Brandon, S., Cowley, P., McDonald, C., Neville, P., Palmer, R., & Wellstood-Eason, S. 1984, 'Electroconvulsive therapy: results in depressive illness from the Leicestershire trial', *Br.Med.J.(Clin.Res.Ed.)*, vol. 288, no. 6410, pp. 22–25.

Brandon, S., Cowley, P., McDonald, C., Neville, P., Palmer, R., & Wellstood-Eason, S. 1985, 'Leicester ECT trial: results in schizophrenia', *Br.J.Psychiatry*, vol. 146, pp. 177–183.

Braslow, J. 1997, *Mental Ills and Bodily Cures.* University of California Press, Berkeley, CA.

Braude, M. 1937, *The Prinicples and Practice of Clinical Psychiatry*, P. Blakiston's Son & Co., Philadelphia.

Breggin, P. R. 1993a, 'Parallels between neuroleptic effects and lethargic encephalitis: the production of dyskinesias and cognitive disorders', *Brain Cogn.*, vol. 23, no. 1, pp. 8–27.

Breggin, P. R. 1993b, *Toxic Psychiatry.* Fontana, London.

Breggin, P. R. 1997, *Brain Disabling Treatments in Psychiatry: Drugs Electroshock and the Role of the FDA.* Springer Publishing Company, New York.

Breggin, P. R. 2001, *Talking Back to Ritalin.* Perseus Publishing, Cambridge, MA.

Breggin, P. R. 2006, 'Intoxicatrion anosognosia: the spellbinding effect of psychiatric drugs', *Ethical Hum.Psychol.Psychiatry*, vol. 8, no. 3, pp. 201–215.

Breier, A. 1989, 'A.E. Bennett award paper. Experimental approaches to human stress research: assessment of neurobiological mechanisms of stress in volunteers and psychiatric patients', *Biol.Psychiatry*, vol. 26, no. 5, pp. 438–462.

Breier, A., Su, T. P., Saunders, R., Carson, R. E., Kolachana, B. S., de Bartolomeis, A., Weinberger, D. R., Weisenfeld, N., Malhotra, A. K., Eckelman, W. C., & Pickar, D. 1997, 'Schizophrenia is associated with elevated amphetamine-induced synaptic dopamine concentrations: evidence from a novel positron emission tomography method', *Proc.Natl.Acad.Sci.U.S.A*, vol. 94, no. 6, pp. 2569–2574.

Brill, H. & Patton, R. 1958, 'Some statistical trends of importance for planning psychiatric programs in New York', *Bull.N.Y.Acad.Med.*, vol. 34, no. 12, pp. 786–793.

Brill, H. & Patton, R. E. 1957, 'Analysis of 1955–1956 population fall in New York State mental hospitals in first year of large-scale use of tranquilizing drugs', *Am.J.Psychiatry*, vol. 114, no. 6, pp. 509–517.

Brill, H. & Patton, R. E. 1962, 'Clinical-statistical analysis of population changes in New York State mental hospitals since introduction of psychotropic drugs', *Am.J.Psychiatry*, vol. 119, pp. 20–35.

British Medical Association and Pharmaceutical Society of Great Britain 1963, *British National Formulary*, Alternative Edition, based on a pharmacological classification edn, British Medical Association and Pharmaceutical Society of Great Britain, London.

Brown, W. A. 2002, 'Are antidepressants as ineffective as they look?', *Prev.Treat.*, vol. 5, www.content.apa.org/journals/pre/5/1/26.

Brugha, T. S., Bebbington, P. E., MacCarthy, B., Sturt, E., & Wykes, T. 1992, 'Antidepressants may not assist recovery in practice: a naturalistic prospective survey', *Acta Psychiatr.Scand.*, vol. 86, no. 1, pp. 5–11.

Burt, D. R., Creese, I., & Snyder, S. H. 1977, 'Antischizophrenic drugs: chronic treatment elevates dopamine receptor binding in brain', *Science*, vol. 196, no. 4287, pp. 326–328.

Busfield, J. 2006, 'Pills, power, people: Sociological understandings of the pharmaceutical industry', *Sociology*, vol. 40, pp. 297–314.

Busto, U. E., Bremner, K. E., Knight, K., terBrugge, K., & Sellers, E. M. 2000, 'Long-term benzodiazepine therapy does not result in brain abnormalities', *J.Clin.Psychopharmacol.*, vol. 20, no. 1, pp. 2–6.

Butler, T. 1985, *Mental Health, Social Policy and the Law.* Macmillan, London.

Cade, J. F. J. 1949, 'Lithium salts in the treatment of psychotic excitement.', *Med.J.Aust.*, vol. 36, pp. 349–352.

Cahn, W., Hulshoff Pol, H. E., Lems, E. B., van Haren, N. E., Schnack, H. G., van der Linden, J. A., Schothorst, P. F., van Engeland, H., & Kahn, R. S. 2002, 'Brain volume changes in first-episode schizophrenia: a 1-year follow-up study', *Arch.Gen.Psychiatry*, vol. 59, no. 11, pp. 1002–1010.

Calabrese, J. R., Bowden, C. L., Sachs, G., Yatham, L. N., Behnke, K., Mehtonen, O. P., Montgomery, P., Ascher, J., Paska, W., Earl, N., & DeVeaugh-Geiss, J. 2003, 'A placebo-controlled 18-month trial of lamotrigine and lithium maintenance treatment in recently depressed patients with bipolar I disorder', *J.Clin.Psychiatry*, vol. 64, no. 9, pp. 1013–1024.

California State Senate 1956, *California 1955/56 Senate Interim Committee on the Treatment of Mental Illness. First Partial Report*. California State Senate, Sacramento CA.

Calil, H. M., Zwicker, A. P., & Klepacz, S. 1990, 'The effects of lithium carbonate on healthy volunteers: mood stabilization?', *Biol.Psychiatry*, vol. 27, no. 7, pp. 711–722.

Carlsson, A. 1988, 'The current status of the dopamine hypothesis of schizophrenia', *Neuropsychopharmacology*, vol. 1, no. 3, pp. 179–186.

Carone, B. J., Harrow, M., & Westermeyer, J. F. 1991, 'Posthospital course and outcome in schizophrenia', *Arch.Gen.Psychiatry*, vol. 48, no. 3, pp. 247–253.

Carpenter, W. T., Jr., Buchanan, R. W., Kirkpatrick, B., & Breier, A. F. 1999, 'Diazepam treatment of early signs of exacerbation in schizophrenia', *Am.J.Psychiatry*, vol. 156, no. 2, pp. 299–303.

Carpenter, W. T., Jr., Hanlon, T. E., Heinrichs, D. W., Summerfelt, A. T., Kirkpatrick, B., Levine, J., & Buchanan, R. W. 1990, 'Continuous versus targeted medication in schizophrenic outpatients: outcome results', *Am.J.Psychiatry*, vol. 147, no. 9, pp. 1138–1148.

Casey, J. F., Bennett, I. F., Lindley, C. J., Hollister, L. E., Gordon, M. H., & Springer, N. N. 1960a, 'Drug therapy in schizophrenia. A controlled study of the relative effectiveness of chlorpromazine, promazine, phenobarbital, and placebo', *Arch.Gen.Psychiatry*, vol. 2, pp. 210–220.

Casey, J. F., Lasky, J. J., Klett, C. J., & Hollister, L. E. 1960b, 'Treatment of schizophrenic reactions with phenothiazine derivatives. A comparative study of chlorpromazine, triflupromazine, mepazine, prochlorperazine, perphenazine, and phenobarbital', *Am.J.Psychiatry*, vol. 117, pp. 97–105.

Cavanagh, J., Smyth, R., & Goodwin, G. M. 2004, 'Relapse into mania or depression following lithium discontinuation: a 7-year follow-up', *Acta Psychiatr.Scand.*, vol. 109, no. 2, pp. 91–95.

Challoner, J. 'Invisible psychosis; a survey of patients with psychosis managed by GPs without input from secondary care'. 2006.

Chessin, M., Kramer, E. R., & Scott, C. C. 1957, 'Modifications of the pharmacology of reserpine and serotonin by iproniazid', *J.Pharmacol.Exp.Ther.*, vol. 119, no. 4, pp. 453–460.

Chouinard, G. 1988, 'The use of benzodiazepines in the treatment of manicdepressive illness', *J.Clin.Psychiatry*, vol. 49, pp. 15–20.

Chouinard, G. & Jones, B. D. 1980, 'Neuroleptic-induced supersensitivity psychosis: clinical and pharmacologic characteristics', *Am.J.Psychiatry*, vol. 137, no. 1, pp. 16–21.

Chouinard, G., Young, S. N., & Annable, L. 1983, 'Antimanic effect of clonazepam', *Biol.Psychiatry*, vol. 18, no. 4, pp. 451–466.

Cleare, A. 2005, 'Unipolar depression', in *Core Psychiatry*, P. Wright, M. Phelan, & J. Stern, eds, Elsevier Saunders, Edinburgh.

Cohen, D. 1997, 'A critique of the use of neuroleptic drugs in psychiatry,' in *From Placebo to Panacea*, S. Fisher & R. P. Greenberg, eds, John Wiley & Sons, New York, pp. 173–228.

Cohen, D. & Jacobs, D. 2007, 'Randomized controlled trials of antidepressants: clinically and scientifically irrelevant', *Debates in Neuroscience*, vol. 1, pp. 44–45.

Cohen, D., McGubbin, M., Collin, J., & Perodeau, G. 2001, 'Medications as social phenomena', *Health*, vol. 5, pp. 441–469.

Cohen, H. & Cohen, D. 1993, 'What may be gained from neuropsychological investigations of tardive dyskinesia?', *Brain Cogn.*, vol. 23, no. 1, pp. 1–7.

Coleman, E. A., Sackeim, H. A., Prudic, J., Devanand, D. P., McElhiney, M. C., & Moody, B. J. 1996, 'Subjective memory complaints prior to and following electroconvulsive therapy', *Biol.Psychiatry*, vol. 39, no. 5, pp. 346–356.

Commission for Healthcare Audit and Inspection. 2007, *Count me in. Results of the 2006 National Census of Inpatients in Mental Health and Learning Disability Services in England and Wales*. Commission for Healthcare Audit and Inspection, London.

Cook, L. 1958, 'Reports of clinical drug investigations in psychiatry with special reference to methodologies', *Psychiatr.Res.Rep.*, vol. 9, pp. 1–4.

Cookson, J. 2005, 'A brief history of psychiatry', in *Core Psychiatry*, Second edn, P. Wright, J. Stern, & M. Phelan, eds, Elsevier Saunders, Edinburgh, pp. 1–12.

Coppen, A. 1967, 'The biochemistry of affective disorders', *Br.J.Psychiatry*, vol. 113, no. 504, pp. 1237–1264.

Coryell, W., Keller, M., Endicott, J., Andreasen, N., Clayton, P., & Hirschfeld, R. 1989, 'Bipolar II illness: course and outcome over a five-year period', *Psychol.Med.*, vol. 19, no. 1, pp. 129–141.

Coryell, W., Winokur, G., Solomon, D., Shea, T., Leon, A., & Keller, M. 1997, 'Lithium and recurrence in a long-term follow-up of bipolar affective disorder', *Psychol.Med.*, vol. 27, no. 2, pp. 281–289.

Costa, E., Garattini, S., & Valzelli, L. 1960, 'Interactions between reserpine, chlor-promazine, and imipramine', *Experientia*, vol. 16, pp. 461–463.

Costall, B. & Naylor, R. J. 1976, 'A comparison of the abilities of typical neu-roleptic agents and of thioridazine, clozapine, sulpiride and metoclopramide to antagonise the hyperactivity induced by dopamine applied intracerebrally to areas of the extrapyramidal and mesolimbic systems', *Eur.J.Pharmacol.*, vol. 40, no. 1, pp. 9–19.

Crane, G. E. 1956, 'Further studies on iproniazid phosphate; isonicotinil-isopropyl-hydrazine phosphate marsilid', *J.Nerv.Ment.Dis.*, vol. 124, no. 3, pp. 322–331.

Crane, G. E. 1957, 'Iproniazid (marsilid) phosphate, a therapeutic agent for mental disorders and debilitating diseases', *Psychiatr.Res.Rep.Am.Psychiatr. Assoc.*, vol. 135, no. 8, pp. 142–152.

Cross, A. J., Crow, T. J., & Owen, F. 1981, '3H-Flupenthixol binding in post-mortem brains of schizophrenics: evidence for a selective increase in dopamine D2 receptors', *Psychopharmacology (Berl)*, vol. 74, no. 2, pp. 122–124.

Crow, T. J., Cross, A. J., Johnstone, E. C., Owen, F., Owens, D. G., & Waddington, J. L. 1982, 'Abnormal involuntary movements in schizophrenia: are they related to the disease process or its treatment? Are they associated with changes in dopamine receptors?', *J.Clin.Psychopharmacol.*, vol. 2, no. 5, pp. 336–340.

Crow, T. J., MacMillan, J. F., Johnson, A. L., & Johnstone, E. C. 1986, 'A randomised controlled trial of prophylactic neuroleptic treatment', *Br.J.Psychiatry*, vol. 148, pp. 120–127.

Cryan, J. F., Markou, A., & Lucki, I. 2002, 'Assessing antidepressant activity in rodents: recent developments and future trends', *Trend Pharmacol.Sci.*, vol. 23, pp. 238–245.

Cundall, R. L., Brooks, P. W., & Murray, L. G. 1972, 'A controlled evaluation of lithium prophylaxis in affective disorders', *Psychol.Med.*, vol. 2, no. 3, pp. 308–311.

D'Aquila, P. S., Panin, F., & Serra, G. 2004, 'Long-term imipramine withdrawal induces a depressive-like behaviour in the forced swimming test', *Eur.J.Pharmacol.*, vol. 492, no. 1, pp. 61–63.

D'Aquila, P. S., Peana, A. T., Panin, F., Grixoni, C., Cossu, M., & Serra, G. 2003, 'Reversal of antidepressant-induced dopaminergic behavioural supersensitivity after long-term chronic imipramine withdrawal', *Eur.J.Pharmacol.*, vol. 458, no. 1–2, pp. 129–134.

Dally, P. 1967, *Chemotherapy of Psychiatric Disorders*. Logos Press, London.

Dally, P. J. & Rohde, P. 1961, 'Comparison of antidepressant drugs in depressive illnesses', *Lancet*, vol. 1, pp. 18–20.

Dao-Castellana, M. H., Paillere-Martinot, M. L., Hantraye, P., Attar-Levy, D., Remy, P., Crouzel, C., Artiges, E., Feline, A., Syrota, A., & Martinot, J. L. 1997, 'Presynaptic dopaminergic function in the striatum of schizophrenic patients', *Schizophr.Res.*, vol. 23, no. 2, pp. 167–174.

David, A. S., Malmberg, A., Brandt, L., Allebeck, P., & Lewis, G. 1997, 'IQ and risk for schizophrenia: a population-based cohort study', *Psychol.Med.*, vol. 27, no. 6, pp. 1311–1323.

Davies, D. L. & Shepherd, M. 1955, 'Reserpine in the treatment of anxious and depressed patients', *Lancet*, vol. 269, no. 6881, pp. 117–120.

Davis, J. M., Chen, N., & Glick, I. D. 2003, 'A meta-analysis of the efficacy of second-generation antipsychotics', *Arch.Gen.Psychiatry*, vol. 60, no. 6, pp. 553–564.

Davis, J. M., Wang, Z., & Janicak, P. G. 1993, 'A quantitative analysis of clinical drug trials for the treatment of affective disorders', *Psychopharmacol.Bull.*, vol. 29, no. 2, pp. 175–181.

Davis, K. L., Kahn, R. S., Ko, G., & Davidson, M. 1991, 'Dopamine in schizophrenia: a review and reconceptualization', *Am.J.Psychiatry*, vol. 148, no. 11, pp. 1474–1486.

Dazzan, P., Morgan, K. D., Orr, K., Hutchinson, G., Chitnis, X., Suckling, J., Fearon, P., McGuire, P. K., Mallett, R. M., Jones, P. B., Leff, J., & Murray, R. M. 2005, 'Different effects of typical and atypical antipsychotics on grey matter in first episode psychosis: the AESOP study', *Neuropsychopharmacology*, vol. 30, no. 4, pp. 765–774.

Deegan, P. E. & Drake, R. E. 2006, 'Shared decision making and medication management in the recovery process', *Psychiatr.Serv.*, vol. 57, no. 11, pp. 1636–1639.

Delay, J. & Buisson, J. F. 1958, 'Psychic action of isoniazid in the treatment of depressive states', *J.Clin.Exp.Psychopathol.*, vol. 19, no. 2, suppl. 1, pp. 51–55.

Delay, J. & Deniker, P. 1952, '38 cas de psychoses traites par la cure prolongee et continue de 4560 R.P.', *C.R.Congres Med.Alien.Neurol.France*, vol. 50, pp. 503–513.

Delgado, P. L., Miller, H. L., Salomon, R. M., Licinio, J., Krystal, J. H., Moreno, F. A., Heninger, G. R., & Charney, D. S. 1999, 'Tryptophan-depletion challenge in depressed patients treated with desipramine or fluoxetine: implications for the role of serotonin in the mechanism of antidepressant action', *Biol.Psychiatry*, vol. 46, no. 2, pp. 212–220.

Delini-Stula, A. & Vassout, A. 1979, 'Modulation of dopamine-mediated behavioural responses by antidepressants: effects of single and repeated treatment', *Eur.J.Pharmacol.*, vol. 58, no. 4, pp. 443–451.

DeLisi, L. E., Hoff, A. L., Schwartz, J. E., Shields, G. W., Halthore, S. N., Gupta, S. M., Henn, F. A., & Anand, A. K. 1991, 'Brain morphology in first-episode schizophrenic-like psychotic patients: a quantitative magnetic resonance imaging study', *Biol.Psychiatry*, vol. 29, no. 2, pp. 159–175.

Denber, H. C. B. 1959, 'Side effects of phenothiazines,' in *Psychopharmacology Frontiers*, N. S. Kline, ed., Little, Brown, Boston, pp. 61–62.

Deniker, P. 1960, 'Experimental neurological syndromes and the new drug therapies in psychiatry', *Compr.Psychiatry*, vol. 1, pp. 92–102.

Deniker, P. 1970a, in *Discoveries in Biological Psychiatry*, F. Ayd & B. Blackwell, eds, JB Lippincott Company, Philadelphia.

Deniker, P. 1970b, 'Introduction of neuroleptic chemotherapy into psychiatry,' in *Discoveries in Biological Psychiatry*, F. Ayd & B. Blackwell, eds, JB Lippincott Company, Philadelphia, pp. 155–164.

Deniker, P. & Lemperiere, T. 1964, 'Drug treatment of depression,' in *Depression: Proceedings of the Symposium held at Cambridge 22 to 26 September 1959.* Cambridge University Press, Cambridge, pp. 214–234.

Deptula, D. & Pomara, N. 1990, 'Effects of antidepressants on human performance: a review', *J.Clin.Psychopharmacol.*, vol. 10, no. 2, pp. 105–111.

Devanand, D. P., Dwork, A. J., Hutchinson, E. R., Bolwig, T. G., & Sackeim, H. A. 1994, 'Does ECT alter brain structure?', *Am.J.Psychiatry*, vol. 151, no. 7, pp. 957–970.

Devanand, D. P., Sackeim, H. A., Decina, P., & Prudic, J. 1988, 'The development of mania and organic euphoria during ECT', *J.Clin.Psychiatry*, vol. 49, no. 2, pp. 69–71.

Dewa, C. S., Hoch, J. S., Lin, E., Paterson, M., & Goering, P. 2003, 'Pattern of antidepressant use and duration of depression-related absence from work', *Br.J.Psychiatry*, vol. 183, pp. 507–513.

Dexedrine advertisement 1960, 'Dexedrine advertisement', *Am.J.Psychiatry*, vol. 117, no. February.

Dielenberg, R. A., Arnold, J. C., & McGregor, I. S. 1999, 'Low-dose midazolam attenuates predatory odor avoidance in rats', *Pharmacol.Biochem.Behav.*, vol. 62, no. 2, pp. 197–201.

Dilsaver, S. C., Greden, J. F., & Snider, R. M. 1987, 'Antidepressant withdrawal syndromes: phenomenology and pathophysiology', *Int.Clin.Psychopharmacol.*, vol. 2, no. 1, pp. 1–19.

Dinan, T. G. 2004, ed., *Sizophrenia and Diabetes 2003: An Expert Consensus Meeting*, *Br.J.Psychiatry*, vol. 184, suppl. 47.

Dolder, C. R. & Jeste, D. V. 2003, 'Incidence of tardive dyskinesia with typical versus atypical antipsychotics in very high risk patients', *Biol.Psychiatry*, vol. 53, no. 12, pp. 1142–1145.

Double, D. 2006, 'The biopsychological approach in psychiatry: the Meyerian legacy,' in *Critical Psychiatry: The Limits of Madness*, D. Double, ed., Palgrave Macmillan, Basingstoke, pp. 165–189.

Drevets, W. C., Frank, E., Price, J. C., Kupfer, D. J., Holt, D., Greer, P. J., Huang, Y., Gautier, C., & Mathis, C. 1999, 'PET imaging of serotonin 1A receptor binding in depression', *Biol.Psychiatry*, vol. 46, no. 10, pp. 1375–1387.

Drinamyl advertisement 1960, 'Drinamyl advertisement', *Am.J.Psychiatry*, vol. 117, no. March, p. XIV.

Drinamyl advertisement 1962, 'Drinamyl advertisement', *Br.Med.J.*, vol. 1, no. January 27th.

Dubicka, B., Hadley, S., & Roberts, C. 2006, 'Suicidal behaviour in youths with depression treated with new-generation antidepressants: meta-analysis', *Br.J.Psychiatry*, vol. 189, pp. 393–398.

Dubovsky, S. L., Davies, R., & Dubovsky, A. N. 2001, 'Mood Disorders', in *Textbook of Clinical Psychiatry*, R. E. Hales & S. C. Yudofsky, eds, American Psychiatric Association, Washington.

Dubovsky, S. L., Davies, R., & Dubovsky, A. N. 2002, 'Mood Disorders', in *Textbook of Clinical Psychiatry*, R. E. Hales & S. C. Yudofsky, eds, American Psychiatric Association, Washington.

Dumont, G. J., de Visser, S. J., Cohen, A. F., & van Gerven, J. M. 2005, 'Biomarkers for the effects of selective serotonin reuptake inhibitors (SSRIs) in healthy subjects', *Br.J.Clin.Pharmacol.*, vol. 59, no. 5, pp. 495–510.

Dunner, D. L., Fleiss, J. L., & Fieve, R. R. 1976, 'Lithium carbonate prophylaxis failure', *Br.J.Psychiatry*, vol. 129, pp. 40–44.

Dunner, D. L., Murphy, D., Stallone, F., & Fieve, R. R. 1979, 'Episode frequency prior to lithium treatment in bipolar manic-depressive patients', *Compr.Psychiatry*, vol. 20, no. 6, pp. 511–515.

Ebaugh, F. G. 1943, 'A review of the drastic shock therapies in the treatment of the psychoses.', *Ann.Int.Med.*, vol. 18, pp. 294–295.

Eberhard, J., Lindstrom, E., & Levander, S. 2006, 'Tardive dyskinesia and antipsychotics: a 5-year longitudinal study of frequency, correlates and course', *Int.Clin.Psychopharmacol.*, vol. 21, no. 1, pp. 35–42.

Ehrhardt, H. 1966, 'Present status of insulin coma and electric convulsive treatment in Germany,' in *Biological Treatment of Mental Illness*, M. Rinkel, ed., Farrar, Straus & Giroux, New York.

Eli Lilly. www.lilly.com. 10.2.2006a.

Eli Lilly. Zyprexa website. www.zyprexa.com/bipolar/treating.asp. 07.12.2006b.

Elkashef, A. M., Doudet, D., Bryant, T., Cohen, R. M., Li, S. H., & Wyatt, R. J. 2000, '6-(18)F-DOPA PET study in patients with schizophrenia. Positron emission tomography', *Psychiatry Res.*, vol. 100, no. 1, pp. 1–11.

Elkes, J. & Elkes, C. 1954, 'Effects of chlorpromazine on the behaviour of chronically overactive psychotic patients', *Br.Med.J.*, vol. ii, pp. 560–565.

Elkin, I., Shea, M. T., Watkins, J. T., Imber, S. D., Sotsky, S. M., Collins, J. F., Glass, D. R., Pilkonis, P. A., Leber, W. R., Docherty, J. P., Fiester, S. J., & Parloff, M. B. 1989, 'National Institute of Mental Health Treatment of Depression Collaborative Research Program. General effectiveness of treatments', *Arch.Gen.Psychiatry*, vol. 46, no. 11, pp. 971–982.

Elvevag, B. & Goldberg, T. E. 2000, 'Cognitive impairment in schizophrenia is the core of the disorder', *Crit.Rev.Neurobiol.*, vol. 14, no. 1, pp. 1–21.

Emrich, H. M., Vogt, P., & Herz, A. 1982, 'Possible antidepressive effects of opioids: action of buprenorphine', *Ann.N.Y.Acad.Sci.*, vol. 398, pp. 108–112.

Engelhardt, D. M., Margolis, R. A., Rudorfer, L., & Paley, H. M. 1969, 'Physician bias and the double-blind', *Arch.Gen.Psychiatry*, vol. 20, no. 3, pp. 315–320.

Engstrom, C., Astrom, M., Nordqvist-Karlsson, B., Adolfsson, R., & Nylander, P. O. 1997, 'Relationship between prophylactic effect of lithium therapy and family history of affective disorders', *Biol.Psychiatry*, vol. 42, no. 6, pp. 425–433.

Ernst, A. M. 1967, 'Mode of action of apomorphine and dexamphetamine on gnawing compulsion in rats', *Psychopharmacologia*, vol. 10, no. 4, pp. 316–323.

Fabre, L. F. 1990, 'Buspirone in the management of major depression: a placebo-controlled comparison', *J.Clin.Psychiatry*, vol. 51, suppl., pp. 55–61.

Faedda, G. L., Tondo, L., & Baldessarini, R. J. 2001, 'Lithium discontinuation: uncovering latent bipolar disorder?', *Am.J.Psychiatry*, vol. 158, no. 8, pp. 1337–1339.

Faedda, G. L., Tondo, L., Baldessarini, R. J., Suppes, T., & Tohen, M. 1993, 'Outcome after rapid vs gradual discontinuation of lithium treatment in bipolar disorders', *Arch.Gen.Psychiatry*, vol. 50, no. 6, pp. 448–455.

Fagan, D., Scott, D. B., Mitchell, M., & Tiplady, B. 1991, 'Effects of remoxipride on measures of psychological performance in healthy volunteers', *Psychopharmacology (Berl)*, vol. 105, no. 2, pp. 225–229.

Fagerlund, B., Mackeprang, T., Gade, A., & Glenthoj, B. Y. 2004, 'Effects of low-dose risperidone and low-dose zuclopenthixol on cognitive functions in first-episode drug-naive schizophrenic patients', *CNS.Spectr.*, vol. 9, no. 5, pp. 364–374.

Farde, L., Wiesel, F. A., Hall, H., Halldin, C., Stone-Elander, S., & Sedvall, G. 1987, 'No D2 receptor increase in PET study of schizophrenia', *Arch.Gen.Psychiatry*, vol. 44, no. 7, pp. 671–672.

Farde, L., Wiesel, F. A., Stone-Elander, S., Halldin, C., Nordstrom, A. L., Hall, H., & Sedvall, G. 1990, 'D2 dopamine receptors in neuroleptic-naive schizophrenic patients. A positron emission tomography study with [11C] raclopride', *Arch.Gen.Psychiatry*, vol. 47, no. 3, pp. 213–219.

Faurbye, A. 1968, 'The role of amines in the etiology of schizophrenia', *Compr.Psychiatry*, vol. 9, no. 2, pp. 155–177.

Feighner, J. P., Aden, G. C., Fabre, L. F., Rickels, K., & Smith, W. T. 1983, 'Comparison of alprazolam, imipramine, and placebo in the treatment of depression', *JAMA*, vol. 249, no. 22, pp. 3057–3064.

Fergusson, D., Doucette, S., Glass, K. C., Shapiro, S., Healy, D., Hebert, P., & Hutton, B. 2005, 'Association between suicide attempts and selective serotonin reuptake inhibitors: systematic review of randomised controlled trials', *Br.Med.J.*, vol. 330, no. 7488, p. 396.

Feyerabend, P. 1975, *Against Method: Outline of an Anarchistic Theory of Knowledge*. Verso, London.

Fink, M. 1979, *Convulsive Therapy: Theory and Practice*. Raven Press, New York.

Fink, M. & Karliner, W. Primary sources: insulin coma therapy. PBS American Experience, www.pbs.org/wgbh/amex/nash/filmmore/ps_ict.html, accessed 13.03.2007.

Finlay, J. M. & Zigmond, M. J. 1997, 'The effects of stress on central dopaminergic neurons: possible clinical implications', *Neurochem.Res.*, vol. 22, no. 11, pp. 1387–1394.

Fisher, S. & Greenberg, R. P. 1993, 'How sound is the double-blind design for evaluating psychotropic drugs?', *J.Nerv.Ment.Dis.*, vol. 181, no. 6, pp. 345–350.

Flugel, F. 1956, 'Therapeutique par medication neuroleptique obtenue en realisant systematiquement des etats parkinsoniformes', in *Colloque international sur la chlorpromazine et les medicaments neuroleptiques en therapeutique psychiatrique, Paris, 20,21,22 Octobre 1955*, G. Douin & Cie, Paris, pp. 790–792.

Flugel, F. 1959, 'Neuroleptic treatment in schizophrenia', in *Psychopharmacology Frontiers*, N. S. Kline, ed., Little, Brown & Co., Boston, pp. 45–47.

Flugel, F. 1966, 'Pharmacotherapy of endogenous psychoses', in *Biological Treatment of Mental Illness*, M. Rinkel, ed., L.C. Page & Co., a division of Farrar, Straus & Giroux, New York, pp. 492–496.

Foucault, M. 1965, *Madness and Civilisation*. Tavistock, London.

Foucault, M. 2006, *Psychiatric power. Lectures at the College de France 1973–1974*. Palgrave Macmillan, Basingstoke, Hampshire, UK.

Frank, L. R. 1978, *The History of Shock Treatment*. Self published, San Fransisco.

Frankenhaeuser, M., Lundberg, U., Rauste, v. W., von Wright, J., & Sedvall, G. 1986, 'Urinary monoamine metabolites as indices of mental stress in healthy males and females', *Pharmacol.Biochem.Behav.*, vol. 24, no. 6, pp. 1521–1525.

Franks, M. A., Macritchie, K. A. N., & Young, A. H. 2005, 'The consequences of suddenly stopping psychotropic medication in bipolar disorder', *Bipolar.Disord.*, vol. 4, no. 1, pp. 11–17.

Frazer, A. & Mendels, J. 1977, 'Do tricyclic antidepressants enhance adrenergic transmission?', *Am.J.Psychiatry*, vol. 134, no. 9, pp. 1040–1042.

Freeman, T. W., Clothier, J. L., Pazzaglia, P., Lesem, M. D., & Swann, A. C. 1992, 'A double-blind comparison of valproate and lithium in the treatment of acute mania', *Am.J.Psychiatry*, vol. 149, no. 1, pp. 108–111.

Freemantle, N., Anderson, I. M., & Young, P. 2000, 'Predictive value of pharmacological activity for the relative efficacy of antidepressant drugs. Meta-regression analysis', *Br.J.Psychiatry*, vol. 177, pp. 292–302.

Furlan, P. M., Kallan, M. J., Have, T. T., Lucki, I., & Katz, I. 2004, 'SSRIs do not cause affective blunting in healthy elderly volunteers', *Am.J.Geriatr.Psychiatry*, vol. 12, no. 3, pp. 323–330.

Gaddum, J. H. & Kwiatkowski, H. 1938, 'The action of ephedrine', *J.Physiol*, vol. 94, no. 1, pp. 87–100.

Gao, W. M., Wang, B., & Zhou, X. Y. 1999, 'Effects of prenatal low-dose beta radiation from tritiated water on learning and memory in rats and their possible mechanisms', *Radiat.Res.*, vol. 152, no. 3, pp. 265–272.

Garattini, S., Giachetti, A., Jori, A., Pieri, L., & Valzelli, L. 1962, 'Effect of imipramine, amitriptyline and their monomethyl derivatives on reserpine activity', *J.Pharm.Pharmacol.*, vol. 14, pp. 509–514.

Garfinkel, P. E., Stancer, H. C., & Persad, E. 1980, 'A comparison of haloperidol, lithium carbonate and their combination in the treatment of mania', *J.Affect.Disord.*, vol. 2, no. 4, pp. 279–288.

Garland, E. J. & Baerg, E. A. 2001, 'A motivational syndrome associated with selective serotonin reuptake inhibitors in children and adolescents', *J.Child Adolesc.Psychopharmacol.*, vol. 11, no. 2, pp. 181–186.

Geddes, J., Freemantle, N., Harrison, P., & Bebbington, P. 2000, 'Atypical antipsychotics in the treatment of schizophrenia: systematic overview and meta-regression analysis', *Br.Med.J.*, vol. 321, no. 7273, pp. 1371–1376.

Geddes, J. R., Burgess, S., Hawton, K., Jamison, K., & Goodwin, G. M. 2004, 'Long-term lithium therapy for bipolar disorder: systematic review and meta-analysis of randomized controlled trials', *Am.J.Psychiatry*, vol. 161, no. 2, pp. 217–222.

Gelder, M., Mayou, R., & Cowen, P. 2001, *Shorter Oxford Textbook of Psychiatry*, 4th edn, Oxford University Press, Oxford.

Gelman, S. 1999, *Medicating Schizophrenia: A History.* Rutgers University Press, New Brunswick, NJ.

Gemperle, A. Y., McAllister, K. H., & Olpe, H. R. 2003, 'Differential effects of iloperidone, clozapine, and haloperidol on working memory of rats in the delayed non-matching-to-position paradigm', *Psychopharmacology (Berl)*, vol. 169, no. 3–4, pp. 354–364.

Gerber, P. E. & Lynd, L. D. 1998, 'Selective serotonin-reuptake inhibitor-induced movement disorders', *Ann.Pharmacother.*, vol. 32, no. 6, pp. 692–698.

Gerlach, J. & Larsen, E. B. 1999, 'Subjective experience and mental side-effects of antipsychotic treatment', *Acta Psychiatr.Scand.Suppl.*, vol. 395, pp. 113–117.

Gershon, S. & Yuwiler, A. 1960, 'Lithium ion: a specific psychopharmacological approach to the treatment of mania', *J.Neuropsychiatr.*, vol. 1, pp. 229–241.

Gharabawi, G. M., Bossie, C. A., Zhu, Y., Mao, L., & Lasser, R. A. 2005, 'An assessment of emergent tardive dyskinesia and existing dyskinesia in patients receiving long-acting, injectable risperidone: results from a long-term study', *Schizophr.Res.*, vol. 77, no. 2–3, pp. 129–139.

Gilbert, P. L., Harris, M. J., McAdams, L. A., & Jeste, D. V. 1995, 'Neuroleptic withdrawal in schizophrenic patients. A review of the literature', *Arch.Gen.Psychiatry*, vol. 52, no. 3, pp. 173–188.

Glowinski, J. & Axelrod, J. 1964, 'Inhibition of uptake of tritiated-noradrenaline in the intact rat brain by imipramine and structurally related compounds', *Nature*, vol. 204, pp. 1318–1319.

Goldberg, D., Privett, M., Ustun, B., Simon, G., & Linden, M. 1998, 'The effects of detection and treatment on the outcome of major depression in primary care: a naturalistic study in 15 cities', *Br.J.Gen.Pract.*, vol. 48, no. 437, pp. 1840–1844.

Goldenberg, M. J. 2006, 'On evidence and evidence-based medicine: lessons from the philosophy of science', *Soc.Sci.Med.*, vol. 62, no. 11, pp. 2621–2632.

Goldman, D. 1966, 'Critical contrasts in psychopharmacology,' in *Biological Treatment of Mental Illness*, M. Rinkel, ed., L.C.Page, New York, pp. 524–533.

Gony, M., Lapeyre-Mestre, M., & Montastruc, J. L. 2003, 'Risk of serious extrapyramidal symptoms in patients with Parkinson's disease receiving antidepressant drugs: a pharmacoepidemiologic study comparing serotonin reuptake inhibitors and other antidepressant drugs', *Clin.Neuropharmacol.*, vol. 26, no. 3, pp. 142–145.

Goodwin, F. K. & Bunney, W. E., Jr. 1971, 'Depressions following reserpine: a reevaluation', *Semin.Psychiatry*, vol. 3, no. 4, pp. 435–448.

Goodwin, G. M. 1994, 'Recurrence of mania after lithium withdrawal. Implications for the use of lithium in the treatment of bipolar affective disorder', *Br.J.Psychiatry*, vol. 164, no. 2, pp. 149–152.

Gottlieb, S. 2002, 'A fifth of Americans contact their doctor as a result of drug advertising', *Br.Med.J. News*, vol. 325, no. 19th October, p. 854.

Grahame-Smith, D. G. & Aronson, J. K. 1992, *Oxford Textbook of Clinical Pharmacology and Drug Therapy.* Oxford University Press, Oxford.

Greenberg, R. P. & Fisher, S. 1989, 'Examining antidepressant effectiveness: Findings, ambiguities and some vexing puzzles', in *The Limits of Biological Treatments for Psychological Distress*, S. Fisher & R. P. Greenberg, eds, Lawrence Erlbaum Associates, Hillsdale, NJ, pp. 1–38.

Greenblatt, M., Levinson, D. J., & Shapiro, A. K. 1959, 'Placebo effect, social milieu, and the evaluation of psychiatric therapies', *J.Chronic.Dis.*, vol. 9, no. 4, pp. 327–333.

Greil, W., Kleindienst, N., Erazo, N., & Muller-Oerlinghausen, B. 1998, 'Differential response to lithium and carbamazepine in the prophylaxis of bipolar disorder', *J.Clin.Psychopharmacol.*, vol. 18, no. 6, pp. 455–460.

Grob, G. 1983, *The Inner World of American Psychiatry 1890–1940.* Rutgers University Press, New Brunswick.

Grob, G. 1994, *The Mad among Us.* The Free Press, New York.

Gronfein, W. 1985, 'Psychotropic drugs and the origins of deinstitutionalisation', *Social Problems*, vol. 32, pp. 437–454.

Gross, G. & Schumann, H. J. 1982, 'Effect of long term treatment with atypical neuroleptic drugs on beta adrenoceptor binding in rat cerebral cortex and myocardium', *Naunyn Schmiedebergs Arch.Pharmacol.*, vol. 321, no. 4, pp. 271–275.

Gunnell, D. & Ashby, D. 2004, 'Antidepressants and suicide: what is the balance of benefit and harm', *Br.Med.J.*, vol. 329, no. 7456, pp. 34–38.

Gunnell, D., Saperia, J., & Ashby, D. 2005, 'Selective serotonin reuptake inhibitors (SSRIs) and suicide in adults: meta-analysis of drug company data from placebo controlled, randomised controlled trials submitted to the MHRA's safety review', *Br.Med.J.*, vol. 330, no. 7488, p. 385.

Gur, R. E., Cowell, P., Turetsky, B. I., Gallacher, F., Cannon, T., Bilker, W., & Gur, R. C. 1998, 'A follow-up magnetic resonance imaging study of schizophrenia. Relationship of neuroanatomical changes to clinical and neurobehavioral measures', *Arch.Gen.Psychiatry*, vol. 55, no. 2, pp. 145–152.

Hall, W. D., Mant, A., Mitchell, P. B., Rendle, V. A., Hickie, I. B., & McManus, P. 2003, 'Association between antidepressant prescribing and suicide in Australia, 1991–2000: trend analysis', *Br.Med.J.*, vol. 326, no. 7397, p. 1008.

Hamilton, M. 1960, 'A rating scale for depression', *J.Neurol.Neurosurg.Psychiatry*, vol. 23, pp. 56–62.

Hankoff, L. D., Rudorfer, L., & Paley, H. M. 1962, 'A reference study of ataraxics. A two-week double blind outpatient evaluation', *J.New Drugs*, vol. 2, pp. 173–178.

Hannigan, B. & Allen, D. 2006, 'Complexity and change in the United Kingdom's system of mental health care', *Soc. Theory Health*, vol. 4, pp. 244–263.

Hare, E. H. 1965, 'Treatment in depressive illness', *Br.Med.J.*, vol. 1, no. 5442, pp. 1125–1126.

Hare, E. H., McCance, C., & McCormick, W. O. 1964, 'Imipramine and 'drinamyl' in depressive illness: a comparative trial', *Br.Med.J.*, vol. 1, no. 5386, pp. 818–820.

Harmer, C. J., Hill, S. A., Taylor, M. J., Cowen, P. J., & Goodwin, G. M. 2003, 'Toward a neuropsychological theory of antidepressant drug action: increase in positive emotional bias after potentiation of norepinephrine activity', *Am.J.Psychiatry*, vol. 160, no. 5, pp. 990–992.

Harmer, C. J., Shelley, N. C., Cowen, P. J., & Goodwin, G. M. 2004, 'Increased positive versus negative affective perception and memory in healthy volunteers following selective serotonin and norepinephrine reuptake inhibition', *Am.J.Psychiatry*, vol. 161, no. 7, pp. 1256–1263.

Haro, J. M., Edgell, E. T., Novick, D., Alonso, J., Kennedy, L., Jones, P. B., Ratcliffe, M., & Breier, A. 2005, 'Effectiveness of antipsychotic treatment for schizophrenia: 6-month results of the Pan-European Schizophrenia Outpatient Health Outcomes (SOHO) study', *Acta Psychiatr.Scand.*, vol. 111, no. 3, pp. 220–231.

Harrington, M., Lelliott, P., Paton, C., Okacha, C., Duffett, R., & Sensky, T. 2002, 'The results of a multicentre audit of the prescribing of antipsychotic drugs for inpatients in the United Kingdom', *Psychiatr.Bull.*, vol. 26, pp. 414–418.

Harris, M., Chandran, S., Chakraborty, N., & Healy, D. 2003, 'Mood-stabilizers: the archaeology of the concept', *Bipolar.Disord.*, vol. 5, no. 6, pp. 446–452.

Harris, M., Chandran, S., Chakraborty, N., & Healy, D. 2005, 'The impact of mood stabilizers on bipolar disorder: the 1890s and 1990s compared', *Hist. Psychiatry*, vol. 16, no. pt 4 (no. 64), pp. 423–434.

Harrow, M., Grossman, L. S., Jobe, T. H., & Herbener, E. S. 2005, 'Do patients with schizophrenia ever show periods of recovery? A 15-year multi-follow-up study', *Schizophr.Bull.*, vol. 31, no. 3, pp. 723–734.

Hartigan, G. P. 1963, 'The use of lithium salts in affective disorders', *Br.J.Psychiatry*, vol. 109, pp. 810–814.

Hartong, E. G., Moleman, P., Hoogduin, C. A., Broekman, T. G., & Nolen, W. A. 2003, 'Prophylactic efficacy of lithium versus carbamazepine in treatment-naive bipolar patients', *J.Clin.Psychiatry*, vol. 64, no. 2, pp. 144–151.

Harvey, P. D., Rabinowitz, J., Eerdekens, M., & Davidson, M. 2005, 'Treatment of cognitive impairment in early psychosis: a comparison of risperidone and haloperidol in a large long-term trial', *Am.J.Psychiatry*, vol. 162, no. 10, pp. 1888–1895.

Harwood, A. J. & Agam, G. 2003, 'Search for a common mechanism of mood stabilizers', *Biochem.Pharmacol.*, vol. 66, no. 2, pp. 179–189.

Healthcare Commission 2007, *Talking about Medicines: The Management of Medicines in Trusts Providing Mental Health Services.* Commission for Healthcare, Audit and Inspection, London.

Healy, D. 1996, *The Psychopharmacologists. Interviews by David Healy. Volume 1.* Chapman and Hall, London.

Healy, D. 1997, *The Antidepressant Era.* Harvard University Press, New York.

Healy, D. 2002, *The Creation of Psychopharmacology.* Harvard University Press, Cambridge, MA.

Healy, D. 2004, 'Shaping the intimate: influences on the experience of everyday nerves', *Soc.Stud.Sci.*, vol. 34, no. 2, pp. 219–245.

Healy, D. 2006, 'The latest mania: selling bipolar disorder', *PLoS.Med.*, vol. 3, no. 4, p. e185.

Healy, D. & Farquhar, G. 1998, 'Immediate effects of droperidol', *Hum.Psychopharmacol.*, vol. 13, pp. 113–120.

Healy, D., Herxheimer, A., & Menkes, D. B. 2006, 'Antidepressants and violence: problems at the interface of medicine and law', *PLoS.Med.*, vol. 3, no. 9, p. e372.

Healy, D. & Whitaker, C. 2003, 'Antidepressants and suicide: risk-benefit conundrums', *J.Psychiatry Neurosci.*, vol. 28, no. 5, pp. 331–337.

Hegarty, J. D., Baldessarini, R. J., Tohen, M., Waternaux, C., & Oepen, G. 1994, 'One hundred years of schizophrenia: a meta-analysis of the outcome literature', *Am.J.Psychiatry*, vol. 151, no. 10, pp. 1409–1416.

Hekimian, L. J. & Friedhoff, A. J. 1967, 'A controlled study of placebo, chlordiazepoxide and chlorpromazine with thirty male schizophrenic patients', *Dis.Nerv.Syst.*, vol. 28, no. 10, pp. 675–678.

Hemphill, R. E. & Reiss, M. 1945, 'Serum gonadotrophin and testis biopsy in the treatment of schizophrenia', *J.Ment.Sci.*, vol. 91, pp. 1–7.

Henderson, D. & Gillespie, R. D. 1927, *Henderson and Gillespie's Textbook of Psychiatry*, First edn, Oxford University Press, Oxford.

Henderson, D. & Gillespie, R. D. 1944, *Henderson and Gillespie's Textbook of Psychiatry*, Sixth edn, Oxford University Press, Oxford.

Henderson, D. & Gillespie, R. D. 1962, *Henderson and Gillespie's Textbook of Psychiatry*, Ninth edn, Oxford, Oxford University Press.

Heninger, G., Dimascio, A., & Klerman, G. L. 1965, 'Personality factors in variability of response to phenothiazines,' *Am.J.Psychiatry*, vol. 121, pp. 1091–1094.

Heres, S., Davis, J., Maino, K., Jetzinger, E., Kissling, W., & . Leucht, S. 2006, 'Why olanzapine beats risperidone, risperidone beats quetiapine, and quetiapine beats olanzapine: an exploratory analysis of head-to-head comparison studies of second-generation antipsychotics', *Am.J.Psychiatry*, vol. 163, no. 2, pp. 185–194.

Herman, Z. S. 1970, 'The effects of noradrenaline on rat's behaviour', *Psychopharmacologia*, vol. 16, no. 5, pp. 369–374.

Herrmann, W. M. & McDonald, R. J. 1978, 'A multidimensional test approach for the description of the CNS activity of drugs in human pharmacology', *Pharmakopsychiatr.Neuropsychopharmakol.*, vol. 11, no. 6, pp. 247–265.

Hess, E. J., Bracha, H. S., Kleinman, J. E., & Creese, I. 1987, 'Dopamine receptor subtype imbalance in schizophrenia', *Life Sci.*, vol. 40, no. 15, pp. 1487–1497.

Heydorn, W., Frazer, A., & Mendels, J. 1980, 'Do tricyclic antidepressants enhance adrenergic transmission? An update', *Am.J.Psychiatry*, vol. 137, no. 1, pp. 113–114.

Hietala, J., Syvalahti, E., Vuorio, K., Rakkolainen, V., Bergman, J., Haaparanta, M., Solin, O., Kuoppamaki, M., Kirvela, O., Ruotsalainen, U., & Salokangas, R. K. R. 1995, 'Presynaptic dopamine function in striatum of neuroleptic-naive schizophrenic patients', *Lancet*, vol. 346, no. 8983, pp. 1130–1131.

Hill, S. K., Beers, S. R., Kmiec, J. A., Keshavan, M. S., & Sweeney, J. A. 2004, 'Impairment of verbal memory and learning in antipsychotic-naive patients with first-episode schizophrenia', *Schizophr.Res.*, vol. 68, no. 2–3, pp. 127–136.

Himmich, H. E. 1958, 'Prospects in psychopharmacology', in *The New Chemotherapy in Mental Illness*, H. L. Gordon, ed., Peter Owen, London.

Hindmarch, I., Kimber, S., & Cockle, S. M. 2000, 'Abrupt and brief discontinuation of antidepressant treatment: effects on cognitive function and psychomotor performance', *Int.Clin.Psychopharmacol.*, vol. 15, no. 6, pp. 305–318.

Hoch, P. H., Lesse, S., & Malitz, S. 1956, 'A two-year evaluation of chlorpromazine in clinical research and practice', *Am.J.Psychiatry*, vol. 113, no. 6, pp. 540–545.

Hogarty, G. E. & Ulrich, R. F. 1998, 'The limitations of antipsychotic medication on schizophrenia relapse and adjustment and the contributions of psychosocial treatment', *J.Psychiatr.Res.*, vol. 32, no. 3–4, pp. 243–250.

Hollister, L. E. 1992, 'Neuroleptic dysphoria: so what's new?', *Biol.Psychiatry*, vol. 31, no. 5, pp. 531–532.

Hollister, L. E., Overall, J. E., Johnson, M., Pennington, V., Katz, G., & Shelton, J. 1964, 'Controlled comparison of amitriptyline, imipramine and placebo in hospitalized depressed patients', *J.Nerv.Ment.Dis.*, vol. 139, pp. 370–375.

Hollister, L. E., Overall, J. E., Shelton, J., Pennington, V., Kimbell, I., & Johnson, M. 1967, 'Drug therapy of depression. Amitriptyline, perphenazine, and their combination in different syndromes', *Arch.Gen.Psychiatry*, vol. 17, no. 4, pp. 486–493.

Honig, A., Arts, B. M., Ponds, R. W., & Riedel, W. J. 1999, 'Lithium induced cognitive side-effects in bipolar disorder: a qualitative analysis and implications for daily practice', *Int.Clin.Psychopharmacol.*, vol. 14, no. 3, pp. 167–171.

Hsieh, M. T. 1982, 'The involvement of monoaminergic and GABAergic systems in locomotor inhibition produced by clobazam and diazepam in rats', *Int.J.Clin.Pharmacol.Ther.Toxicol.*, vol. 20, no. 5, pp. 227–235.

Hutton, I. E. 1940, *Mental Disorders in Modern Life: An Outline of Hopeful Treatment.* William Heinman (Medical Books), London.

Huttunen, M. 1995, 'The evolution of the serotonin-dopamine antagonist concept', *J.Clin.Psychopharmacol.*, vol. 15, no. 1, suppl. 1, pp. 4S–10S.

Hyman, S. E. & Nestler, E. J. 1996, 'Initiation and adaptation: a paradigm for understanding psychotropic drug action', *Am.J.Psychiatry*, vol. 153, no. 2, pp. 151–162.

Hyman, S. E. & Nestler, E. J. 1997, 'Drs Hyman and Nestler reply', *Am.J.Psychiatry*, vol. 154, pp. 440–441.

Imlah, N. W. 1985, 'An evaluation of alprazolam in the treatment of reactive or neurotic (secondary) depression', *Br.J.Psychiatry*, vol. 146, pp. 515–519.

Ingelby, D. 1982, 'The social construction of mental illness,' in *The Problem of Medical Knowledge*, P. Wright & A. Treacher, eds, Edinburgh University Press, Edinburgh, pp. 123–143.

Jablensky, A., Sartorius, N., Ernberg, G., Anker, M., Korten, A., Cooper, J. E., Day, R., & Bertelsen, A. 1992, 'Schizophrenia: manifestations, incidence and course in different cultures. A World Health Organization ten-country study', *Psychol.Med.Monogr Suppl.*, vol. 20, pp. 1–97.

Jackson, G. E. 2005, *Rethinking Psychiatric Drugs*. AuthorHouse, Bloomington, Indiana.

Jacobsen, E. 1964, 'The theoretical basis of the chemotherapy of depression,' in *Depression: Proceedings of the Symposium Held at Cambridge 22 to 26 September 1959*, Cambridge University Press, Cambridge, pp. 208–213.

Jacyna, L. S. 1982, 'Somatic theories of mind and the interests of medicine in Britain 1850–1879', *Medical History*, vol. 16, pp. 233–258.

Jenner, F. A. Interview with Alec Jenner. 06.05.1997a.

Jessner, L. & Ryan, V. G. 1943, *Shock Treatment in Psychiatry*. William Heinman, London.

Jeste, D. V., Caligiuri, M. P., Paulsen, J. S., Heaton, R. K., Lacro, J. P., Harris, M. J., Bailey, A., Fell, R. L., & McAdams, L. A. 1995, 'Risk of tardive dyskinesia in older patients. A prospective longitudinal study of 266 outpatients', *Arch.Gen.Psychiatry*, vol. 52, no. 9, pp. 756–765.

Jick, H., Kaye, J. A., & Jick, S. S. 2004, 'Antidepressants and the risk of suicidal behaviors', *JAMA*, vol. 292, no. 3, pp. 338–343.

Jick, S. S., Dean, A. D., & Jick, H. 1995, 'Antidepressants and suicide', *Br.Med.J.*, vol. 310, no. 6974, pp. 215–218.

Johnson, F. N. 1984, *The History of Lithium Therapy*. Macmillan, London.

Johnson, R. E. & McFarland, B. H. 1996, 'Lithium use and discontinuation in a health maintenance organization', *Am.J.Psychiatry*, vol. 153, no. 8, pp. 993–1000.

Johnstone, E. C., Crow, T. J., Frith, C. D., Carney, M. W., & Price, J. S. 1978, 'Mechanism of the antipsychotic effect in the treatment of acute schizophrenia', *Lancet*, vol. 1, no. 8069, pp. 848–851.

Johnstone, E. C., Crow, T. J., Frith, C. D., & Owens, D. G. 1988, 'The Northwick Park 'functional' psychosis study: diagnosis and treatment response', *Lancet*, vol. 2, no. 8603, pp. 119–125.

Johnstone, E. C., Deakin, J. F., Lawler, P., Frith, C. D., Stevens, M., McPherson, K., & Crow, T. J. 1980, 'The Northwick Park electroconvulsive therapy trial', *Lancet*, vol. 2, no. 8208–8209, pp. 1317–1320.

Johnstone, E. C., MacMillan, J. F., Frith, C. D., Benn, D. K., & Crow, T. J. 1990, 'Further investigation of the predictors of outcome following first schizophrenic episodes', *Br.J.Psychiatry*, vol. 157, pp. 182–189.

Johnstone, L. 2003, 'A shocking treatment', *The Psychologist*, vol. 16, no. May, pp. 236–239.

Joint Commission on Mental Illness and Mental Health 1961, *Action for Mental Health: Final Report, 1961*. Basic Books, New York.

Jones, P. B., Barnes, T. R., Davies, L., Dunn, G., Lloyd, H., Hayhurst, K. P., Murray, R. M., Markwick, A., & Lewis, S. W. 2006, 'Randomized controlled trial of the effect on quality of Life of second- vs first-generation antipsychotic drugs in schizophrenia: Cost utility of the latest antipsychotic drugs in schizophrenia study (Cutlass 1)', *Arch.Gen.Psychiatry*, vol. 63, no. 10, pp. 1079–1087.

Joseph, J. 2003, *The Gene Illusion: Genetic Research in Psychiatry and Psychology under the Microscope*. PCCS Books, Ross-on-Wye, Herefordshire.

Joukamaa, M., Heliovaara, M., Knekt, P., Aromaa, A., Raitasalo, R., & Lehtinen, V. 2006, 'Schizophrenia, neuroleptic medication and mortality', *Br.J.Psychiatry*, vol. 188, pp. 122–127.

Joyce, P. R. & Paykel, E. S. 1989, 'Predictors of drug response in depression', *Arch.Gen.Psychiatry*, vol. 46, no. 1, pp. 89–99.

Judd, L. L., Hubbard, B., Janowsky, D. S., Huey, L. Y., & Attewell, P. A. 1977a, 'The effect of lithium carbonate on affect, mood, and personality of normal subjects', *Arch.Gen.Psychiatry*, vol. 34, no. 3, pp. 346–351.

Judd, L. L., Hubbard, B., Janowsky, D. S., Huey, L. Y., & Takahashi, K. I. 1977b, 'The effect of lithium carbonate on the cognitive functions of normal subjects', *Arch.Gen.Psychiatry*, vol. 34, no. 3, pp. 355–357.

Judge, R., Parry, M. G., Quail, D., & Jacobson, J. G. 2002, 'Discontinuation symptoms: comparison of brief interruption in fluoxetine and paroxetine treatment', *Int.Clin.Psychopharmacol.*, vol. 17, no. 5, pp. 217–225.

Kalinowsky, L. & Hoch, P. 1950, *Shock Treatments and Other Somatic Procedures in Psychiatry*. Grune & Stratton, New York.

Kalinowsky, L. & Worthing, H. J. 1943, 'Results with electric convulsive therapy in 200 cases of schizophrenia', *Psychiatr.Quarterly*, vol. 17, pp. 144–153.

Kane, J. M., Honigfeld, G., Singer, J., & Meltzer, H. 1988, 'Clozapine in treatment-resistant schizophrenics', *Psychopharmacol.Bull.*, vol. 24, no. 1, pp. 62–67.

Kane, J. M., Quitkin, F. M., Rifkin, A., Ramos-Lorenzi, J. R., Nayak, D. D., & Howard, A. 1982, 'Lithium carbonate and imipramine in the prophylaxis of unipolar and bipolar II illness: a prospective, placebo-controlled comparison', *Arch.Gen.Psychiatry*, vol. 39, no. 9, pp. 1065–1069.

Kaptchuk, T. J. 2001, 'The double-blind, randomized, placebo-controlled trial: gold standard or golden calf?', *J.Clin.Epidemiol.*, vol. 54, no. 6, pp. 541–549.

Kapur, S. 2003, 'Psychosis as a state of aberrant salience: a framework linking biology, phenomenology, and pharmacology in schizophrenia', *Am.J. Psychiatry*, vol. 160, no. 1, pp. 13–23.

Kasper, S., Anghelescu, I. G., Szegedi, A., Dienel, A., & Kieser, M. 2006, 'Superior efficacy of St John's wort extract WS 5570 compared to placebo in patients with major depression: a randomized, double-blind, placebo-controlled, multi-center trial [ISRCTN77277298]', *BMC.Med.*, vol. 4, p. 14.

Kasper, S. & Resinger, E. 2003, 'Cognitive effects and antipsychotic treatment', *Psychoneuroendocrinology*, vol. 28, suppl. 1, pp. 27–38.

Kawai, N., Yamakawa, Y., Baba, A., Nemoto, K., Tachikawa, H., Hori, T., Asada, T., & Iidaka, T. 2006, 'High-dose of multiple antipsychotics and cognitive function in schizophrenia: the effect of dose-reduction', *Prog.Neuropsychopharmacol. Biol.Psychiatry*, vol. 30, no. 6, pp. 1009–1014.

Keefe, R. S., Seidman, L. J., Christensen, B. K., Hamer, R. M., Sharma, T., Sitskoorn, M. M., Rock, S. L., Woolson, S., Tohen, M., Tollefson, G. D., Sanger, T. M., & Lieberman, J. A. 2006, 'Long-term neurocognitive effects of olanzapine or low-dose haloperidol in first-episode psychosis', *Biol.Psychiatry*, vol. 59, no. 2, pp. 97–105.

Keller, M., Montgomery, S., Ball, W., Morrison, M., Snavely, D., Liu, G., Hargreaves, R., Hietala, J., Lines, C., Beebe, K., & Reines, S. 2006, 'Lack of efficacy of the substance p (neurokinin1 receptor) antagonist aprepitant in the treatment of major depressive disorder', *Biol.Psychiatry*, vol. 59, no. 3, pp. 216–223.

Kelly, R. E., Jr., Cohen, L. J., Semple, R. J., Bialer, P., Lau, A., Bodenheimer, A., Neustadter, E., Barenboim, A., & Galynker, I. I. 2006, 'Relationship between drug company funding and outcomes of clinical psychiatric research', *Psychol.Med.*, vol. 36, no. 11, pp. 1647–1656.

Kennedy, A. 1937, 'Convulsion therapy in schizophrenia', *JMent.Sci.*, vol. 83, pp. 609–629.

Kennedy, J. 1963, *Message from the President of the US Relative to Mental Illness and Mental Retardation*, 88–1 Congress, House document No 58, House document No 58.

Kessler, R. C., Coccaro, E. F., Fava, M., Jaeger, S., Jin, R., & Walters, E. 2006, 'The prevalence and correlates of DSM-IV intermittent explosive disorder in the National Comorbidity Survey Replication', *Arch.Gen.Psychiatry*, vol. 63, no. 6, pp. 669–678.

Kety, S. S. 1972, 'Toward hypotheses for a biochemical component in the vulnerability to schizophrenia', *Semin.Psychiatry*, vol. 4, no. 3, pp. 233–238.

Khan, A., Khan, S., Kolts, R., & Brown, W. A. 2003, 'Suicide rates in clinical trials of SSRIs, other antidepressants, and placebo: analysis of FDA reports', *Am.J.Psychiatry*, vol. 160, no. 4, pp. 790–792.

Khan, A., Khan, S. R., Leventhal, R. M., & Brown, W. A. 2001, 'Symptom reduction and suicide risk in patients treated with placebo in antidepressant clinical trials: a replication analysis of the Food and Drug Administration database', *Int.J.Neuropsychopharmacol.*, vol. 4, no. 2, pp. 113–118.

Khan, A., Leventhal, R. M., Khan, S. R., & Brown, W. A. 2002, 'Severity of depression and response to antidepressants and placebo: an analysis of the Food and Drug Administration database', *J.Clin.Psychopharmacol.*, vol. 22, no. 1, pp. 40–45.

Khan, A., Warner, H. A., & Brown, W. A. 2000, 'Symptom reduction and suicide risk in patients treated with placebo in antidepressant clinical trials: an analysis of the Food and Drug Administration database', *Arch.Gen.Psychiatry*, vol. 57, no. 4, pp. 311–317.

Khan, A. U. How do psychotropic drugs really work? *Psychiatric Times* 16 [10]. 1999, pp. 1–12.

King, D. J. 1990, 'The effect of neuroleptics on cognitive and psychomotor function', *Br.J.Psychiatry*, vol. 157, pp. 799–811.

King, D. J. 1994, 'Psychomotor impairment and cognitive disturbances induced by neuroleptics', *Acta Psychiatr.Scand.Suppl.*, vol. 380, pp. 53–58.

King, D. J., Burke, M., & Lucas, R. A. 1995, 'Antipsychotic drug-induced dysphoria', *Br.J.Psychiatry*, vol. 167, no. 4, pp. 480–482.

Kirsch, I., Deacon, B. J., Moore, T. J., & Scoboria, A. 2007, 'Initial severity and antidepressant benefits: a pooled analysis of data submitted to the FDA', *PLoS.Med.*, in press.

Kirsch, I., Moore, T. J., Scoboria, A., & Nicholls, S. S. 2002, 'The emperor's new drugs: an analysis of antidepressant medication data submitted to the US Food and Drug Administration', *Prev. Treat.*, vol. 5, www.content.apa.org/journals/pre/5/1/23.

Klawans, H. L., Jr., Goetz, C., & Westheimer, R. 1972, 'Pathophysiology of schizophrenia and the striatum', *Dis.Nerv.Syst.*, vol. 33, no. 11, pp. 711–719.

Klawans, H. L., Jr. & Rubovits, R. 1972, 'An experimental model of tardive dyskinesia', *J.Neural Transm.*, vol. 33, no. 3, pp. 235–246.

Klimek, V. & Maj, J. 1989, 'Repeated administration of antidepressants enhances agonist affinity for mesolimbic D2-receptors', *J.Pharm.Pharmacol.*, vol. 41, no. 8, pp. 555–558.

Kline, N. S. 1970, 'Monoamine oxidase inhibitors: an unfinished picaresque tale,' in *Discoveries in Biological Psychiatry*, F. Ayd & B. Blackwell, eds, JB Lippincott Company, Philadelphia, pp. 194–204.

Kocsis, J. H., Croughan, J. L., Katz, M. M., Butler, T. P., Secunda, S., Bowden, C. L., & Davis, J. M. 1990, 'Response to treatment with antidepressants of patients with severe or moderate nonpsychotic depression and of patients with psychotic depression', *Am.J.Psychiatry*, vol. 147, no. 5, pp. 621–624.

Kocsis, J. H., Shaw, E. D., Stokes, P. E., Wilner, P., Elliot, A. S., Sikes, C., Myers, B., Manevitz, A., & Parides, M. 1993, 'Neuropsychologic effects of lithium discontinuation', *J.Clin.Psychopharmacol.*, vol. 13, no. 4, pp. 268–275.

Koerner, B. 'Disorders made to order'. *Mother Jones*, 27 [July/August] 2002, pp. 58–63.

Koran, L. M., Chuong, H. W., Bullock, K. D., & Smith, S. C. 2003, 'Citalopram for compulsive shopping disorder: an open-label study followed by double-blind discontinuation', *J.Clin.Psychiatry*, vol. 64, no. 7, pp. 793–798.

Kornhuber, J., Riederer, P., Reynolds, G. P., Beckmann, H., Jellinger, K., & Gabriel, E. 1989, '3H-spiperone binding sites in post-mortem brains from schizophrenic patients: relationship to neuroleptic drug treatment, abnormal movements, and positive symptoms', *J.Neural Transm.*, vol. 75, no. 1, pp. 1–10.

Kropf, D. & Muller-Oerlinghausen, B. 1979, 'Changes in learning, memory, and mood during lithium treatment. Approach to a research strategy', *Acta Psychiatr.Scand.*, vol. 59, no. 1, pp. 97–124.

Kuhn, R. 1958, 'The treatment of depressive states with G 22355 (imipramine hydrochloride)', *Am.J.Psychiatry*, vol. 115, no. 5, pp. 459–464.

Kuhn, R. 1970, 'The imipramine story', in *Discoveries in Biological Psychiatry*, F. Ayd & B. Blackwell, eds, JB Lippincott Company, Philadelphia, pp. 205–217.

Lacasse, J. R. & Leo, J. 2005, 'Serotonin and depression: a disconnect between the advertisements and the scientific literature', *PLoS.Med.*, vol. 2, no. 12, p. e392.

Lader, M. 1994, 'Neuroleptic-induced deficit syndrome. Historical introduction', *Acta Psychiatr.Scand.Suppl.*, vol. 380, pp. 6–7.

Lader, M., Melhuish, A., Frcka, G., Fredricson, O. K., & Christensen, V. 1986, 'The effects of citalopram in single and repeated doses and with alcohol on physiological and psychological measures in healthy subjects', *Eur.J.Clin.Pharmacol.*, vol. 31, no. 2, pp. 183–190.

Lader, M. H., Ron, M., & Petursson, H. 1984, 'Computed axial brain tomography in long-term benzodiazepine users', *Psychol.Med.*, vol. 14, no. 1, pp. 203–206.

Lahti, R. A. & Maickel, R. P. 1971, 'The tricyclic antidepressants – inhibition of norepinephrine uptake as related to potentiation of norepinephrine and clinical efficacy', *Biochemical Pharmacology*, vol. 20, pp. 482–486.

Laing, R. D. 1965, *The Divided Self*. Pelican Books, Harmondsworth.

Laing, R. D. 1967, *The Politics of Experience and the Bird of Paradise*. Penguin Books, Harmondsworth.

Lambourn, J. & Gill, D. 1978, 'A controlled comparison of simulated and real ECT', *Br.J.Psychiatry*, vol. 133, pp. 514–519.

Lapin, I. P., Osipova, S. V., Uskova, N. V., & Stabrovski, E. M. 1968, 'Synergism of imipramine and desmethylimipramine with reserpine in teh frog. Interaction with 5-hydroxytryptophan and 2-bromolysergid diethylamide (BOL-148)', *Arch.Int.Pharmacodyn.Ther.*, vol. 174, no. 1, pp. 37–49.

Largactil advertisement 1962, 'Largactil advertisement', *Br.Med.J.*, vol. 1, no. February 17th.

Largactil advertisement 1964, *Br.Med.J.*, vol. 2, no. 5th Sept.

Laroxyl advertisement 1962, 'Laroxyl advertisement', *Br.Med.J.*, vol. 1, no. January 20th.

Larsen, T. K., Melle, I., Auestad, B., Friis, S., Haahr, U., Johannessen, J. O., Opjordsmoen, S., Rund, B. R., Simonsen, E., Vaglum, P., & McGlashan, T. 2006, 'Early detection of first-episode psychosis: the effect on 1-year outcome', *Schizophr.Bull.*, vol. 32, no. 4, pp. 758–764.

Laruelle, M., Abi-Dargham, A., Gil, R., Kegeles, L., & Innis, R. 1999, 'Increased dopamine transmission in schizophrenia: relationship to illness phases', *Biol.Psychiatry*, vol. 46, no. 1, pp. 56–72.

Laruelle, M., Abi-Dargham, A., van Dyck, C. H., Gil, R., D'Souza, C. D., Erdos, J., McCance, E., Rosenblatt, W., Fingado, C., Zoghbi, S. S., Baldwin, R. M., Seibyl, J. P., Krystal, J. H., Charney, D. S., & Innis, R. B. 1996, 'Single photon emission computerized tomography imaging of amphetamine-induced dopamine release in drug-free schizophrenic subjects', *Proc.Natl.Acad.Sci.U.S.A*, vol. 93, no. 17, pp. 9235–9240.

Lee, J. & Park, S. 2005, 'Working memory impairments in schizophrenia: a meta-analysis', *J.Abnorm.Psychol.*, vol. 114, no. 4, pp. 599–611.

Lee, T., Seeman, P., Tourtellotte, W. W., Farley, I. J., & Hornykeiwicz, O. 1978, 'Binding of 3H-neuroleptics and 3H-apomorphine in schizophrenic brains', *Nature*, vol. 274, no. 5674, pp. 897–900.

Leff, J., Sartorius, N., Jablensky, A., Korten, A., & Ernberg, G. 1992, 'The international pilot study of schizophrenia: five-year follow-up findings', *Psychol.Med.*, vol. 22, no. 1, pp. 131–145.

Legangneux, E., McEwen, J., Wesnes, K. A., Bergougnan, L., Miget, N., Canal, M., L'Heritier, C., Pinquier, J. L., & Rosenzweig, P. 2000, 'The acute effects of amisulpride (50 mg and 200 mg) and haloperidol (2 mg) on cognitive function in healthy elderly volunteers', *J.Psychopharmacol.*, vol. 14, no. 2, pp. 164–171.

Lehmann, H. 1975, 'Psychopharmacological treatment of schizophrenia', *Schizophr.Bull.*, vol. 13, pp. 27–45.

Lehmann, H. 1996, 'Psychopharmacotherapy', in *The Psychopharmacologists*, D. Healy, ed., Chapman & Hall, London, pp. 159–186.

Lehmann, H. E. 1955, 'Therapeutic results with chlorpromazine (largactil) in psychiatric conditions', *Can.Med.Assoc.J.*, vol. 72, no. 2, pp. 91–99.

Lehmann, H. E., Cahn, C. H., & de Verteuil, R. L. 1958, 'The treatment of depressive conditions with imipramine (G 22355)', *Can.Psychiatr.Assoc.J.*, vol. 3, no. 4, pp. 155–164.

Lehmann, H. E. & Hanrahan, G. E. 1954, 'Chlorpromazine; new inhibiting agent for psychomotor excitement and manic states', *AMA.Arch.Neurol.Psychiatry*, vol. 71, no. 2, pp. 227–237.

Lehmann, H. E. & Kline, N. S. 1983, 'Clinical discoveries with antidepressant drugs. Volume 1,' in *Discoveries in Pharmacology, Volume 1*, M. J. Parnham & J. Bruinvels, eds, Elsevier Science Publishers B.V., London, pp. 209–247.

Lehtinen, V., Aaltonen, J., Koffert, T., Rakkolainen, V., & Syvalahti, E. 2000, 'Two-year outcome in first-episode psychosis treated according to an integrated model. Is immediate neuroleptisation always needed?', *Eur.Psychiatry*, vol. 15, no. 5, pp. 312–320.

Lerer, B., Moore, N., Meyendorff, E., Cho, S. R., & Gershon, S. 1987, 'Carbamazepine versus lithium in mania: a double-blind study', *J.Clin. Psychiatry*, vol. 48, no. 3, pp. 89–93.

Lerman, P. 1982, *Deinstitutionalisation and the Welfare State*. Rutgers University Press, New Brunswick.

Leucht, S., Arbter, D., Engel, R. R., Kissling, W., & Davis, J. M. 2007, 'How effective are new generation antipsychotic drugs? A meta-analysis of placebo controlled trials', *Br.J.Psychiatry*, in press.

Levin, E. D. & Christopher, N. C. 2006, 'Effects of clozapine on memory function in the rat neonatal hippocampal lesion model of schizophrenia', *Prog.Neuropsychopharmacol.Biol.Psychiatry*, vol. 30, no. 2, pp. 223–229.

Lewis, S. E. 2002, 'European first-episode schizophrenia network', *Br.J.Psychiatry Suppl.*, vol. 181, suppl. no. 43.

Lieberman, J. A., Stroup, T. S., McEvoy, J. P., Swartz, M. S., Rosenheck, R. A., Perkins, D. O., Keefe, R. S., Davis, S. M., Davis, C. E., Lebowitz, B. D., Severe, J., & Hsiao, J. K. 2005, 'Effectiveness of antipsychotic drugs in patients with chronic schizophrenia', *N.Engl.J.Med.*, vol. 353, no. 12, pp. 1209–1223.

Lieberman, J. A., Tollefson, G. D., Charles, C., Zipursky, R., Sharma, T., Kahn, R. S., Keefe, R. S., Green, A. I., Gur, R. E., McEvoy, J., Perkins, D., Hamer, R. M., Gu, H., & Tohen, M. 2005f, 'Antipsychotic drug effects on brain morphology in first-episode psychosis', *Arch.Gen.Psychiatry*, vol. 62, no. 4, pp. 361–370.

Lindstrom, L. H., Gefvert, O., Hagberg, G., Lundberg, T., Bergstrom, M., Hartvig, P., & Langstrom, B. 1999, 'Increased dopamine synthesis rate in medial pre-frontal cortex and striatum in schizophrenia indicated by L-(beta-11C) DOPA and PET', *Biol.Psychiatry*, vol. 46, no. 5, pp. 681–688.

Linn, L. A. 1955, *Handbook of Hospital Psychiatry*. International Universities Press, New York.

Lisanby, S. H., Maddox, J. H., Prudic, J., Devanand, D. P., & Sackeim, H. A. 2000, 'The effects of electroconvulsive therapy on memory of autobiographical and public events', *Arch.Gen.Psychiatry*, vol. 57, no. 6, pp. 581–590.

Lohr, J. B., Kuczenski, R., & Niculescu, A. B. 2003, 'Oxidative mechanisms and tardive dyskinesia', *CNS.Drugs*, vol. 17, no. 1, pp. 47–62.

Loomer, H. P., Saunders, J. C., & Kline, N. S. 1957, 'A clinical and pharmacody-namic evaluation of iproniazid as a psychic energizer', *Psychiatr.Res.Rep.Am. Psychiatr.Assoc.*, vol. 135, no. 8, pp. 129–141.

Lowther, S., De Paermentier, F., Cheetham, S. C., Crompton, M. R., Katona, C. L., & Horton, R. W. 1997, '5-HT1A receptor binding sites in post-mortem brain samples from depressed suicides and controls', *J.Affect.Disord.*, vol. 42, no. 2–3, pp. 199–207.

Lu, M. L., Pan, J. J., Teng, H. W., Su, K. P., & Shen, W. W. 2002, 'Metoclopramide-induced supersensitivity psychosis', *Ann.Pharmacother.*, vol. 36, no. 9, pp. 1387–1390.

Lundquist, G. 1945, 'Prognosis and course in manic depressive psychosis', *Acta Psychiatr.Neurol.Scand. Suppl.*, vol. 35, pp. 1–96.

Mackay, A. V., Iversen, L. L., Rossor, M., Spokes, E., Bird, E., Arregui, A., Creese, I., & Synder, S. H. 1982, 'Increased brain dopamine and dopamine receptors in schizophrenia', *Arch.Gen.Psychiatry*, vol. 39, no. 9, pp. 991–997.

Maculans, G. A. 1964, 'Comparison of diazepam, chlorprothixene and chlorpromazine in chronic schizophrenic patients', *Dis.Nerv.Syst.*, vol. 25, pp. 164–168.

Maj, J., Dziedzicka-Wasylewska, M., Rogoz, R., Rogoz, Z., & Skuza, G. 1996, 'Antidepressant drugs given repeatedly change the binding of the dopamine D2 receptor agonist, [3H]N-0437, to dopamine D2 receptors in the rat brain', *Eur.J.Pharmacol.*, vol. 304, no. 1–3, pp. 49–54.

Maj, M., Pirozzi, R., Magliano, L., & Bartoli, L. 1998, 'Long-term outcome of lithium prophylaxis in bipolar disorder: a 5-year prospective study of 402 patients at a lithium clinic', *Am.J.Psychiatry*, vol. 155, no. 1, pp. 30–35.

Malamud, W. 1960, 'Psychiatric research and motivation.', *Am.J.Psychiatry*, vol. 117, pp. 1–10.

Malhi, G. S., Parker, G. B., & Greenwood, J. 2005, 'Structural and functional models of depression: from sub-types to substrates', *Acta Psychiatr.Scand.*, vol. 111, no. 2, pp. 94–105.

Malt, U. F., Robak, O. H., Madsbu, H. P., Bakke, O., & Loeb, M. 1999, 'The Norwegian naturalistic treatment study of depression in general practice (NORDEP)-I: randomised double blind study', *Br.Med.J.*, vol. 318, no. 7192, pp. 1180–1184.

Malzberg, B. 1938, 'Outcome of insulin treatment of one thousand patients with Dementia Praecox.', *Psychiatr.Quarterly*, vol. 12, pp. 528–553.

Mapp, Y. & Nodine, J. H. 1962, 'Psychopharmacology II. Tranquillisers and antipsychotic drugs', *Psychosomatics*, vol. 3, pp. 458–463.

Marangell, L. B., Silver, J. M., Goff, D. C., & Yudofsky, S. C. 2001, 'Psychopharmacology and ECT', in *Textbook of Clinical Psychiatry*, R. E. Hales & S. C. Yudofsky, eds, American Psychiatric Association, pp. 1047–1149.

Margolese, H. C., Chouinard, G., Kolivakis, T. T., Beauclair, L., Miller, R., & Annable, L. 2005, 'Tardive dyskinesia in the era of typical and atypical antipsychotics. Part 2: Incidence and management strategies in patients with schizophrenia', *Can.J.Psychiatry*, vol. 50, no. 11, pp. 703–714.

Margraf, J., Ehlers, A., Roth, W. T., Clark, D. B., Sheikh, J., Agras, W. S., & Taylor, C. B. 1991, 'How 'blind' are double-blind studies?', *J.Consult.Clin.Psychol.*, vol. 59, no. 1, pp. 184–187.

Markar, H. R. & Mander, A. J. 1989, 'Efficacy of lithium prophylaxis in clinical practice', *Br.J.Psychiatry*, vol. 155, pp. 496–500.

Marshall, M., Lewis, S., Lockwood, A., Drake, R., Jones, P., & Croudace, T. 2005, 'Association between duration of untreated psychosis and outcome in cohorts of first-episode patients: a systematic review', *Arch.Gen.Psychiatry*, vol. 62, no. 9, pp. 975–983.

Martinez, C., Rietbrock, S., Wise, L., Ashby, D., Chick, J., Moseley, J., Evans, S., & Gunnell, D. 2005, 'Antidepressant treatment and the risk of fatal and non-fatal self harm in first episode depression: nested case-control study', *Br.Med.J.*, vol. 330, no. 7488, p. 389.

Marx, K. 1990, *Capital Volume 1*. Penguin Books, London.

Marx, K. & Engels, F. 1970, *The German Ideology*. Lawrence & Wishart, London.

Matsubara, S., Arora, R. C., & Meltzer, H. Y. 1991, 'Serotonergic measures in suicide brain: 5-HT1A binding sites in frontal cortex of suicide victims', *J.Neural Transm.Gen.Sect.*, vol. 85, no. 3, pp. 181–194.

Matthysse, S. 1973, 'Antipsychotic drug actions: a clue to the neuropathology of schizophrenia?', *Fed.Proc.*, vol. 32, no. 2, pp. 200–205.

Matthysse, S. 1974, 'Dopamine and the pharmacology of schizophrenia: the state of the evidence', *J.Psychiatr.Res.*, vol. 11, pp. 107–113.

May, P. R., Tuma, A. H., Dixon, W. J., Yale, C., Thiele, D. A., & Kraude, W. H. 1981, 'Schizophrenia. A follow-up study of the results of five forms of treatment', *Arch.Gen.Psychiatry*, vol. 38, no. 7, pp. 776–784.

Mayer-Gross, W., Slater, E., & Roth, M. 1954, *Clinical Psychiatry*, First edn, Cassell & Co., London.

Mayer-Gross, W., Slater, E., & Roth, M. 1960, *Clinical Psychiatry*, Second edn, Cassell & Co., London.

Mayers, A. G. & Baldwin, D. S. 2005, 'Antidepressants and their effect on sleep', *Hum.Psychopharmacol.*, vol. 20, no. 8, pp. 533–559.

McClelland, G. R., Cooper, S. M., & Pilgrim, A. J. 1990, 'A comparison of the central nervous system effects of haloperidol, chlorpromazine and sulpiride in normal volunteers', *Br.J.Clin.Pharmacol.*, vol. 30, no. 6, pp. 795–803.

McDonald, C., Bullmore, E., Sham, P., Chitnis, X., Suckling, J., MacCabe, J., Walshe, M., & Murray, R. M. 2005, 'Regional volume deviations of brain structure in schizophrenia and psychotic bipolar disorder: computational morphometry study', *Br.J.Psychiatry*, vol. 186, pp. 369–377.

McGlashan, T. H., Zipursky, R. B., Perkins, D., Addington, J., Miller, T., Woods, S. W., Hawkins, K. A., Hoffman, R. E., Preda, A., Epstein, I., Addington, D., Lindborg, S., Trzaskoma, Q., Tohen, M., & Breier, A. 2006, 'Randomized, double-blind trial of olanzapine versus placebo in patients prodromally symptomatic for psychosis', *Am.J.Psychiatry*, vol. 163, no. 5, pp. 790–799.

McGorry, P., Nordentoft, M., & Simonsen, E. E. 2005, 'Early Psychosis; a bridge to the future', *Br.J.Psychiatry Suppl.*, vol. 187, suppl. no. 48.

McGorry, P. D., Yung, A. R., Phillips, L. J., Yuen, H. P., Francey, S., Cosgrave, E. M., Germano, D., Bravin, J., McDonald, T., Blair, A., Adlard, S., & Jackson, H. 2002, 'Randomized controlled trial of interventions designed to reduce the risk of progression to first-episode psychosis in a clinical sample with subthreshold symptoms', *Arch.Gen.Psychiatry*, vol. 59, no. 10, pp. 921–928.

McGurk, S. R., Carter, C., Goldman, R., Green, M. F., Marder, S. R., Xie, H., Schooler, N. R., & Kane, J. M. 2005, 'The effects of clozapine and risperidone on spatial working memory in schizophrenia', *Am.J.Psychiatry*, vol. 162, no. 5, pp. 1013–1016.

Medawar, C. 2001, *Health, Pharma and the EU. A Briefing for Members of the European Parliament on Direct to Consumer Advertising*, www.socialaudit.org.uk/5111–005.htm#HEALTH.

Medical Research Council 1965, 'Clinical trial of the treatment of depressive illness.', *Br.Med.J.*, vol. 1, pp. 881–886.

Meek, C. 'SSRI ads questioned'. *Can.Med.Assoc.J. News*, 174 [6], 754, 2006.

Mehta, M. A., Sahakian, B. J., McKenna, P. J., & Robbins, T. W. 1999, 'Systemic sulpiride in young adult volunteers simulates the profile of cognitive deficits in Parkinson's disease', *Psychopharmacology (Berl)*, vol. 146, no. 2, pp. 162–174.

Melander, H., Ahlqvist-Rastad, J., Meijer, G., & Beermann, B. 2003, 'Evidence b(i)ased medicine – selective reporting from studies sponsored by pharmaceutical industry: review of studies in new drug applications', *Br.Med.J.*, vol. 326, no. 7400, pp. 1171–1173.

Melleril advertisement 1962, 'Melleril advertisement', *Br.Med.J.*, vol. 1, no. 20th January.

Meltzer, H. Y. 1976, 'Biochemical studies in schizophrenia', *Schizophr.Bull.*, vol. 2, no. 1, pp. 10–18.

Meltzer, H. Y. & Stahl, S. M. 1976, 'The dopamine hypothesis of schizophrenia: a review', *Schizophr.Bull.*, vol. 2, no. 1, pp. 19–76.

Mendels, J. & Frazer, A. 1974, 'Brain biogenic amine depletion and mood', *Arch.Gen.Psychiatry*, vol. 30, no. 4, pp. 447–451.

Mendels, J., Stinnett, J. L., Burns, D., & Frazer, A. 1975, 'Amine precursors and depression', *Arch.Gen.Psychiatry*, vol. 32, no. 1, pp. 22–30.

Merlis, S., Turner, W. J., & Krumholz, W. 1962, 'A double-blind comparison of diazepam, chlordiazepoxide and chlorpromazine in psychotic patients', *J.Neuropsychiatr.*, vol. 3, suppl. 1, p. S8.

Meyer, J. H., Houle, S., Sagrati, S., Carella, A., Hussey, D. F., Ginovart, N., Goulding, V., Kennedy, J., & Wilson, A. A. 2004, 'Brain serotonin transporter binding potential measured with carbon 11-labeled DASB positron emission tomography: effects of major depressive episodes and severity of dysfunctional attitudes', *Arch.Gen.Psychiatry*, vol. 61, no. 12, pp. 1271–1279.

Meyer-Lindenberg, A., Miletich, R. S., Kohn, P. D., Esposito, G., Carson, R. E., Quarantelli, M., Weinberger, D. R., & Berman, K. F. 2002, 'Reduced prefrontal activity predicts exaggerated striatal dopaminergic function in schizophrenia', *Nat.Neurosci.*, vol. 5, no. 3, pp. 267–271.

Mizrahi, R., Bagby, R. M., Zipursky, R. B., & Kapur, S. 2005, 'How antipsychotics work: the patients' perspective', *Prog.Neuropsychopharmacol.Biol.Psychiatry*, vol. 29, no. 5, pp. 859–864.

Monahan, J., Redlich, A. D., Swanson, J., Robbins, P. C., Appelbaum, P. S., Petrila, J., Steadman, H. J., Swartz, M., Angell, B., & McNiel, D. E. 2005, 'Use of leverage to improve adherence to psychiatric treatment in the community', *Psychiatr.Serv.*, vol. 56, no. 1, pp. 37–44.

Moncrieff, J. 1995, 'Lithium revisited. A re-examination of the placebo-controlled trials of lithium prophylaxis in manic-depressive disorder', *Br.J.Psychiatry*, vol. 167, no. 5, pp. 569–573.

Moncrieff, J. 1997, 'Lithium: evidence reconsidered', *Br.J.Psychiatry*, vol. 171, pp. 113–119.

Moncrieff, J. 1999, 'An investigation into the precedents of modern drug treatment in psychiatry', *Hist. Psychiatry*, vol. 10, no. 40, Pt 4, pp. 475–490.

Moncrieff, J. 2003a, 'A comparison of antidepressant trials using active and inert placebos', *Int.J.Methods Psychiatr.Res.*, vol. 12, no. 3, pp. 117–127.

Moncrieff, J. 2003b, 'Antidepressant prescribing and suicide: analysis is misleading', *Br.Med.J.*, vol. 327, no. 7409, p. 288.

Moncrieff, J. 2003c, *Is Psychiatry for Sale?* Institute of Psychiatry, London.

Moncrieff, J. 2006, 'Does antipsychotic withdrawal provoke psychosis? Review of the literature on rapid onset psychosis (supersensitivity psychosis) and withdrawal-related relapse', *Acta Psychiatr.Scand.*, vol. 114, no. 1, pp. 3–13.

Moncrieff, J. 2007, 'Neoliberalism and biopsychiatry: a marriage of convenience,' in *Liberatory Psychiatry*, C. Cohen & S. Timimi, eds, Cambridge University Press, Cambridge.

Moncrieff, J. & Cohen, D. 2005, 'Rethinking models of psychotropic drug action', *Psychother.Psychosom.*, vol. 74, no. 3, pp. 145–153.

Moncrieff, J. & Crawford, M. J. 2001, 'British psychiatry in the 20th century – observations from a psychiatric journal', *Soc.Sci.Med.*, vol. 53, no. 3, pp. 349–356.

Moncrieff, J. & Kirsch, I. 2005, 'Efficacy of antidepressants in adults', *Br.Med.J.*, vol. 331, no. 7509, pp. 155–157.

Moncrieff, J. & Pomerleau, J. 2000, 'Trends in sickness benefits in Great Britain and the contribution of mental disorders', *J.Public Health Med.*, vol. 22, no. 1, pp. 59–67.

Moncrieff, J., Wessely, S., & Hardy, R. 1998, 'Meta-analysis of trials comparing antidepressants with active placebos', *Br.J.Psychiatry*, vol. 172, pp. 227–231.

Montgomery, A. J., Mehta, M. A., & Grasby, P. M. 2006, 'Is psychological stress in man associated with increased striatal dopamine levels?: A [11C]raclopride PET study', *Synapse*, vol. 60, no. 2, pp. 124–131.

Montgomery, S. A. & Asberg, M. 1979, 'A new depression scale designed to be sensitive to change', *Br.J.Psychiatry*, vol. 134, pp. 382–389.

Moss, B. F. J., Thigpen, C. H., & Robinson, W. P. 1953, 'Report on the use of succinyl choline dichloride (a curare-like drug) in electroconvulsive therapy.', *Am.J.Psychiatry*, vol. 109, pp. 895–898.

Moynihan, R. & Cassels, A. 2005, *Selling Sickness: How the World's Biggest Pharmaceutical Companies are Turning Us All into Patients*. Nation Books, New York.

Moynihan, R., Heath, I., & Henry, D. 2002, 'Selling sickness: the pharmaceutical industry and disease mongering', *Br.Med.J.*, vol. 324, no. 7342, pp. 886–891.

Mueller, T. I., Leon, A. C., Keller, M. B., Solomon, D. A., Endicott, J., Coryell, W., Warshaw, M., & Maser, J. D. 1999, 'Recurrence after recovery from major depressive disorder during 15 years of observational follow-up', *Am.J.Psychiatry*, vol. 156, no. 7, pp. 1000–1006.

Muller, P. & Seeman, P. 1977, 'Brain neurotransmitter receptors after long-term haloperidol: dopamine, acetylcholine, serotonin, alpha-noradrenergic and naloxone receptors', *Life Sci.*, vol. 21, no. 12, pp. 1751–1758.

Muller, P. & Seeman, P. 1978, 'Dopaminergic supersensitivity after neuroleptics: time-course and specificity', *Psychopharmacology (Berl)*, vol. 60, no. 1, pp. 1–11.

Muller-Oerlinghausen, B., Hamann, S., Herrmann, W. M., & Kropf, D. 1979, 'Effects of lithium on vigilance, psychomotoric performance and mood', *Pharmakopsychiatr.Neuropsychopharmakol.*, vol. 12, no. 5, pp. 388–396.

Murphy, F. C., Smith, K. A., Cowen, P. J., Robbins, T. W., & Sahakian, B. J. 2002, 'The effects of tryptophan depletion on cognitive and affective processing in healthy volunteers', *Psychopharmacology (Berl)*, vol. 163, no. 1, pp. 42–53.

Murphy, G. E. & Wetzel, R. D. 1980, 'Suicide risk by birth cohort in the United States, 1949 to 1974', *Arch.Gen.Psychiatry*, vol. 37, no. 5, pp. 519–523.

Myslobodsky, M. S. 1993, 'Central determinants of attention and mood disorder in tardive dyskinesia ('tardive dysmentia')', *Brain Cogn.*, vol. 23, no. 1, pp. 88–101.

Nardil advertisement. 1960, *Am.J.Psychiatry*, no. March, p. XII.

Nardil advertisement. 1961, *Br.Med.J.*, no. Jan 14th.

National Institute for Clinical Excellence. 2002, *Schizophrenia: Core interventions in the Treatment and Management of Schizophrenia in Primary and Secondary Care*. National Institute for Clinical Excellence, London.

National Institute for Clinical Excellence. 2004, *Depression: Management of Depression in Primary and Secondary Care. Clinical Practice Guideline Number 23*, National Institute for Clinical Excellence, London.

National Institute for Clinical Excellence. 2006, *Bipolar Disorder. The Management of Bipolar Disorder in Adults, Children and Adolescents, in Primary and Secondary Care*. National Institute for Clinical Excellence, London, NICE Clinical Guideline 38.

National Institute for Health Care Management. 2002, *Prescription Drug Expenditures in 2001*, National Institute for Health Care Management, Washington, DC.

Nemeroff, C. B. 1997, 'Dosing the antipsychotic medication olanzapine', *J.Clin.Psychiatry*, vol. 58, suppl. 10, pp. 45–49.

New York Times. Mind is mapped in cure of insane. *New York Times*, 15.05.1937.

New York Times. President seeks funds to to reduce mental illness. *New York Times*, 06.02. 1963.

Newcomer, J. W., Haupt, D. W., Fucetola, R., Melson, A. K., Schweiger, J. A., Cooper, B. P., & Selke, G. 2002, 'Abnormalities in glucose regulation during antipsychotic treatment of schizophrenia', *Arch.Gen.Psychiatry*, vol. 59, no. 4, pp. 337–345.

Niamid advertisement. 1962, *Br.Med.J.*, vol. 1, no. Jan 27th.

Nishikawa, T., Tsuda, A., Tanaka, M., Koga, I., & Uchida, Y. 1982, 'Prophylactic effect of neuroleptics in symptom-free schizophrenics', *Psychopharmacology (Berl)*, vol. 77, no. 4, pp. 301–304.

Nordstrom, A. L., Farde, L., Eriksson, L., & Halldin, C. 1995, 'No elevated D2 dopamine receptors in neuroleptic-naive schizophrenic patients revealed by positron emission tomography and [11C]N-methylspiperone', *Psychiatry Res.*, vol. 61, no. 2, pp. 67–83.

Norton, B. & Whalley, L. J. 1984, 'Mortality of a lithium-treated population', *Br.J.Psychiatry*, vol. 145, pp. 277–282.

Noyes, A. P. & Kolb, L. C. 1958, *Modern Clinical Psychiatry*. Saunders, Philadelphia.

O'Connell, R. A., Mayo, J. A., Flatow, L., Cuthbertson, B., & O'Brien, B. E. 1991, 'Outcome of bipolar disorder on long-term treatment with lithium', *Br.J.Psychiatry*, vol. 159, pp. 123–129.

Odegaard, O. 1964, 'Pattern of discharge from Norwegian psychiatric hospitals before and after the introduction of psychiatric drugs', *Am.J.Psychiatry*, vol. 70, pp. 772–778.

Olfson, M., Blanco, C., Liu, L., Moreno, C., & Laje, G. 2006, 'National trends in the outpatient treatment of children and adolescents with antipsychotic drugs', *Arch.Gen.Psychiatry*, vol. 63, no. 6, pp. 679–685.

Olfson, M., Marcus, S. C., & Shaffer, D. 2006, 'Antidepressant drug therapy and suicide in severely depressed children and adults: a case-control study', *Arch.Gen.Psychiatry*, vol. 63, no. 8, pp. 865–872.

Opbroek, A., Delgado, P. L., Laukes, C., McGahuey, C., Katsanis, J., Moreno, F. A., & Manber, R. 2002, 'Emotional blunting associated with SSRI-induced sexual dysfunction. Do SSRIs inhibit emotional responses?', *Int.J.Neuropsychopharmacol.*, vol. 5, no. 2, pp. 147–151.

Osborn, D. P., Levy, G., Nazareth, I., Petersen, I., Islam, A., & King, M. B. 2007, 'Relative risk of cardiovascular and cancer mortality in people with severe mental illness from the United Kingdom's General Practice Rsearch Database', *Arch.Gen.Psychiatry*, vol. 64, no. 2, pp. 242–249.

Osby, U., Correia, N., Brandt, L., Ekbom, A., & Sparen, P. 2000, 'Mortality and causes of death in schizophrenia in Stockholm county, Sweden', *Schizophr.Res.*, vol. 45, no. 1–2, pp. 21–28.

Overall, J. E., Hollister, L. E., Meyer, F., Kimbell, I., Jr., & Shelton, J. 1964, 'Imipramine and thioridazine in depressed and schizophrenic patients. Are there specific antidepressant drugs?', *JAMA*, vol. 189, pp. 605–608.

Overholser, W. 1956, 'Has chlorpromazine inaugurated a new era in mental hospitals?', *J.Clin.Exp.Psychopathology*, vol. 17, pp. 197–201.

Palisa, Ch. 1938, 'The awakening from hypoglycaemic shock', *Am.J.Psychiatry Suppl.*, vol. 94, pp. 96–108.

Pariante, C. M., Vassilopoulou, K., Velakoulis, D., Phillips, L., Soulsby, B., Wood, S. J., Brewer, W., Smith, D. J., Dazzan, P., Yung, A. R., Zervas, I. M., Christodoulou, G. N., Murray, R., McGorry, P. D., & Pantelis, C. 2004, 'Pituitary volume in psychosis', *Br.J.Psychiatry*, vol. 185, pp. 5–10.

Parker, I. 1992, *Discourse Dynamics: Critical Analysis for Social and Individual Psychology*. Routledge, London.

Parra, A. 2003, 'A common role for psychotropic medications: memory impairment', *Med.Hypotheses*, vol. 60, pp. 133–142.

Parsey, R. V., Oquendo, M. A., Ogden, R. T., Olvet, D. M., Simpson, N., Huang, Y. Y., Van Heertum, R. L., Arango, V., & Mann, J. J. 2006, 'Altered Serotonin 1A Binding in Major Depression: A [carbonyl-C-11]WAY100635 Positron Emission Tomography Study', *Biol.Psychiatry*, vol. 59, no. 2, pp. 106–113.

Parstellin advertisement. 1962, *Br.Med.J.*, vol. 1, no. Feb 10th.

Paterson, A. S. 1963, *Electrical and Drug Treatments in Psychiatry*. Elsevier, London.

Patten, S. B. 2004, 'The impact of antidepressant treatment on population health: synthesis of data from two national data sources in Canada', *Popul.Health Metr.*, vol. 2, no. 1, p. 9.

Paykel, E. S., Hollyman, J. A., Freeling, P., & Sedgwick, P. 1988, 'Predictors of therapeutic benefit from amitriptyline in mild depression: a general practice placebo-controlled trial', *J.Affect.Disord.*, vol. 14, no. 1, pp. 83–95.

Paykel, E. S. & Priest, R. G. 1992, 'Recognition and management of depression in general practice: consensus statement', *Br.Med.J.*, vol. 305, no. 6863, pp. 1198–1202.

Pearson, I. B. & Jenner, F. A. 1971, 'Lithium in psychiatry', *Nature*, vol. 232, no. 5312, pp. 532–533.

Pellegrino, E. D. 1979, 'The socio-cultural impact of twentieth century therapeutics,' in *The Therapeutic Revolution*, M. J. Vogel & C. E. Rosenberg, eds, University of Pennsylvania Press, Philadelphia, PA, pp. 245–266.

Perera, K. M., Powell, T., & Jenner, F. A. 1987, 'Computerized axial tomographic studies following long-term use of benzodiazepines', *Psychol.Med.*, vol. 17, no. 3, pp. 775–777.

Peretti, C. S., Danion, J. M., Kauffmann-Muller, F., Grange, D., Patat, A., & Rosenzweig, P. 1997, 'Effects of haloperidol and amisulpride on motor and cognitive skill learning in healthy volunteers', *Psychopharmacology (Berl)*, vol. 131, no. 4, pp. 329–338.

Perlis, R. H., Sachs, G. S., Lafer, B., Otto, M. W., Faraone, S. V., Kane, J. M., & Rosenbaum, J. F. 2002, 'Effect of abrupt change from standard to low serum levels of lithium: a reanalysis of double-blind lithium maintenance data', *Am.J.Psychiatry*, vol. 159, no. 7, pp. 1155–1159.

Perlis, R. H., Welge, J. A., Vornik, L. A., Hirschfeld, R. M., & Keck, P. E., Jr. 2006, 'Atypical antipsychotics in the treatment of mania: a meta-analysis of randomized, placebo-controlled trials', *J.Clin.Psychiatry*, vol. 67, no. 4, pp. 509–516.

Petrie, A. A. W. 1945, 'Psychiatric developments. The presidential address delivered at one hundred and third annual meeting of the Association on Wednesday November 29, 1944', *J.Ment.Sci.*, vol. 91, pp. 267–280.

Pfizer. Pfizer website . 06.02.2006. www.geodon.com/s_WhatCauses.asp.

Philipp, M., Kohnen, R., & Hiller, K. O. 1999, 'Hypericum extract versus imipramine or placebo in patients with moderate depression: randomised multicentre study of treatment for eight weeks', *Br.Med.J.*, vol. 319, no. 7224, pp. 1534–1538.

Pilowsky, L. S., Costa, D. C., Ell, P. J., Verhoeff, N. P., Murray, R. M., & Kerwin, R. W. 1994, 'D2 dopamine receptor binding in the basal ganglia of antipsychotic-free schizophrenic patients. An 123I-IBZM single photon emission computerised tomography study', *Br.J.Psychiatry*, vol. 164, no. 1, pp. 16–26.

Pincus, H. A., Tanielian, T. L., Marcus, S. C., Olfson, M., Zarin, D. A., Thompson, J., & Magno, Z. J. 1998, 'Prescribing trends in psychotropic medications: primary care, psychiatry, and other medical specialties', *JAMA*, vol. 279, no. 7, pp. 526–531.

Pollock, H. 1939, 'A statistical study of 1,140 Dementia Praecox patients treated with metrazol', *Psychiatr.Q.*, vol. 13, pp. 558–568.

Post, R. M., Denicoff, K. D., Frye, M. A., Dunn, R. T., Leverich, G. S., Osuch, E., & Speer, A. 1998, 'A history of the use of anticonvulsants as mood stabilizers in the last two decades of the 20th century', *Neuropsychobiology*, vol. 38, no. 3, pp. 152–166.

Posternak, M. A., Solomon, D. A., Leon, A. C., Mueller, T. I., Shea, M. T., Endicott, J., & Keller, M. B. 2006, 'The naturalistic course of unipolar major depression in the absence of somatic therapy', *J.Nerv.Ment.Dis.*, vol. 194, no. 5, pp. 324–329.

Prien, R. F., Caffey, E. M., Jr., & Klett, C. J. 1972, 'Comparison of lithium carbonate and chlorpromazine in the treatment of mania. Report of the Veterans Administration and National Institute of Mental Health Collaborative Study Group', *Arch.Gen.Psychiatry*, vol. 26, no. 2, pp. 146–153.

Prien, R. F., Caffey, E. M., Jr., & Klett, C. J. 1973, 'Prophylactic efficacy of lithium carbonate in manic-depressive illness. Report of the Veterans Administration and National Institute of Mental Health collaborative study group', *Arch.Gen.Psychiatry*, vol. 28, no. 3, pp. 337–341.

Priest, R. G., Vize, C., Roberts, A., Roberts, M., & Tylee, A. 1996, 'Lay people's attitudes to treatment of depression: results of opinion poll for Defeat Depression Campaign just before its launch', *Br.Med.J.*, vol. 313, no. 7061, pp. 858–859.

Proceedings held under the auspices of Smith Kline & French laboratories, J. 6. 1. 1955, 'Chlorpormazine and Mental Health', Lea & Febiger.

Prolixen advertisement. 1960, 'Prolixen advertisement', *Am.J.Psychiatry*, vol. 117, no. March, p. X.

Pruessner, J. C., Champagne, F., Meaney, M. J., & Dagher, A. 2004, 'Dopamine release in response to a psychological stress in humans and its relationship to early life maternal care: a positron emission tomography study using [11C]raclopride', *J.Neurosci.*, vol. 24, no. 11, pp. 2825–2831.

Pycock, C., Tarsy, D., & Marsden, C. D. 1975c, 'Inhibition of circling behavior by neuroleptic drugs in mice with unilateral 6-hydroxydopamine lesions of the striatum', *Psychopharmacologia.*, vol. 45, no. 2, pp. 211–219.

Quality Assurance Project 1983, 'A treatment outline for depressive disorders. The Quality Assurance Project', *Aust.N.Z.J.Psychiatry*, vol. 17, no. 2, pp. 129–146.

Quitkin, F. M., Rabkin, J. G., Gerald, J., Davis, J. M., & Klein, D. F. 2000, 'Validity of clinical trials of antidepressants', *Am.J.Psychiatry*, vol. 157, no. 3, pp. 327–337.

Ramaekers, J. G., Louwerens, J. W., Muntjewerff, N. D., Milius, H., de Bie, A., Rosenzweig, P., Patat, A., & O'Hanlon, J. F. 1999, 'Psychomotor, cognitive, extrapyramidal, and affective functions of healthy volunteers during treatment with an atypical (amisulpride) and a classic (haloperidol) antipsychotic', *J.Clin.Psychopharmacol.*, vol. 19, no. 3, pp. 209–221.

Ramaekers, J. G., Muntjewerff, N. D., & O'Hanlon, J. F. 1995, 'A comparative study of acute and subchronic effects of dothiepin, fluoxetine and placebo on psychomotor and actual driving performance', *Br.J.Clin.Pharmacol.*, vol. 39, no. 4, pp. 397–404.

Rammsayer, T. & Gallhofer, B. 1995, 'Remoxipride versus haloperidol in healthy volunteers: psychometric performance and subjective tolerance profiles', *Int.Clin.Psychopharmacol.*, vol. 10, no. 1, pp. 31–37.

Rappaport, M., Hopkins, H. K., Hall, K., Belleza, T., & Silverman, J. 1978, 'Are there schizophrenics for whom drugs may be unnecessary or contraindicated?', *Int.Pharmacopsychiatry*, vol. 13, no. 2, pp. 100–111.

Raptopoulos, P., McClelland, G. R., & Jackson, D. 1989, 'The clinical pharmacology of paroxetine in healthy subjects', *Acta Psychiatr.Scand.Suppl.*, vol. 350, pp. 46–48.

Raskin, A. & Crook, T. H. 1975, 'Antidepressants in black and white inpatients. Differential response to a controlled trial of chlorpromazine and imipramine', *Arch.Gen.Psychiatry*, vol. 32, no. 5, pp. 643–649.

Raskin, A. & Crook, T. H. 1976, 'The endogenous-neurotic distinction as a predictor of response to antidepressant drugs', *Psychol.Med.*, vol. 6, no. 1, pp. 59–70.

Raskin, A., Schulterbrandt, J. G., Reatig, N., & McKeon, J. J. 1970, 'Differential response to chlorpromazine, imipramine, and placebo. A study of subgroups of hospitalized depressed patients', *Arch.Gen.Psychiatry*, vol. 23, no. 2, pp. 164–173.

Rauste-von Wright, M. & Frankenhaeuser, M. 1989, 'Females' emotionality as reflected in the excretion of the dopamine metabolite HVA during mental stress', *Psychol.Rep.*, vol. 64, no. 3, Pt 1, pp. 856–858.

Rees, L. 1960, 'Treatment of depression by drugs and other means', *Nature*, vol. 186, pp. 114–120.

Rees, L., Brown, A. C., & Benaim, S. 1961, 'A controlled trial of imipramine ('Tofranil') in the treatment of severe depressive states', *J.Ment.Sci.*, vol. 107, pp. 552–559.

Reichenberg, A., Weiser, M., Caspi, A., Knobler, H. Y., Lubin, G., Harvey, P. D., Rabinowitz, J., & Davidson, M. 2006, 'Premorbid intellectual functioning and risk of schizophrenia and spectrum disorders', *J.Clin.Exp.Neuropsychol.*, vol. 28, no. 2, pp. 193–207.

Reichenberg, A., Weiser, M., Rapp, M. A., Rabinowitz, J., Caspi, A., Schmeidler, J., Knobler, H. Y., Lubin, G., Nahon, D., Harvey, P. D., & Davidson, M. 2005, 'Elaboration on premorbid intellectual performance in schizophrenia: premorbid intellectual decline and risk for schizophrenia', *Arch.Gen.Psychiatry*, vol. 62, no. 12, pp. 1297–1304.

Reilly, J. L., Harris, M. S., Keshavan, M. S., & Sweeney, J. A. 2006, 'Adverse effects of risperidone on spatial working memory in first-episode schizophrenia', *Arch.Gen.Psychiatry*, vol. 63, no. 11, pp. 1189–1197.

Reith, J., Benkelfat, C., Sherwin, A., Yasuhara, Y., Kuwabara, H., Andermann, F., Bachneff, S., Cumming, P., Diksic, M., Dyve, S. E., Etienne, P., Evans, A. C., Lal, S., Shevell, M., Savard, G., Wong, D. F., Chouinard, G., & Gjedde, A. 1994, 'Elevated dopa decarboxylase activity in living brain of patients with psychosis', *Proc.Natl.Acad.Sci.U.S.A*, vol. 91, no. 24, pp. 11651–11654.

Reivich, M., Amsterdam, J. D., Brunswick, D. J., & Shiue, C. Y. 2004, 'PET brain imaging with [11C](+)McN5652 shows increased serotonin transporter availability in major depression', *J.Affect.Disord.*, vol. 82, no. 2, pp. 321–327.

Reynolds, G. P. 1989, 'Beyond the dopamine hypothesis. The neurochemical pathology of schizophrenia', *Br.J.Psychiatry*, vol. 155, pp. 305–316.

Reynolds, G. P. & Czudek, C. 1988, 'Status of the dopaminergic system in postmortem brain in schizophrenia', *Psychopharmacol.Bull.*, vol. 24, no. 3, pp. 345–347.

Reynolds, G. P., Riederer, P., Jellinger, K., & Gabriel, E. 1981, 'Dopamine receptors and schizophrenia: the neuroleptic drug problem', *Neuropharmacology*, vol. 20, no. 12B, pp. 1319–1320.

Rickels, K., Gordon, P. E., Gansman, D. H., Weise, C. C., Pereira-Ogan, J. A., & Hesbacher, P. T. 1970, 'Pemoline and methylphenidate in mildy depressed outpatients', *Clin.Pharmacol.Ther.*, vol. 11, no. 5, pp. 698–710.

Rifkin, A., Quitkin, F. M., & Klein, D. F. 1975, 'Akinesia: a poorly recognised disorder', *Arch.Gen.Psychiatry*, vol. 32, p. 672.

Risperidol Consta advertisment. *Br.Med.J.*, 334, 03.03.2007.

Ritalin advertisement. 1964, *Br.Med.J.*, vol. 2, no. 24th Oct.

Robertson, M. M. & Trimble, M. R. 1982, 'Major tranquillisers used as antidepressants. A review', *J.Affect.Disord.*, vol. 4, no. 3, pp. 173–193.

Robinson, D. G., Woerner, M. G., McMeniman, M., Mendelowitz, A., & Bilder, R. M. 2004, 'Symptomatic and functional recovery from a first episode of schizophrenia or schizoaffective disorder', *Am.J.Psychiatry*, vol. 161, no. 3, pp. 473–479.

Robinson, D. G., Woerner, M. G., Napolitano, B., Patel, R. C., Sevy, S. M., Gunduz-Bruce, H., Soto-Perello, J. M., Mendelowitz, A., Khadivi, A., Miller, R., McCormack, J., Lorell, B. S., Lesser, M. L., Schooler, N. R., & Kane, J. M. 2006, 'Randomized comparison of olanzapine versus risperidone for the treatment of first-episode schizophrenia: 4-month outcomes', *Am.J.Psychiatry*, vol. 163, no. 12, pp. 2096–2102.

Robinson, D. S., Rickels, K., Feighner, J., Fabre, L. F., Jr., Gammans, R. E., Shrotriya, R. C., Alms, D. R., Andary, J. J., & Messina, M. E. 1990, 'Clinical effects of the 5-HT1A partial agonists in depression: a composite analysis of buspirone in the treatment of depression', *J.Clin.Psychopharmacol.*, vol. 51, no. 3, pp. 67S–76S.

Rochon, P. A., Stukel, T. A., Sykora, K., Gill, S., Garfinkel, S., Anderson, G. M., Normand, S. L., Mamdani, M., Lee, P. E., Li, P., Bronskill, S. E., Marras, C., & Gurwitz, J. H. 2005, 'Atypical antipsychotics and parkinsonism', *Arch.Intern.Med.*, vol. 165, no. 16, pp. 1882–1888.

Rogers, A. & Pilgrim, D. 2001, 'Mental Health Policy in Britan', Basingstoke, Hampshire: Palgrave Macmillan.

Rogers, S. C. & Clay, P. M. 1975, 'A statistical review of controlled trials of imipramine and placebo in the treatment of depressive illnesses', *Br.J.Psychiatry*, vol. 127, pp. 599–603.

Rollin, H. R. 1990, 'The dark before the dawn', *J.Psychopharmacol.*, vol. 4, no. 3, pp. 109–114.

Ronalds, C., Creed, F., Stone, K., Webb, S., & Tomenson, B. 1997, 'Outcome of anxiety and depressive disorders in primary care', *Br.J.Psychiatry*, vol. 171, pp. 427–433.

Rosanoff, A. D. o. I. 1941, *Report for Governor's Council on Activities during June 1941*, California State Printing Office, Sacramento, CA.

Rose, D., Fleischmann, P., Wykes, T., Leese, M., & Bindman, J. 2003, 'Patients' perspectives on electroconvulsive therapy: systematic review', *Br.Med.J.*, vol. 326, no. 7403, p. 1363.

Rose, N. 2004, 'Becoming neurochemical selves,' in *Biotechnology, Commerce and Civil Society*, N. Stehr, ed., Transaction Publishers, New Brunswick, New Jersey, pp. 89–128.

Rose, S., Lewontin, R. C., & Kamin, L. J. 1984, *Not in Our Genes. Biology, Ideology and Human Nature*. Pantheon Books, New York.

Rosenberg, C. E. 1977, 'The therapeutic revolution: medicine, meaning and social change in 19th century America,' J. W. Leavitt & R. L. Numbers, eds, University of Wisconsin Press, Wisconsin.

Rosenberg, C. E. 1986, 'Disease and social order in America: perceptions and expectations', *Milbank Quarterly*, vol. 64, pp. 34–55.

Rosengarten, H. & Quartermain, D. 2002, 'Effect of prenatal administration of haloperidol, risperidone, quetiapine and olanzapine on spatial learning and retention in adult rats', *Pharmacol.Biochem.Behav.*, vol. 72, no. 3, pp. 575–579.

Rosenhan, D. L. 1973, 'On being sane in insane places', *Science*, vol. 179, no. 70, pp. 250–258.

Rosenheck, R., Perlick, D., Bingham, S., Liu-Mares, W., Collins, J., Warren, S., Leslie, D., Allan, E., Campbell, E. C., Caroff, S., Corwin, J., Davis, L., Douyon, R., Dunn, L., Evans, D., Frecska, E., Grabowski, J., Graeber, D., Herz, L., Kwon, K., Lawson, W., Mena, F., Sheikh, J., Smelson, D., & Smith-Gamble, V. 2003, 'Effectiveness and cost of olanzapine and haloperidol in the treatment of schizophrenia: a randomized controlled trial', *JAMA*, vol. 290, no. 20, pp. 2693–2702.

Rosenzweig, P., Canal, M., Patat, A., Bergougnan, L., Zieleniuk, I., & Bianchetti, G. 2002, 'A review of the pharmacokinetics, tolerability and pharmacodynamics of amisulpride in healthy volunteers', *Hum.Psychopharmacol.*, vol. 17, no. 1, pp. 1–13.

Ross, C. A. 2006, 'The sham ECT literature: implications for consent to ECT', *Ethical Hum. Psychol.Psychiatry*, vol. 8, no. 1, pp. 17–28.

Ross, J. & Malzberg, B. 1939, 'A review of the results of the pharmacological shock therapy and the metrazol convulsive therapy in New York State.', *Am.J.Psychiatry*, vol. 96, pp. 297–316.

Rossum J.M.Van 1966, 'The significance of dopamine receptor blockade for the action of neuroleptic drugs', in *Neuro-psycho-pharmacology*, H. Brill, ed., Excerpta Medica Foundation, Amsterdam, pp. 321–329.

Rossum, J. M. Van1966a, 'The significance of dopamine-receptor blockade for the mechanism of action of neuroleptic drugs', *Arch.Int.Pharmacodyn.Ther.*, vol. 160, no. 2, pp. 492–494.

Roth, M. 1973, 'Psychiatry and its critics.', *Br.J.Psychiatry*, vol. 122, pp. 373–378.

Rothschild, A. J. & Locke, C. A. 1991, 'Reexposure to fluoxetine after serious suicide attempts by three patients: the role of akathisia', *J.Clin.Psychiatry*, vol. 52, no. 12, pp. 491–493.

Royal College of Psychiatrists. 'Mental health and growing up'. 2004.

Royal College of Psychiatrists. Depression. www.rcpsych.ac.uk/mentalhealth information/mentalhealthproblems/depression/depression.aspx.22.12.2006.

Royal College of Psychiatrists. Antidepressants. 2007. London, Royal College of Psychiatrists.

Royal Commission. 1926, *Report of the Royal Commission on Lunacy and Mental Disorders*, Stationery Office, London, Cmd. 2700.

Royal Commission 1957, *Royal Commission on the Law Relating to Mental Illness and Mental Deficiency 1954–1957*, HMSO, London.

Rubin, E. H., Kinscherf, D. A., Figiel, G. S., & Zorumski, C. F. 1993, 'The nature and time course of cognitive side effects during electroconvulsive therapy in the elderly', *J.Geriatr.Psychiatry Neurol.*, vol. 6, no. 2, pp. 78–83.

Saarialho-Kere, U., Mattila, M. J., Paloheimo, M., & Seppala, T. 1987, 'Psychomotor, respiratory and neuroendocrinological effects of buprenorphine and amitripty-line in healthy volunteers', *Eur.J.Clin.Pharmacol.*, vol. 33, no. 2, pp. 139–146.

Sabshin, M. 1990, 'Turning points in twentieth-century American psychiatry', *Am.J.Psychiatry*, vol. 147, no. 10, pp. 1267–1274.

Sachs, G. S., Nierenberg, A. A., Calabrese, J. R., Marangell, L. B., Wisniewski, S. R., Gyulai, L., Friedman, E. S., Bowden, C. L., Fossey, M. D., Ostacher, M. J., Ketter, T. A., Patel, J., Hauser, P., Rapport, D., Martinez, J. M., Allen, M. H., Miklowitz, D. J., Otto, M. W., Dennehy, E. B., & Thase, M. E. 2007, 'Effectiveness of adjunctive antidepressant treatment for bipolar depression', *N.Engl.J.Med.*, vol. 356, pp. 1711–1722.

Sackeim, H. A., Prudic, J., Devanand, D. P., Kiersky, J. E., Fitzsimons, L., Moody, B. J., McElhiney, M. C., Coleman, E. A., & Settembrino, J. M. 1993, 'Effects of stimulus intensity and electrode placement on the efficacy and cognitive effects of electroconvulsive therapy', *N.Engl.J.Med.*, vol. 328, no. 12, pp. 839–846.

Sacks, O. 1999, *Awakenings*. Vintage Books, Random House, New York.

Sadler, W. S. 1953, *Practice of Psychiatry*. Henry Kimpton, London.

Sakel, M. 1937, 'A new treatment of schizophrenia', *Am.J.Psychiatry*, vol. 93, pp. 829–841.

Sakel, M. 1958, *Schizophrenia*. Philosophical Library, New York.

Saletu, B., Frey, R., Krupka, M., Anderer, P., Grunberger, J., & See, W. R. 1991, 'Sleep laboratory studies on the single-dose effects of serotonin reuptake inhibitors paroxetine and fluoxetine on human sleep and awakening qualities', *Sleep*, vol. 14, no. 5, pp. 439–447.

Samaha, A. N., Seeman, P., Stewart, J., Rajabi, H., & Kapur, S. 2007, ''Breakthrough' dopamine supersensitivity during ongoing antipsychotic treatment leads to treatment failure over time', *J.Neurosci.*, vol. 27, no. 11, pp. 2979–2986.

Saran, B. M. 1969, 'Lithium', *Lancet*, vol. 1, no. 7607, pp. 1208–1209.

Sargant, W. & Slater, E. 1944, *An Introduction to Physical Methods of Treatment in Psychiatry.* Churchill Livingstone, Edinburgh.

Sargent, P. A., Kjaer, K. H., Bench, C. J., Rabiner, E. A., Messa, C., Meyer, J., Gunn, R. N., Grasby, P. M., & Cowen, P. J. 2000, 'Brain serotonin1A receptor binding measured by positron emission tomography with [11C]WAY-100635: effects of depression and antidepressant treatment', *Arch.Gen.Psychiatry*, vol. 57, no. 2, pp. 174–180.

Saroten advertisement. 1962, 'Saroten advertisement', *Br.Med.J.*, vol. 2, no. July 7th, p. 19.

Saykin, A. J., Shtasel, D. L., Gur, R. E., Kester, D. B., Mozley, L. H., Stafiniak, P., & Gur, R. C. 1994, 'Neuropsychological deficits in neuroleptic naive patients with first-episode schizophrenia', *Arch.Gen.Psychiatry*, vol. 51, no. 2, pp. 124–131.

Schachter, H. M., Pham, B., King, J., Langford, S., & Moher, D. 2001, 'How efficacious and safe is short-acting methylphenidate for the treatment of attention-deficit disorder in children and adolescents? A meta-analysis', *CMAJ.*, vol. 165, no. 11, pp. 1475–1488.

Schatzberg, A. F. & Cole, J. O. 1978, 'Benzodiazepines in depressive disorders', *Arch.Gen.Psychiatry*, vol. 35, no. 11, pp. 1359–1365.

Scherer, H., Bedard, M. A., Stip, E., Paquet, F., Richer, F., Beriault, M., Rodriguez, J. P., & Motard, J. P. 2004, 'Procedural learning in schizophrenia can reflect the pharmacologic properties of the antipsychotic treatments', *Cogn.Behav.Neurol.*, vol. 17, no. 1, pp. 32–40.

Scherk, H. & Falkai, P. 2006, 'Effects of antipsychotics on brain structure', *Curr.Opin.Psychiatry*, vol. 19, no. 2, pp. 145–150.

Scherk, H., Pajonk, F. G., & Leucht, S. 2007, 'Second-generation antipsychotic agents in the treatment of acute mania: a systematic review and meta-analysis of randomized controlled trials', *Arch.Gen.Psychiatry*, vol. 64, no. 4, pp. 442–455.

Schildkraut, J. J. 1965, 'The catecholamine hypothesis of affective disorders: a review of supporting evidence', *Am.J.Psychiatry*, vol. 122, no. 5, pp. 509–522.

Schildkraut, J. J., Winokur, A., & Applegate, C. W. 1970, 'Norepinephrine turnover and metabolism in rat brain after long-term administration of imipramine', *Science*, vol. 168, no. 933, pp. 867–869.

Schillevoort, I., van Puijenbroek, E. P., de Boer, A., Roos, R. A., Jansen, P. A., & Leufkens, H. G. 2002, 'Extrapyramidal syndromes associated with selective serotonin reuptake inhibitors: a case-control study using spontaneous reports', *Int.Clin.Psychopharmacol.*, vol. 17, no. 2, pp. 75–79.

Schmauss, C. & Krieg, J. C. 1987, 'Enlargement of cerebrospinal fluid spaces in long-term benzodiazepine abusers', *Psychol.Med.*, vol. 17, no. 4, pp. 869–873.

Schmitt, J. A., Riedel, W. J., Vuurman, E. F., Kruizinga, M., & Ramaekers, J. G. 2002, 'Modulation of the critical flicker fusion effects of serotonin reuptake inhibitors by concomitant pupillary changes', *Psychopharmacology (Berl)*, vol. 160, no. 4, pp. 381–386.

Schooler, N., Rabinowitz, J., Davidson, M., Emsley, R., Harvey, P. D., Kopala, L., McGorry, P. D., Van, H., I, Eerdekens, M., Swyzen, W., & De Smedt, G. 2005, 'Risperidone and haloperidol in first-episode psychosis: a long-term randomized trial', *Am.J.Psychiatry*, vol. 162, no. 5, pp. 947–953.

Schooler, N. R., Goldberg, S. C., Boothe, H., & Cole, J. O. 1967, 'One year after discharge: community adjustment of schizophrenic patients', *Am.J.Psychiatry*, vol. 123, no. 8, pp. 986–995.

Schou, M. 1963, 'Normothymotics, 'mood-normalizers': are lithium and the imipramine drugs specific for affective disorders?', *Br.J.Psychiatry*, vol. 109, pp. 803–809.

Schou, M. 2001, 'Lithium treatment at 52', *J.Affect.Disord.*, vol. 67, no. 1–3, pp. 21–32.

Schou, M., Juel-Nielsen, N., Stromgren, E., & Voldby, H. 1954, 'The treatment of manic psychoses by the administration of lithium salts', *J.Neurol.Neurosurg. Psychiatry*, vol. 17, no. 4, pp. 250–260.

Schultz, J. 1976, 'Psychoactive drug effects on a system which generates cyclic AMP in brain', *Nature*, vol. 261, no. 5559, pp. 417–418.

Schwartz, T. L., Saba, M., Hardoby, W., Virk, S., & Masand, P. S. 2002, 'Use of atypical antipsychotics in a Veterans Affairs hospital', *Prog.Neuropsychopharmacol. Biol.Psychiatry*, vol. 26, no. 6, pp. 1207–1210.

Scott, J., Paykel, E., Morriss, R., Bentall, R., Kinderman, P., Johnson, T., Abbott, R., & Hayhurst, H. 2006, 'Cognitive-behavioural therapy for severe and recurrent bipolar disorders: randomised controlled trial', *Br.J.Psychiatry*, vol. 188, pp. 313–320.

Scott, T. 2006, *America Fooled: The Truth About Antidepressants, Antipsychotics and How We've been Deceived*. Argo Publishing, LLC, Victoria, Texas.

Scull, A. 1977, *Decarceration: Community Treatment and the Deviant – a Radical View*. Prentice Hall, Englewood Cliffs, NJ.

Scull, A. 1993, *The Most Solitary of Afflictions*. Yale University Press, New Haven.

Scull, A. 1994, 'Somatic treatments and the historiography of psychiatry', *Hist.Psychiatry*, vol. 5, pp. 1–12.

Sedgwick, P. 1982, *Psychopolitics*. Harper & Row, London.

Seeman, P. 1995, 'Dopamine receptors and psychosis', *Sci.Am.*, vol. 2, pp. 28–37.

Seeman, P. & Kapur, S. 2000, 'Schizophrenia: more dopamine, more D2 receptors', *Proc.Natl.Acad.Sci.U.S.A*, vol. 97, no. 14, pp. 7673–7675.

Seidman, L. J., Pepple, J. R., Faraone, S. V., Kremen, W. S., Green, A. I., Brown, W. A., & Tsuang, M. T. 1993, 'Neuropsychological performance in chronic schizophrenia in response to neuroleptic dose reduction', *Biol.Psychiatry*, vol. 33, no. 8–9, pp. 575–584.

Sernyak, M. J., Leslie, D. L., Alarcon, R. D., Losonczy, M. F., & Rosenheck, R. 2002, 'Association of diabetes mellitus with use of atypical neuroleptics in the treatment of schizophrenia', *Am.J.Psychiatry*, vol. 159, no. 4, pp. 561–566.

Sharp, L. I., Gabriel, A. R., & Impastato, D. J. 1953, 'Management of the acutely disturbed patient by sedative electroshock therapy', *Dis.Nerv.Syst.*, vol. 14, no. 1, pp. 21–24.

Shepherd, M. 1994, 'Neurolepsis and the psychopharmacological revolution: myth and reality', *Hist.Psychiatry*, vol. 5, no. 17, Pt 1, pp. 89–96.

Shepherd, M., Goodman, N. & Watt, D. C. 1961, 'The application of hospital statistics in the evaluation of pharmacotherapy in a psychiatric population', *Comprehensive Psychiatry*, vol. 2, pp. 11–19.

Shirzadi, A. A. & Ghaemi, S. N. 2006, 'Side effects of atypical antipsychotics: extrapyramidal symptoms and the metabolic syndrome', *Harv.Rev.Psychiatry*, vol. 14, no. 3, pp. 152–164.

Shorter, E. 1997, *A History of Psychiatry. From the Era of the Asylum to the Age of Prozac*. John Wiley & Sons, New York.

Shukakidze, A., Lazriev, I., & Mitagvariya, N. 2003, 'Behavioral impairments in acute and chronic manganese poisoning in white rats', *Neurosci.Behav.Physiol*, vol. 33, no. 3, pp. 263–267.

Silvestri, S., Seeman, M. V., Negrete, J. C., Houle, S., Shammi, C. M., Remington, G. J., Kapur, S., Zipursky, R. B., Wilson, A. A., Christensen, B. K., & Seeman, P. 2000, 'Increased dopamine D2 receptor binding after long-term treatment with antipsychotics in humans: a clinical PET study', *Psychopharmacology (Berl)*, vol. 152, no. 2, pp. 174–180.

Simpson, S. H., Eurich, D. T., Majumdar, S. R., Padwal, R. S., Tsuyuki, R. T., Varney, J., & Johnson, J. A. 2006, 'A meta-analysis of the association between adherence to drug therapy and mortality', *Br.Med.J.*, vol. 333, no. 7557, p. 15.

Sixseal.com. www.sixseal.com/2005/01/zyprexa_olanzapine_experience.html. 2007.

Skarsfeldt, T. 1996, 'Differential effect of antipsychotics on place navigation of rats in the Morris water maze. A comparative study between novel and reference antipsychotics', *Psychopharmacology (Berl)*, vol. 124, no. 1–2, pp. 126–133.

Small, J. G., Klapper, M. H., Milstein, V., Kellams, J. J., Miller, M. J., Marhenke, J. D., & Small, I. F. 1991, 'Carbamazepine compared with lithium in the treatment of mania', *Arch.Gen.Psychiatry*, vol. 48, no. 10, pp. 915–921.

Smialowski, A. 1991, 'Dopamine D2 receptor blocking effect of imipramine in the rat hippocampus', *Pharmacol.Biochem.Behav.*, vol. 39, no. 1, pp. 105–108.

Smith, A., Li, M., Becker, S., & Kapur, S. 2004, 'A model of antipsychotic action in conditioned avoidance: a computational approach', *Neuropsychopharmacology*, vol. 29, no. 6, pp. 1040–1049.

Smith, A., Traganza, E., & Harrison, G. 1969, 'Studies on the effectiveness of antidepressant drugs', *Psychopharmacol.Bull.*, p. Suppl-53.

Smith, M. E. 1961, 'A clinical study of chlorpromazine and chlordiazepoxide', *Conn.Med.*, vol. 25, pp. 153–157.

Smith, T. D., Kuczenski, R., George-Friedman, K., Malley, J. D., & Foote, S. L. 2000, 'In vivo microdialysis assessment of extracellular serotonin and dopamine levels in awake monkeys during sustained fluoxetine administration', *Synapse*, vol. 38, no. 4, pp. 460–470.

Snyder, S. H. 1972, 'Catecholamines in the brain as mediators of amphetamine psychosis', *Arch.Gen.Psychiatry*, vol. 27, no. 2, pp. 169–179.

Snyder, S. H., Taylor, K. M., Coyle, J. T., & Meyerhoff, J. L. 1970, 'The role of brain dopamine in behavioral regulation and the actions of psychotropic drugs', *Am.J.Psychiatry*, vol. 127, no. 2, pp. 199–207.

Soares, J. C. & Gershon, S. 2000, 'The psychopharmacologic specificity of the lithium ion: origins and trajectory', *J.Clin.Psychiatry*, vol. 61, suppl. 9, pp. 16–22.

Sobin, C., Sackeim, H. A., Prudic, J., Devanand, D. P., Moody, B. J., & McElhiney, M. C. 1995, 'Predictors of retrograde amnesia following ECT', *Am.J.Psychiatry*, vol. 152, no. 7, pp. 995–1001.

Spitzer, R. L. 1975, 'On pseudoscience in science, logic in remission, and psychiatric diagnosis: a critique of Rosenhan's "On Being Sane in Insane Places"', *J.Abnorm.Psychol.*, vol. 84, no. 5, pp. 442–452.

Spitzer, R. L. 1976, 'More on pseudoscience in science and the case for psychiatric diagnosis. A critique of D.L. Rosenhan's 'On Being Sane in Insane Places' and 'The Contestual Nature of Psychiatric Diagnosis'', *Arch.Gen.Psychiatry*, vol. 33, no. 4, pp. 459–470.

Squire, L. R., Judd, L. L., Janowsky, D. S., & Huey, L. Y. 1980, 'Effects of lithium carbonate on memory and other cognitive functions', *Am.J.Psychiatry*, vol. 137, no. 9, pp. 1042–1046.

Stagnitti, M. 2005, *Antidepressant Use in the US Civilian Non-Institutionalised Population, 2002. Statistical Brief #77*, Medical Expenditure Panel, Agency for Healthcare Research and Quality, Rockville,MD.

Stagnitti, M. N. 2007, *Trends in the Use and Expenditures for the Therapeutic Class Prescribed Psychotherapeutic Agents and All Subclasses, 1997 and 2004*, Agency for Healthcare Research and Quality, Rockville, Statistical brief #163.

Stahl, S. M. 1984, 'Regulation of neurotransmitter receptors by desipramine and other antidepressant drugs: the neurotransmitter receptor hypothesis of antidepressant action', *J.Clin.Psychiatry*, vol. 45, no. 10, Pt 2, pp. 37–45.

Stahl, S. M. 2000, *Essential Psychopharmacology*. Cambridge University Press, Cambridge.

Steck, H. 1954, 'Le syndrome extra-pyramidal et di-encephalique au cours des traitments au Largactil at au Serpasil [The extra-pyradmial and di-encephalic syndrome during treatment with largactil and serpasil]', *Annales Medico-psychologiques*, vol. 112, pp. 737–743.

Steen, R. G., Mull, C., McClure, R., Hamer, R. M., & Lieberman, J. A. 2006, 'Brain volume in first-episode schizophrenia: systematic review and meta-analysis of magnetic resonance imaging studies', *Br.J.Psychiatry*, vol. 188, pp. 510–518.

Stelazine advertisement. 1960, 'Stelazine advertisement', *Am.J.Psychiatry*, vol. 117, no. 3, p. XV.

Stern, J. M. & Simes, R. J. 1997, 'Publication bias: evidence of delayed publication in a cohort study of clinical research projects', *Br.Med.J.*, vol. 315, no. 7109, pp. 640–645.

Stip, E., Dufresne, J., Lussier, I., & Yatham, L. 2000, 'A double-blind, placebo-controlled study of the effects of lithium on cognition in healthy subjects: mild and selective effects on learning', *J.Affect.Disord.*, vol. 60, no. 3, pp. 147–157.

Stockmeier, C. A., Dilley, G. E., Shapiro, L. A., Overholser, J. C., Thompson, P. A., & Meltzer, H. Y. 1997, 'Serotonin receptors in suicide victims with major depression', *Neuropsychopharmacology*, vol. 16, no. 2, pp. 162–173.

Stokes, P. E., Shamoian, C. A., Stoll, P. M., & Patton, M. J. 1971, 'Efficacy of lithium as acute treatment of manic-depressive illness', *Lancet*, vol. 1, no. 7713, pp. 1319–1325.

Storosum, J. G., van Zwieten, B. J., van den, B. W., Gersons, B. P., & Broekmans, A. W. 2001, 'Suicide risk in placebo-controlled studies of major depression', *Am.J.Psychiatry*, vol. 158, no. 8, pp. 1271–1275.

Storosum, J. G., Wohlfarth, T., Gispen-de Wied, C. C., Linszen, D. H., Gersons, B. P., van Zwieten, B. J., & van den, B. W. 2005, 'Suicide risk in placebo-controlled trials of treatment for acute manic episode and prevention of manic-depressive episode', *Am.J.Psychiatry*, vol. 162, no. 4, pp. 799–802.

Struve, F. A. & Willner, A. E. 1983, 'Cognitive dysfunction and tardive dyskinesia', *Br.J.Psychiatry*, vol. 143, pp. 597–600.

Suppes, T., Baldessarini, R. J., Faedda, G. L., & Tohen, M. 1991, 'Risk of recurrence following discontinuation of lithium treatment in bipolar disorder', *Arch.Gen.Psychiatry*, vol. 48, no. 12, pp. 1082–1088.

Sussman, N. 2002, 'Choosing an atypical antipsychotic', *Int.Clin.Psychopharmacol.*, vol. 17, suppl. 3, pp. S29–S33.

Swazey, J. 1974, *Chlorpromazine in Psychiatry*. Massachusetts Institute of Technology, Cambridge, MA.

Szasz, T. 1970, *Ideology and Insanity; Essays on the psychiatric dehumanization of man*. Anchor Books, New York.

Szasz, T. 1994, *Cruel Compassion. Psychiatric control of society's unwanted*. John Wiley & Sons, New York.

Szegedi, A., Kohnen, R., Dienel, A., & Kieser, M. 2005, 'Acute treatment of moderate to severe depression with hypericum extract WS 5570 (St John's wort): randomised controlled double blind non-inferiority trial versus paroxetine', *Br.Med.J.*, vol. 330, no. 7490, p. 503.

Takahashi, R., Sakuma, A., Itoh, K., Itoh, H., & Kurihara, M. 1975, 'Comparison of efficacy of lithium carbonate and chlorpromazine in mania. Report of collaborative study group on treatment of mania in Japan', *Arch.Gen.Psychiatry*, vol. 32, no. 10, pp. 1310–1318.

Tandon, R., Mazzara, C., DeQuardo, J., Craig, K. A., Meador-Woodruff, J. H., Goldman, R., & Greden, J. F. 1991, 'Dexamethasone suppression test in schizophrenia: relationship to symptomatology, ventricular enlargement, and outcome', *Biol.Psychiatry*, vol. 29, no. 10, pp. 953–964.

Tasaka, K., Kamei, C., Akahori, H., & Kitazumi, K. 1985, 'The effects of histamine and some related compounds on conditioned avoidance response in rats', *Life Sci.*, vol. 37, no. 21, pp. 2005–2014.

Tegler, J., Strauss, W. H., Luthcke, H., & Bertling, R. 1988, 'Cognitive functions in schizophrenic patients with tardive dyskinesia', *Pharmacopsychiatry*, vol. 21, pp. 308–309.

Teicher, M. H., Glod, C., & Cole, J. O. 1990, 'Emergence of intense suicidal preoccupation during fluoxetine treatment', *Am.J.Psychiatry*, vol. 147, no. 2, pp. 207–210.

Terry, A. V., Jr., Hill, W. D., Parikh, V., Evans, D. R., Waller, J. L., & Mahadik, S. P. 2002, 'Differential effects of chronic haloperidol and olanzapine exposure on brain cholinergic markers and spatial learning in rats', *Psychopharmacology (Berl)*, vol. 164, no. 4, pp. 360–368.

Teulie, M., Follin, & Begoin 1955, '[Study of the action of lithium salts in states of psychomotor excitation.]', *Encephale*, vol. 44, no. 3, pp. 266–285.

Tharyan, P. & Adams, C. E. 2005, 'Electroconvulsive therapy for schizophrenia', *Cochrane.Database.Syst.Rev.*, issue. 2, article no. CD000076.

The National Institute of Mental Health Psychopharmacology Service Center Collaborative Study Group. 1964, 'Phenothiazine treatment in acute schizophrenia', *Arch.Gen.Psychiatry*, vol. 10, pp. 246–258.

Thiebot, M. H., Kloczko, J., Chermat, R., Simon, P., & Soubrie, P. 1980, 'Oxolinic acid and diazepam: their reciprocal antagonism in rodents', *Psychopharmacology (Berl)*, vol. 67, no. 1, pp. 91–95.

Thomas, A., Katsabouris, G., & Bouras, N. 1997, 'Staff perception on reduction of medication in patients with chronic schizophrenia', *Psychiatric Bulletin*, vol. 21, pp. 692–694.

Thomson, R. 1982, 'Side effects and placebo amplification', *Br.J.Psychiatry*, vol. 140, pp. 64–68.

Thorazine advertisement. 1960, 'Thorazine advertisement', *Am.J.Psychiatry*, vol. 117, no. February, p. IXX.

Tiihonen, J., Walhbeck, K., Lonnqvist, J., Klaukka, T., Ioannidis, J. P., Volavka, J., & Haukka, J. 2006, 'Effectiveness of antipsychotic treatments in a nationwide cohort of patients in community care after first hospitalisation due to schizophrenia and schizoaffective disorder: observational follow-up study', *Br.Med.J.*, vol. 333, no. 7561, p. 224.

Time (1954) 'Wonderdrug of 1954,' 14th June 1954.

Time (1955) 'Pills for the Mind,' 7th March 1955.

Timimi, S. 2002, *Pathological Child Psychiatry and the Medicalisation of Childhood*. Brunner-Routledge, Hove, Esat Sussex.

Titmuss, R. M. 1968, 'Community care: fact or fiction?', in *Commitment to Welfare*, R. M. Titmuss, ed., Allen & Unwin, London.

Tofranil advertisement. 1961, *Br.Med.J.*, vol. 1, no. Jan 14th.

Tohen, M., Calabrese, J. R., Sachs, G. S., Banov, M. D., Detke, H. C., Risser, R., Baker, R. W., Chou, J. C., & Bowden, C. L. 2006, 'Randomized, placebo-controlled trial of olanzapine as maintenance therapy in patients with bipolar I disorder responding to acute treatment with olanzapine', *Am.J.Psychiatry*, vol. 163, no. 2, pp. 247–256.

Tohen, M., Greil, W., Calabrese, J. R., Sachs, G. S., Yatham, L. N., Oerlinghausen, B. M., Koukopoulos, A., Cassano, G. B., Grunze, H., Licht, R. W., Dell'Osso, L., Evans, A. R., Risser, R., Baker, R. W., Crane, H., Dossenbach, M. R., & Bowden, C. L. 2005, 'Olanzapine versus lithium in the maintenance treatment of bipolar disorder: a 12-month, randomized, double-blind, controlled clinical trial', *Am.J.Psychiatry*, vol. 162, no. 7, pp. 1281–1290.

Tollefson, G. D., Beasley, C. M., Jr., Tamura, R. N., Tran, P. V., & Potvin, J. H. 1997, 'Blind, controlled, long-term study of the comparative incidence of treatment-emergent tardive dyskinesia with olanzapine or haloperidol', *Am.J.Psychiatry*, vol. 154, no. 9, pp. 1248–1254.

Tondo, L., Baldessarini, R. J., & Floris, G. 2001, 'Long-term clinical effectiveness of lithium maintenance treatment in types I and II bipolar disorders', *Br.J.Psychiatry Suppl.*, vol. 41, p. s184–s190.

Tondo, L., Baldessarini, R. J., Hennen, J., Floris, G., Silvetti, F., & Tohen, M. 1998, 'Lithium treatment and risk of suicidal behavior in bipolar disorder patients', *J.Clin.Psychiatry*, vol. 59, no. 8, pp. 405–414.

Tranter, R., Healy, H., Cattell, D., & Healy, D. 2002, 'Functional effects of agents differentially selective to noradrenergic or serotonergic systems', *Psychol.Med.*, vol. 32, no. 3, pp. 517–524.

Trilafon advertisement. 1960, 'Trilafon advertisement', *Am.J.Psychiatry*, vol. 117, no. November, p. IX.

Tryptizol advertisement. 1964, 'Tryptizol advertisement', *Br.Med.J.*, vol. 2, no. Sept 12th.

Tschanz, J. T. & Rebec, G. V. 1988, 'Atypical antipsychotic drugs block selective components of amphetamine-induced stereotypy', *Pharmacol.Biochem.Behav.*, vol. 31, no. 3, pp. 519–522.

Tuckwell, H. C. & Koziol, J. A. 1993, 'A meta-analysis of homovanillic acid concentrations in schizophrenia', *Int.J.Neurosci.*, vol. 73, no. 1–2, pp. 109–114.

Tuma, T. A. 2000, 'Outcome of hospital-treated depression at 4.5 years. An elderly and a younger adult cohort compared', *Br.J.Psychiatry*, vol. 176, pp. 224–228.

Uhlenhuth, E. H. & Park, L. C. 1963, 'The influence of medication (imipramine) and doctor in relieving depressed psychoneurotic outpatients', *J.Psychiatr.Res.*, vol. 2, pp. 101–122.

UK ECT review group 2003, 'Efficacy and safety of electroconvulsive therapy in depressive disorders: a systematic review and meta-analysis', *Lancet*, vol. 361, no. 9360, pp. 799–808.

Unsworth, C. 1987, *The Politics of Mental Health Legislation*. Oxford University Press, Oxford.

USSenate Subcommittee on Antitrust and Monopoly 1961, *Report of the Study of Administered Prices in the Drug Industry*, 87th Congress, 1st Session, Washington.

Valenstein, E. 1988, *Blaming the Brain*. Free Press, New York.

Van Putten, T. 1974, 'Why do schizophrenic patients refuse to take their drugs?', *Arch.Gen.Psychiatry*, vol. 31, pp. 67–72.

Van Putten, T. 1975, 'The many faces of akathisia', *Compr.Psychiatry*, vol. 16, pp. 43–47.

Van Putten, T. & May, P. R. A. 1978, 'Subjective response as a predictor of outcome in pharmacotherapy; the consumer has a point', *Arch.Gen.Psychiatry*, vol. 35, pp. 477–480.

Vandel, P., Bonin, B., Leveque, E., Sechter, D., & Bizouard, P. 1997, 'Tricyclic antidepressant-induced extrapyramidal side effects', *Eur.Neuropsychopharmacol.*, vol. 7, no. 3, pp. 207–212.

Vartanian, M. E. 1959, '[Result of lithium carbonate therapy of the agitation states.]', *Zh.Nevropatol.Psikhiatr.Im S.S.Korsakova*, vol. 59, no. 5, pp. 586–589.

Varvel, S. A., Vann, R. E., Wise, L. E., Philibin, S. D., & Porter, J. H. 2002, 'Effects of antipsychotic drugs on operant responding after acute and repeated administration', *Psychopharmacology (Berl)*, vol. 160, no. 2, pp. 182–191.

Verdoux, H. & Bourgeois, M. 1993, 'Short-term sequelae of lithium discontinuation', *Encephale*, vol. 19, no. 6, pp. 645–650.

Vetulani, J. & Sulser, F. 1975, 'Action of various antidepressant treatments reduces reactivity of noradrenergic cyclic AMP-generating system in limbic forebrain', *Nature*, vol. 257, no. 5526, pp. 495–496.

Viguera, A. C., Baldessarini, R. J., & Friedberg, J. 1998, 'Discontinuing antidepressant treatment in major depression', *Harv.Rev.Psychiatry*, vol. 5, no. 6, pp. 293–306.

Viguera, A. C., Baldessarini, R. J., Hegarty, J. D., van Kammen, D. P., & Tohen, M. 1997, 'Clinical risk following abrupt and gradual withdrawal of maintenance neuroleptic treatment', *Arch.Gen.Psychiatry*, vol. 54, no. 1, pp. 49–55.

Visser, H. M. & van der Mast, R. C. 2005, 'Bipolar disorder, antidepressants and induction of hypomania or mania. A systematic review', *World J.Biol.Psychiatry*, vol. 6, no. 4, pp. 231–241.

von Meduna, L. 1938, 'General discussion of the cardiazol therapy', *Am.J.Psychiatry*, vol. 94, pp. 41–50.

Von Voigtlander, P. F. & Moore, K. E. 1973, 'Turning behavior of mice with unilateral 6-hydroxydopamine lesions in the striatum: effects of apomorphine, L-DOPA, amanthadine, amphetamine and other psychomotor stimulants', *Neuropharmacology*, vol. 12, no. 5, pp. 451–462.

Waddington, J. L., O'Callaghan, E., Larkin, C., & Kinsella, A. 1993, 'Cognitive dysfunction in schizophrenia: organic vulnerability factor or state marker for tardive dyskinesia?', *Brain Cogn.*, vol. 23, no. 1, pp. 56–70.

Waddington, J. L., Youssef, H. A., & Kinsella, A. 1990, 'Cognitive dysfunction in schizophrenia followed up over 5 years, and its longitudinal relationship to the emergence of tardive dyskinesia', *Psychol.Med.*, vol. 20, no. 4, pp. 835–842.

Waddington, J. L., Youssef, H. A., & Kinsella, A. 1998, 'Mortality in schizophrenia. Antipsychotic polypharmacy and absence of adjunctive anticholinergics over the course of a 10-year prospective study', *Br.J.Psychiatry*, vol. 173, pp. 325–329.

Wadsworth, E. J., Moss, S. C., Simpson, S. A., & Smith, A. P. 2005, 'SSRIs and cognitive performance in a working sample', *Hum.Psychopharmacol.*, vol. 20, no. 8, pp. 561–572.

Wallace, M. 1994, 'Schizophrenia – a national emergency: preliminary observations on SANELINE', *Acta Psychiatr.Scand.Suppl.*, vol. 380, pp. 33–35.

Walsh, B. T., Seidman, S. N., Sysko, R., & Gould, M. 2002, 'Placebo response in studies of major depression: variable, substantial, and growing', *JAMA*, vol. 287, no. 14, pp. 1840–1847.

Wegner, J. T., Kane, J. M., Weinhold, P., Woerner, M., Kinon, B., & Lieberman, J. 1985, 'Cognitive impairment in tardive dyskinesia', *Psychiatry Res.*, vol. 16, no. 4, pp. 331–337.

Weickert, T. W., Goldberg, T. E., Marenco, S., Bigelow, L. B., Egan, M. F., & Weinberger, D. R. 2003, 'Comparison of cognitive performances during a placebo period and an atypical antipsychotic treatment period in schizophrenia: critical examination of confounds', *Neuropsychopharmacology*, vol. 28, no. 8, pp. 1491–1500.

Weil, P. L. 1950, ''Regressive' electroplexy in schizophrenics', *J.Ment.Sci.*, vol. 96, pp. 514–520.

Weinstein, E. A., Linn, L., & Kahn, R. L. 1952, 'Psychosis during electroshock therapy: its relation to the theory of shock therapy', *Am.J.Psychiatry*, vol. 109, pp. 22–26.

Weintraub, W. & Aronson, H. 1963, 'Clinical judgement in psychopharmacological research', *J.Neuropsychiatry*, vol. 5, pp. 65–70.

Weissman, M. M., Prusoff, B., Sholomskas, A. J., & Greenwald, S. 1992, 'A double-blind clinical trial of alprazolam, imipramine, or placebo in the depressed elderly', *J.Clin.Psychopharmacol.*, vol. 12, no. 3, pp. 175–182.

Wescott, P. 1979, 'One man's schizophrenic illness', *Br.Med.J.*, vol. 1, no. 6169, pp. 989–990.

Whitaker, R. 2002, *Mad in America*. Perseus Publishing, Cambridge, MA.

White, H. S. 2003, 'Mechanism of action of newer anticonvulsants', *J.Clin.Psychiatry*, vol. 64, suppl. 8, pp. 5–8.

Whittington, C. J., Kendall, T., Fonagy, P., Cottrell, D., Cotgrove, A., & Boddington, E. 2004, 'Selective serotonin reuptake inhibitors in childhood depression: systematic review of published versus unpublished data', *Lancet*, vol. 363, no. 9418, pp. 1341–1345.

Wikler, A. 1957, *The Relation of Psychiatry to Pharmacology*. Williams & Wilkins, Baltimore.

Williamson, B. 1966, 'Psychiatry since lithium', *Dis.Nerv.Syst.*, vol. 27, no. 12, pp. 775–782.

Wilson, I. C., Garbutt, J. C., Lanier, C. F., Moylan, J., Nelson, W., & Prange, A. J., Jr. 1983, 'Is there a tardive dysmentia?', *Schizophr.Bull.*, vol. 9, no. 2, pp. 187–192.

Wilson, M. 1993, 'DSM-III and the transformation of American psychiatry: a history', *Am.J.Psychiatry*, vol. 150, no. 3, pp. 399–410.

Winkelman, N. W., Jr. 1954, 'Chlorpromazine in the treatment of neuropsychiatric disorders', *J.Am.Med.Assoc.*, vol. 155, no. 1, pp. 18–21.

Winkelman, N. W., Jr. 1957, 'An appraisal of chlorpromazine; general principles for administration of chlorpromazine, based on experience with 1,090 patients', *Am.J.Psychiatry*, vol. 113, no. 11, pp. 961–971.

Winokur, A., Gary, K. A., Rodner, S., Rae-Red, C., Fernando, A. T., & Szuba, M. P. 2001, 'Depression, sleep physiology, and antidepressant drugs', *Depress.Anxiety*, vol. 14, no. 1, pp. 19–28.

Winokur, G. 1975, 'The Iowa 500: heterogeneity and course in manic-depressive illness (bipolar)', *Compr.Psychiatry*, vol. 16, no. 2, pp. 125–131.

Woerner, M. G., Alvir, J. M., Saltz, B. L., Lieberman, J. A., & Kane, J. M. 1998, 'Prospective study of tardive dyskinesia in the elderly: rates and risk factors', *Am.J.Psychiatry*, vol. 155, no. 11, pp. 1521–1528.

Wohlfarth, T. D., van Zwieten, B. J., Lekkerkerker, F. J., Gispen-de Wied, C. C., Ruis, J. R., Elferink, A. J., & Storosum, J. G. 2006, 'Antidepressants use in children and adolescents and the risk of suicide', *Eur.Neuropsychopharmacol.*, vol. 16, no. 2, pp. 79–83.

Wolf, M. E., Ryan, J. J., & Mosnaim, A. D. 1983, 'Cognitive functions in tardive dyskinesia', *Psychol.Med.*, vol. 13, no. 3, pp. 671–674.

Wolkowitz, O. M. & Pickar, D. 1991, 'Benzodiazepines in the treatment of schizophrenia: a review and reappraisal', *Am.J.Psychiatry*, vol. 148, no. 6, pp. 714–726.

Wong, D. F., Wagner, H. N., Jr., Tune, L. E., Dannals, R. F., Pearlson, G. D., Links, J. M., Tamminga, C. A., Broussolle, E. P., Ravert, H. T., Wilson, A. A., Toung, J. K., Malat, J., Williams, J. A., O'Tuama, L. A., Snyder, S. H., Kuhar, M. J., & Gjedde, A. 1986, 'Positron emission tomography reveals elevated D2 dopamine receptors in drug-naive schizophrenics', *Science*, vol. 234, no. 4783, pp. 1558–1563.

Wonodi, I., Hong, L. E., & Thaker, G. K. 2005, 'Psychopathological and cognitive correlates of tardive dyskinesia in patients treated with neuroleptics', *Adv.Neurol.*, vol. 96, pp. 336–349.

Woodward, N. D., Purdon, S. E., Meltzer, H. Y., & Zald, D. H. 2005, 'A meta-analysis of neuropsychological change to clozapine, olanzapine, quetiapine, and risperidone in schizophrenia', *Int.J.Neuropsychopharmacol.*, vol. 8, no. 3, pp. 457–472.

World Health Organisation. Suicide rates (per 100,000) by gender, Ireland, 1950–2002. www.who.int/entity/mental_health/media/irel.pdf. 2006.

Wyeth. www.effexorxr.com/condition.asp. 21.09.2006.

Yazici, O., Kora, K., Polat, A., & Saylan, M. 2004, 'Controlled lithium discontinuation in bipolar patients with good response to long-term lithium prophylaxis', *J.Affect.Disord.*, vol. 80, no. 2–3, pp. 269–271.

Young, A. H. & Newham, J. I. 2006, 'Lithium in maintenance therapy for bipolar disorder', *J.Psychopharmacol.*, vol. 20, suppl. 2, pp. 17–22.

Youssef, H. A. & Waddington, J. L. 1988, 'Involuntary orofacial movements in hospitalised patients with mental handicap or epilepsy: relationship to developmental/intellectual deficit and presence or absence of long-term exposure to neuroleptics', *J.Neurol.Neurosurg.Psychiatry*, vol. 51, no. 6, pp. 863–865.

Zakzanis, K. K. & Hansen, K. T. 1998, 'Dopamine D2 densities and the schizophrenic brain', *Schizophr.Res.*, vol. 32, no. 3, pp. 201–206.

Zeller, E. A. & Barsky, J. 1952, 'In vivo inhibition of liver and brain monoamine oxidase by 1-Isonicotinyl-2-isopropyl hydrazine', *Proc.Soc.Exp.Biol.Med.*, vol. 81, no. 2, pp. 459–461.

Index